RadCases

All the key Radiology cases for your rounds, rotations, and exams—in print and online!

Simply visit http://RadCases.thieme.com and, when prompted during the registration process, enter the scratch-off code below to get started today.

This book can no longer be returned once this panel is scratched off.

Access and search 250 must-know cases online!

Each book in the RadCases series contains 100 cases plus a scratch-off code that allows 12 months of online access to all of the cases from the book plus 150 additional cases—250 cases in all—related to that book's subspecialty via **RadCases.thieme.com.**

Features of RadCases online include:

- A user-friendly way to study the most commonly encountered cases in each subspecialty
- Diagnostic videos and color images enhance selected subspecialties
- A flexible search function that lets you locate specific cases by age, differential diagnosis, modality, and more
- The ability to bookmark cases you want to return to and to 'hide' the cases you've already learned
- The same user-friendly organization as your ***RadCases*** book
- Clearly labeled, high-quality radiographs to help you absorb key findings at-a-glance

System requirements for optimal use of RadCases online

	WINDOWS	MAC
Recommended Browser(s)**	Microsoft Internet Explorer 7.0 or later, Firefox 2.x, Firefox 3.x *** all browsers should have JavaScript enabled*	Firefox 2.x, Firefox 3.x, Safari 3.x, Safari 4.x
Flash Player Plug-in	Flash Player 8 or Higher* ** Mac users: ATI Rage 128 GPU does not support full-screen mode with hardware scaling*	
Minimum Hardware Configurations	Intel® Pentium® II 450 MHz, AMD Athlon™ 600 MHz or faster processor (or equivalent) 128 MB of RAM	PowerPC® G3 500 MHz or faster processor Intel Core™ Duo 1.33 GHz or faster processor 128 MB of RAM
Recommended for optimal usage experience	Monitor resolutions: • Normal (4:3) 1024×768 or Higher • Widescreen (16:9) 1280×720 or Higher • Widescreen (16:10) 1440×900 or Higher DSL/Cable internet connection at a minimum speed of 384.0 Kbps or faster	

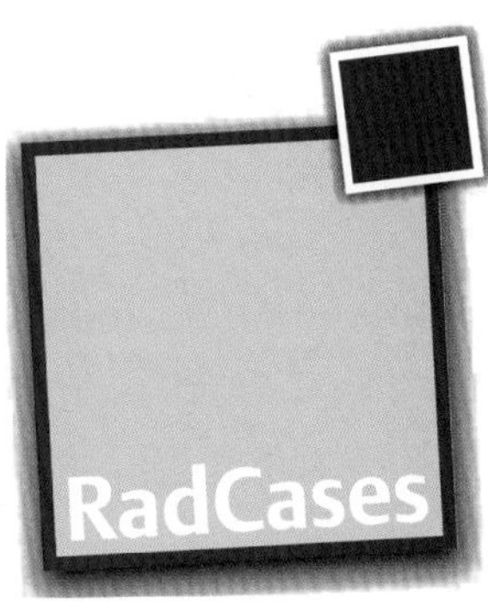

Cardiac Imaging

Edited by

Carlos Santiago Restrepo, MD
Professor of Radiology
Chief of Chest Radiology
Department of Radiology
University of Texas Health Science Center at San Antonio
San Antonio, Texas

Dianna M. E. Bardo, MD
Associate Professor of Radiology
Director of Cardiac Radiology
Oregon Health & Science University
Portland, Oregon

Series Editors

Jonathan Lorenz, MD
Associate Professor of Radiology
Department of Radiology
The University of Chicago
Chicago, Illinois

Hector Ferral, MD
Professor of Radiology
Section Chief, Interventional Radiology
RUSH University Medical Center, Chicago
Chicago, Illinois

Thieme
New York • Stuttgart

Thieme Medical Publishers, Inc.
333 Seventh Ave.
New York, NY 10001

Executive Editor: Timothy Hiscock
Editorial Director: Michael Wachinger
Editorial Assistant: Adriana di Giorgio
International Production Director: Andreas Schabert
Production Editor: Heidi Grauel, Maryland Composition
Vice President, International Marketing and Sales: Cornelia Schulze
Chief Financial Officer: James W. Mitos
President: Brian D. Scanlan
Compositor: MPS Content Services
Printer: Everbest Printing Co.

Library of Congress Cataloging-in-Publication Data

Radcases cardiac imaging / edited by Carlos Santiago Restrepo, Dianna M.E. Bardo.
p. ; cm.
Includes bibliographical references and index.
ISBN 978-1-60406-185-7
1. Heart—Imaging—Case studies. 2. Heart—Diseases—Diagnosis—Case studies. I. Restrepo, Carlos Santiago. II. Bardo, Dianna M. E.
[DNLM: 1. Heart Diseases—diagnosis—Case Reports. 2. Diagnostic Imagin—methods—Case Reports. WG 141 R312 2010]
RC683.5.I42R33 2010
616.1'20754—dc22

2009031579

Important note: Medical knowledge is ever-changing. As new research and clinical experience broaden our knowledge, changes in treatment and drug therapy may be required. The authors and editors of the material herein have consulted sources believed to be reliable in their efforts to provide information that is complete and in accord with the standards accepted at the time of publication. However, in view of the possibility of human error by the authors, editors, or publisher of the work herein or changes in medical knowledge, neither the authors, editors, nor publisher, nor any other party who has been involved in the preparation of this work, warrants that the information contained herein is in every respect accurate or complete, and they are not responsible for any errors or omissions or for the results obtained from use of such information. Readers are encouraged to confirm the information contained herein with other sources. For example, readers are advised to check the product information sheet included in the package of each drug they plan to administer to be certain that the information contained in this publication is accurate and that changes have not been made in the recommended dose or in the contraindications for administration. This recommendation is of particular importance in connection with new or infrequently used drugs.

Printed in China

978-1-60406-185-7

Dedication

To my husband John, who makes it possible to work with passion and makes the rewards of that work worthwhile.

—Dianna M. E. Bardo

To my parents, Ovidio and Marielena, with all my love. And to my wife, Marta, and my children, Catalina, Juan, and Alejandro, the joy of my life.

—Carlos Santiago Restrepo

Series Preface

The ability to assimilate detailed information across the entire spectrum of radiology is the Holy Grail sought by those preparing for their trip to Louisville. As enthusiastic partners in the Thieme RadCases series who formerly took the examination, we understand the exhaustion and frustration shared by residents and the families of residents engaged in this quest. It has been our observation that despite ongoing efforts to improve Web-based interactive databases, residents still find themselves searching for material they can review while preparing for the radiology board examinations and remain frustrated by the fact that only a few printed guidebooks are available, which are limited in both format and image quality. Perhaps their greatest source of frustration is the inability to easily locate groups of cases across all subspecialties of radiology that are organized and tailored for their immediate study needs. Imagine being able to immediately access groups of high-quality cases to arrange study sessions, quickly extract and master information, and prepare for theme-based radiology conferences. Our goal in creating the RadCases series was to combine the popularity and portability of printed books with the adaptability, exceptional quality, and interactive features of an electronic case-based format.

The intent of the printed book is to encourage repeated priming in the use of critical information by providing a portable group of exceptional core cases that the resident can master. The best way to determine the format for these cases was to ask residents from around the country to weigh in. Overwhelmingly, the residents said that they would prefer a concise, point-by-point presentation of the Essential Facts of each case in an easy-to-read, bulleted format. Differentials are limited to a maximum of three, and the first is always the actual diagnosis. This approach is easy on exhausted eyes and provides a quick review of Pearls and Pitfalls as information is absorbed during repeated study sessions. We worked hard to choose cases that could be presented well in this format, recognizing the limitations inherent in reproducing high-quality images in print. Unlike other case-based radiology review books, we removed the guesswork by providing clear annotations and descriptions for all images. In our opinion, there is nothing worse than being unable to locate a subtle finding on a poorly reproduced image even after one knows the final diagnosis.

The electronic cases expand on the printed book and provide a comprehensive review of the entire subspecialty. Thousands of cases are strategically designed to increase the resident's knowledge by providing exposure to additional case examples—from basic to advanced—and by exploring "Aunt Minnie's," unusual diagnoses, and variability within a single diagnosis. The search engine gives the resident a fighting chance to find the Holy Grail by creating individualized, daily study lists that are not limited by factors such as radiology subsection. For example, tailor today's study list to cases involving tuberculosis and include cases in every subspecialty and every system of the body. Or study only thoracic cases, including those with links to cardiology, nuclear medicine, and pediatrics. Or study only musculoskeletal cases. The choice is yours.

As enthusiastic partners in this project, we started small and, with the encouragement, talent, and guidance of Tim Hiscock at Thieme, we have continued to raise the bar in our effort to assist residents in tackling the daunting task of assimilating massive amounts of information. We are passionate about continuing this journey, planning to expand the cases in our electronic series, adapt cases based on direct feedback from residents, and increase the features intended for board review and self-assessment. As the National Board of Medical Examiners converts the American Board of Radiology examination from an oral to an electronic format, our series will be the one best suited to meet the needs of the next generation of overworked and exhausted residents in radiology.

Jonathan Lorenz, MD
Hector Ferral, MD
Chicago, IL

Preface

The opportunity to present a large group of cases to you in Cardiac Imaging, part of the RadCases series, is a real privilege for us. Working in academic medicine provides us the ability to teach and learn from residents and fellows as well as the chance to diagnose a broad range of common and uncommon cardiac diseases, and also further advance cardiac imaging modalities through research.

The high prevalence of cardiovascular diseases in the western world, as well as the amazing evolution of imaging technology available to us makes this book more relevant today than ever before. It is critical that radiologists are capable of diagnosing cardiovascular diseases.

The power of this cardiac case base is the presentation of strengths of both CT and MRI through 100 printed and an additional 150 electronic cases. The 250 cases we have prepared include not only common presentations, but uncommon presentations of common problems and examples of cases you must diagnosis immediately to avert potential disaster. The cases we have written prepare you for your opportunities to shine when confronted with cardiac cases whether that is on a board examination or in practice.

We hope this case base review series will be beneficial for you as you prepare for medical board examinations. This case base series and the learning experiences during your training are the foundation for a lifetime of learning you will experience throughout your career.

Dianna M.E. Bardo, MD
Carlos Santiago Restrepo, MD

Acknowledgments

I wish to acknowledge my colleagues Craig S. Broberg, MD; Michael D. Shapiro, DO; and Thanjavur Bragadeesh, MB, ChB, who generously shared their cases for this text and who teach and inspire excellence in cardiac imaging.

Dianna M. E. Bardo, MD

I want to thank Santiago Martinez, MD (Duke University); Terry Bauch, MD (The University of Texas HSC, San Antonio); Jorge Carrillo, MD (Universidad Nacional, Bogota, Colombia); Ramon Reina, MD (Clinica de Marly, Bogota, Colombia); Julio Lemos, MD (University of Vermont); and Eric Kimura, MD (Instituto Nacional de Cardiologia Ignacio Chavez, Mexico), for their valuable contributions.

Carlos Santiago Restrepo, MD

Case 1

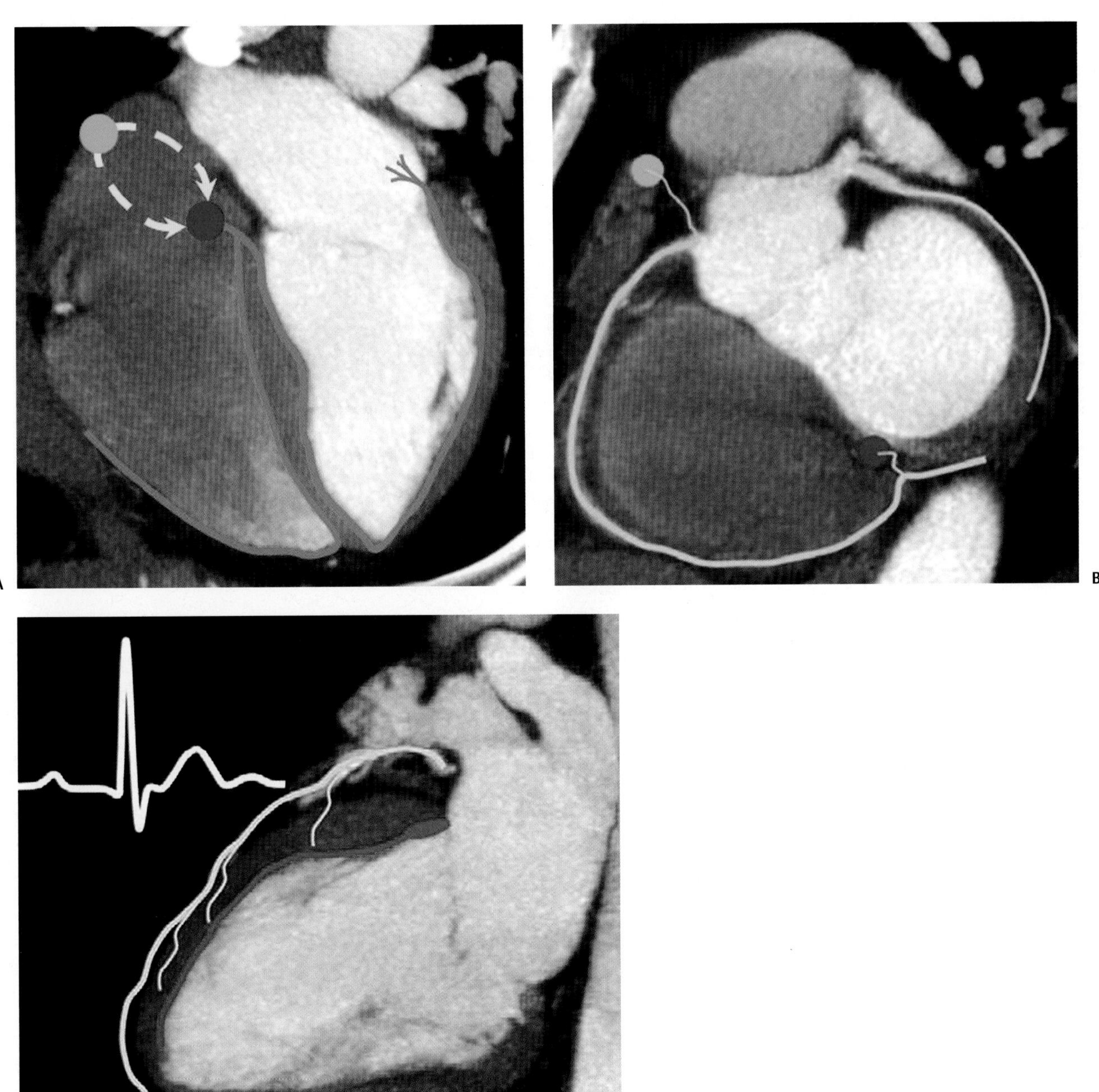

Clinical Presentation

The electrical system of the heart performs critical functions in synchronized depolarization, resulting in contraction of the atria and ventricles and ejection of blood into the pulmonary and systemic vascular beds. The important structures and events in cardiac electrical activity and the usual vascular supply to these structures are described.

Imaging Findings

Components of the electrical conduction system and coronary arteries have been drawn over four-chamber, short-axis, and two-chamber views of the heart.

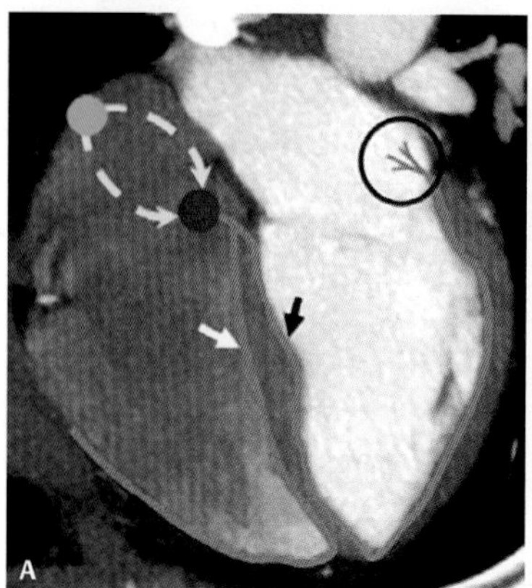

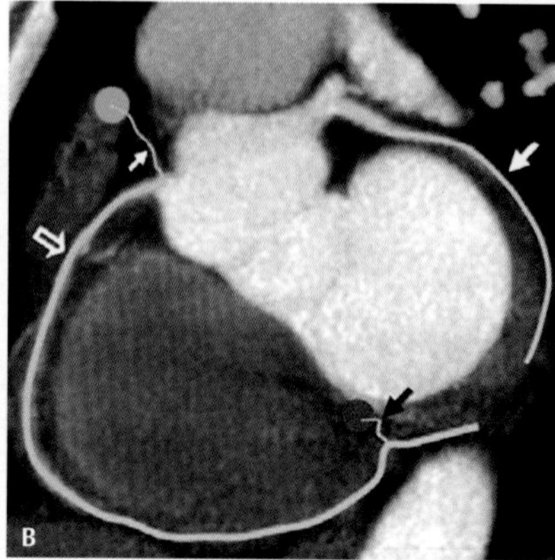

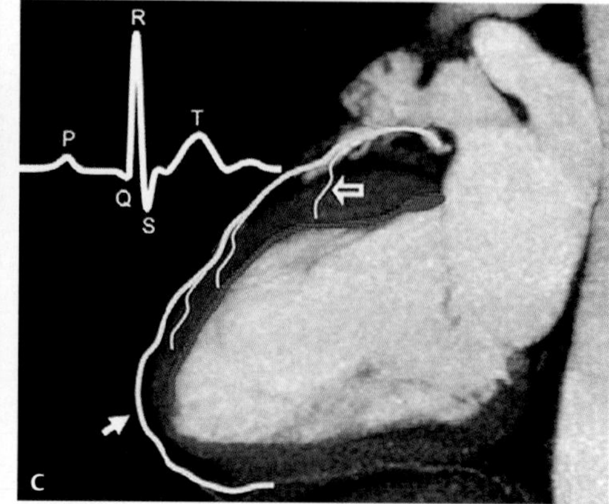

(A) The sinoatrial (SA) node (*green dot*) is at the superior and posterior margin of the right atrium. Internodal pathways (*dotted yellow arrows*) span the SA and the atrioventricular (AV) nodes (*red dot*). The right (*white arrow*) and left (*black arrow*) bundle branches (*orange lines*) and Purkinje fibers (*black circle*) propagate depolarization through the ventricles. **(B)** The SA (*green dot*) and AV (*red dot*) nodes are supplied by the SA nodal (*small white arrow*) and AV nodal (*black arrow*) arteries; both are usually branches of the right coronary artery (*open white arrow*). Occasionally, the AV nodal branch arises from the left circumflex artery (*white arrow*). **(C)** The left anterior descending artery supplies septal branches that perforate the interventricular septum to supply the bundle branches (*orange line*). The P and T waves and the QRS complex of the electrocardiogram (ECG) trace are described below.

Differential Diagnosis

- ***Normal cardiac conduction system:*** The myocardial muscle cells and tissue of a specialized conduction system allow conduction of electrical impulses. Specialized cells in the conductive tissue depolarize spontaneously.

Essential Facts

- Components of the conduction system include the following:
  - The SA node suppresses depolarization of other pacing cells and is therefore the dominant pacemaker of the heart. It excites the internodal pathways and the atrial myocardium.
  - Anterior, middle, and posterior internodal tracts are activated by the SA node, propagating the electrical signal to the AV node, the His bundle, the bundle branches, the Purkinje network, and the ventricular myocardium.
  - The AV node, located at the crux cordis, depolarizes to assist in propagating conduction of electrical activity to the His bundle.
  - The His bundle and the right and left bundle branches are organized groups of cells that propagate electrical activity through the ventricles in an organized manner.
  - Anterosuperior and posteroinferior divisions of the left bundle and the Purkinje network increase the speed of depolarization through the ventricles.
- The main components of the ECG trace are the following:
  - *P wave:* The P wave represents the combination of right atrial activation and the slightly delayed activation of the left atrium; resulting in atrial systole.
  - *QRS complex:* The electrical representation of ventricular muscle depolarization; resulting in ventricular systole.
  - *T wave:* Recovery of the ventricular myocardium; ventricular diastole begins as the ventricles relax.

Other Imaging Findings

- In patients with arrhythmia, look for thrombus in the left atrial appendage.

✔ Pearls & ✘ Pitfalls

✔ Myocardial infarction and ischemia can result in arrhythmia.

✘ Variability of coronary artery dominance results in a minor inconsistency in the vascular supply of the conduction system.

Case 2

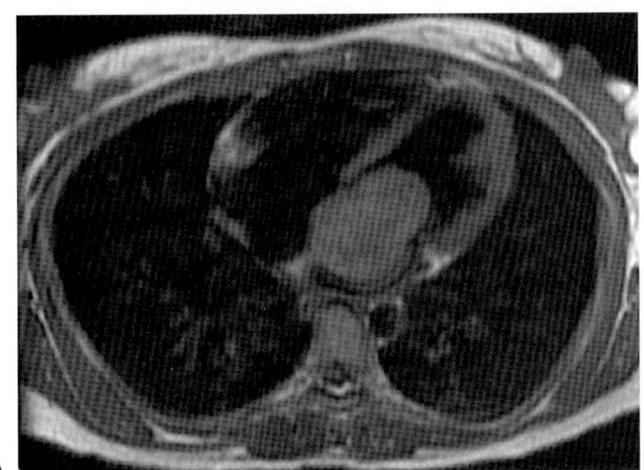
A

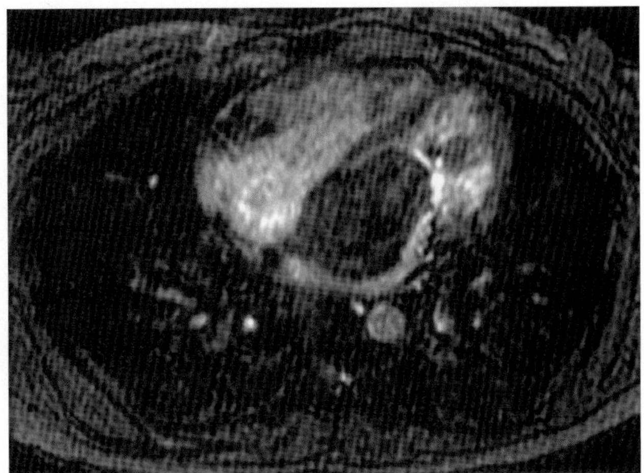
B

■ Clinical Presentation

Shortness of breath and chest pain in a 45-year-old man

Imaging Findings

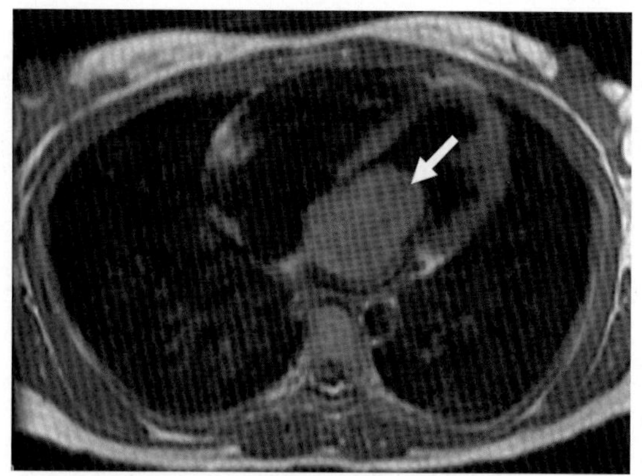

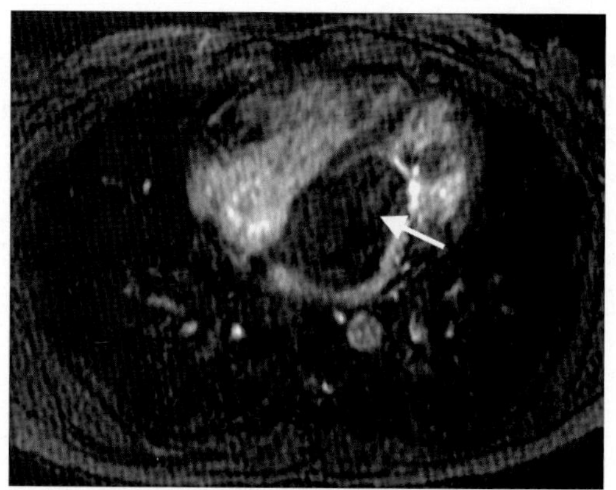

(A) Axial T1-weighted and **(B)** gradient echo (GRE) images at the level of the heart demonstrate a large mass in the left atrium (*white arrow*, Fig. A) attached to the interatrial septum and protruding through the mitral valve into the upper left ventricle.

Differential Diagnosis

- ***Atrial myxoma:*** A well-delineated, smooth, oval left atrial mass attached to the interatrial septum is characteristic of an atrial myxoma. When large enough, an atrial myxoma may protrude into the left ventricle through the mitral valve.
- *Atrial thrombus:* An atrial thrombus more commonly arises from the posterior or lateral wall of an enlarged left atrium.
- *Sarcoma:* An atrial sarcoma typically involves the right atrium and presents as an irregular infiltrative mass of soft-tissue density.

Essential Facts

- Myxomas account for one half of all primary cardiac tumors and are the most common primary cardiac neoplasms.
- Women are affected more than men. The mean age at diagnosis is 50 years.
- Large left atrial myxomas commonly cause mitral valve obstruction (60%).
- Constitutional symptoms (fever, malaise, and weight loss), cardiac arrhythmias, and embolic manifestations are the most common clinical complaints.
- Myxomas are attached to the endocardium, and origin from the fossa ovalis of the interatrial septum is characteristic.
- Seventy-five percent of myxomas arise in the left atrium and 20% in the right atrium.
- On computed tomography, > 50% exhibit calcification.

Other Imaging Findings

- On magnetic resonance imaging (MRI), atrial myxomas have heterogeneous signal intensity.
- On T1-weighted images, they have low signal intensity.
- On cine GRE images, atrial myxomas exhibit contrast enhancement after gadolinium injection.

✔ Pearls & ✘ Pitfalls

✔ The majority of atrial myxomas are sporadic, but 7% are associated with a familial predisposition or manifest as multicentric myxomas with skin pigmentation, endocrine disorders, and other tumors (Carney complex).

✘ Atrial myxomas and thrombi can have a similar appearance on MRI. Contrast-enhanced MRI can help differentiate between these two conditions because myxomas exhibit enhancement and thrombi do not.

Case 3

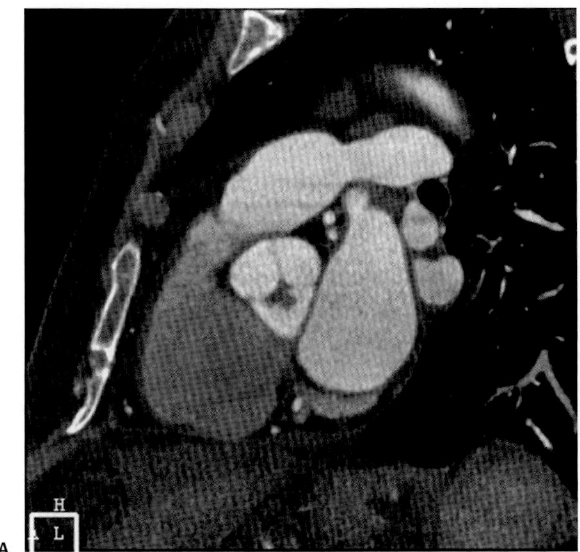

A

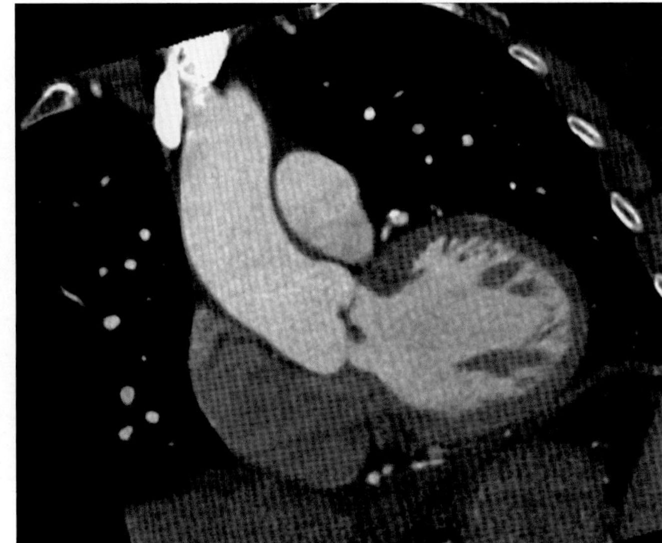

B

Clinical Presentation

A 50-year-old woman presents with a stroke and a heart murmur on physical examination.

Imaging Findings

On cardiac-gated multidetector computed tomography angiography:

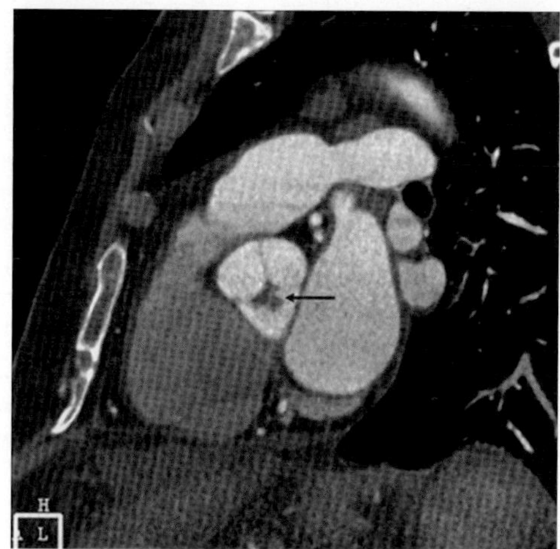

A

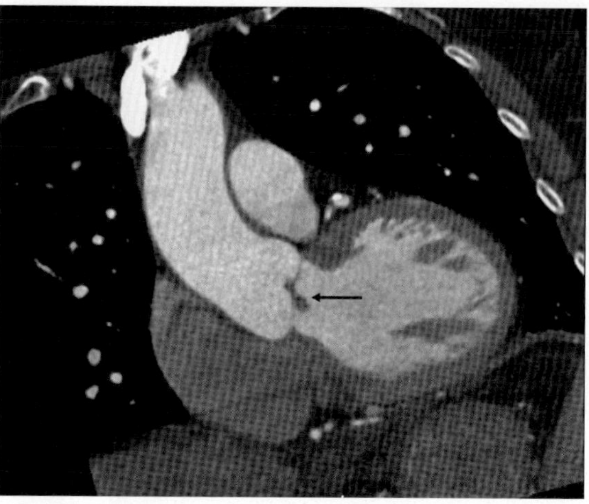

B

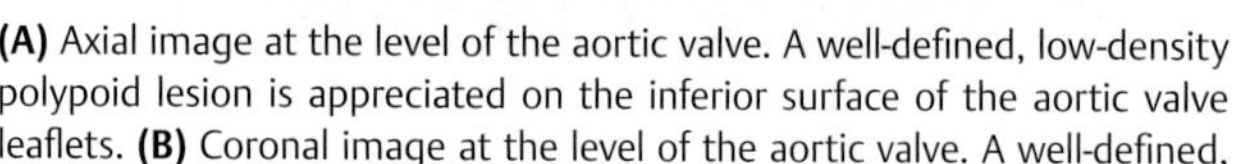

(A) Axial image at the level of the aortic valve. A well-defined, low-density polypoid lesion is appreciated on the inferior surface of the aortic valve leaflets. **(B)** Coronal image at the level of the aortic valve. A well-defined, low-density polypoid lesion is appreciated on the inferior surface of the aortic valve leaflets.

Differential Diagnosis

- ***Papillary fibroelastoma:*** Contrast-enhanced cardiac-gated computed tomography (CT) shows a soft-tissue-density polypoid mass arising from an aortic valve leaflet. The lesion exhibits smooth contour, consistent with the typical appearance and location of a papillary fibroelastoma.
- *Endocarditis vegetation:* Infective and noninfective endocarditis can present with a similar appearance as a result of an aortic valve vegetation. In cases of infective endocarditis, typically more significant damage and dysfunction of the involved valve are present, and the clinical history and presentation favor an infectious process.
- *Other valvular tumors:* In general, valvular tumors other than papillary fibroelastomas are rare. Myxomas, lipomas, and hematic cysts have been reported originating from cardiac valves.

Essential Facts

- Despite being an uncommon tumor, papillary fibroelastoma is the most common valvular neoplasm. More than 90% are attached to valves.
  - The most common location is in the aortic valve (45%), followed by the mitral valve (36%).
  - Papillary fibroelastoma is the third most common benign cardiac tumor, after myxoma and lipoma.
  - Papillary fibroelastomas are usually small (< 20 mm in diameter), mobile, single lesions.
  - The mean age at the time of diagnosis is 60 years.
  - Papillary fibroelastomas can be an incidental finding in asymptomatic patients evaluated for unrelated conditions, or they can be associated with a distal arterial embolization (e.g., stroke and transient ischemic attack) or valvular dysfunction.

Other Imaging Findings

- On echocardiography, a papillary fibroelastoma appears as a small round or oval echogenic polypoid lesion < 2 cm in diameter with a homogeneous echotexture. It is usually mobile and has a small stalk attached to the commissure of a cardiac valve.

✔ Pearls & ✘ Pitfalls

✔ Papillary fibroelastomas are benign, rare gelatinous tumors derived from the endocardium, primarily of the left-sided cardiac valves, with the potential for embolization.

✘ These small lesions can be easily overlooked in a nongated cross-sectional imaging examination.

Case 4

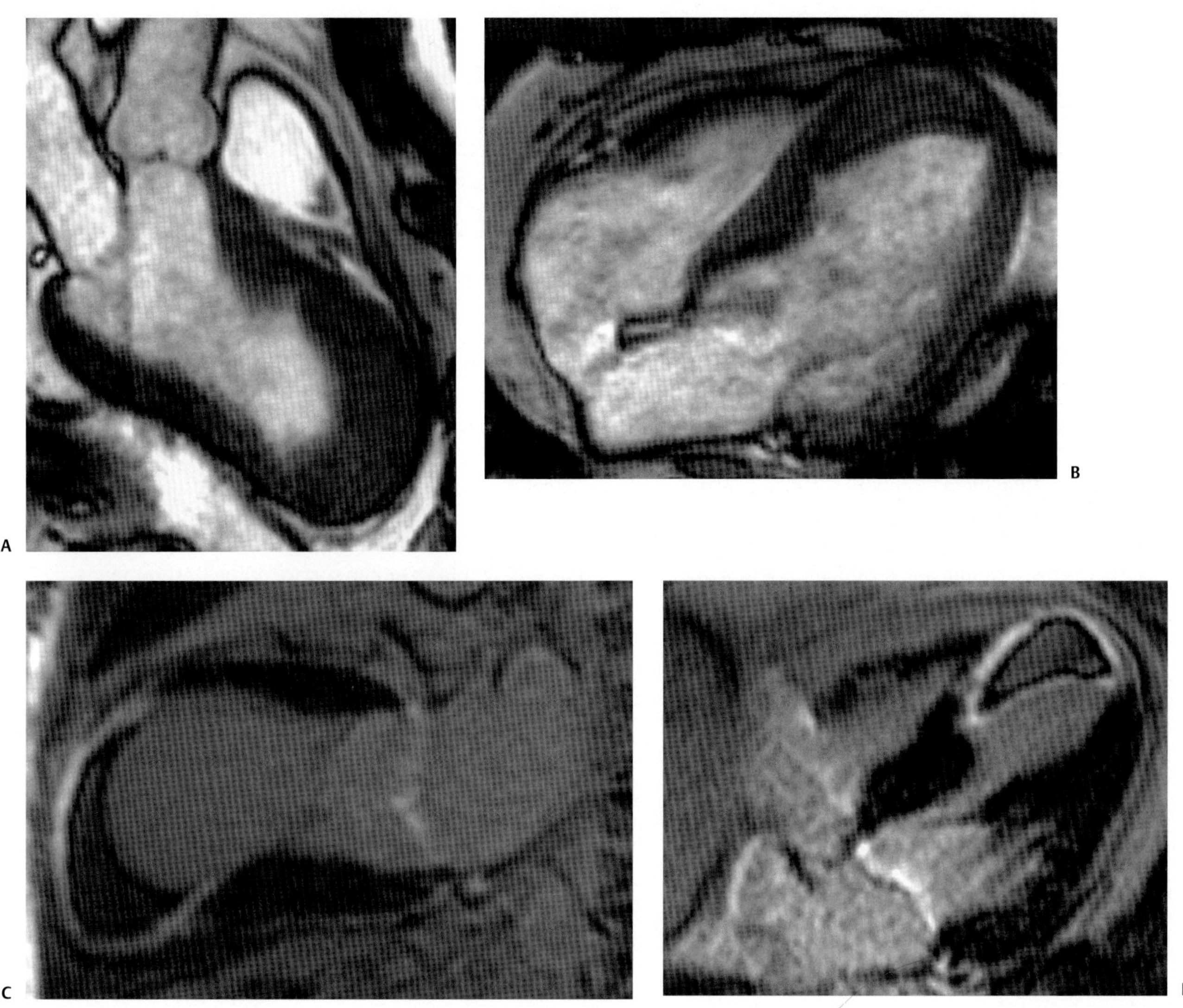

Clinical Presentation

A 57-year-old man presents with a history of recent myocardial infarction with ST wave elevation on electrocardiogram. The apex was not moving normally on echo, and the ejection fraction was measured at 17%.

Imaging Findings

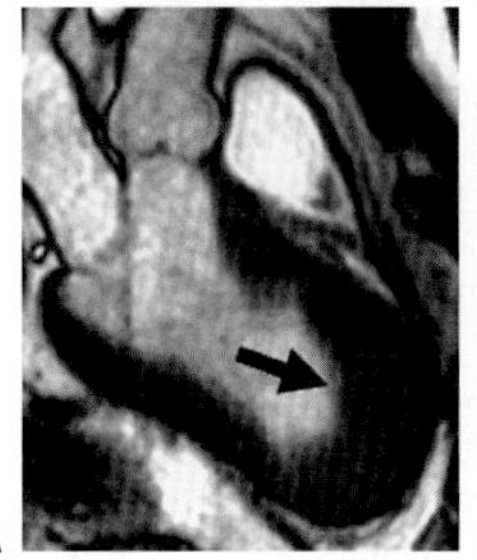
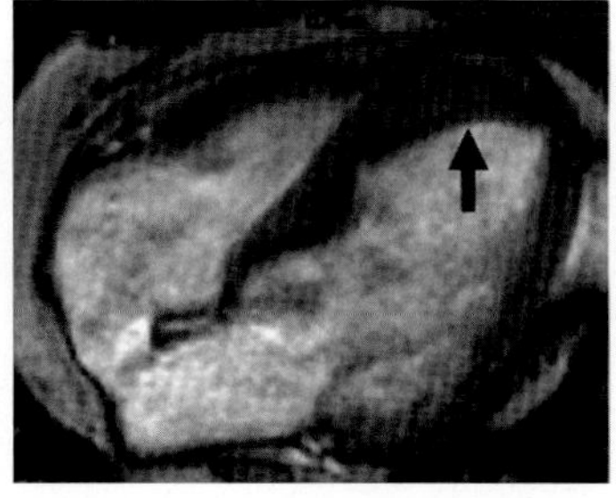
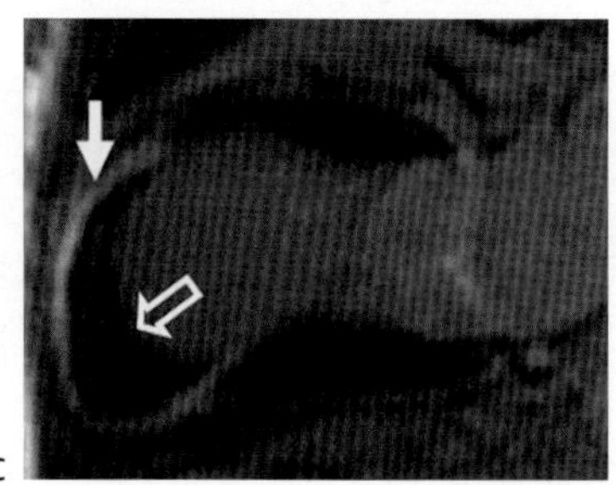
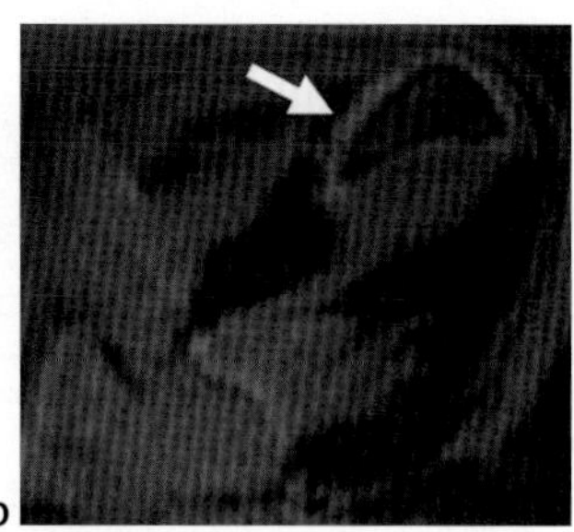

(A) A left ventricular (LV) outflow tract view shows a rounded shape and apparent thickening of the LV apex (*black arrow*). **(B)** This four-chamber white blood image of the heart shows apparent thickening of the rounded apex (*black arrow*). **(C,D)** Following intravenous administration of gadolinium, delayed images in a four-chamber and a two-chamber view show rim enhancement of a mass in the apex (*white arrows*), a thrombus that has formed on the endocardial surface of the infarcted myocardium. The thrombus does not enhance (*open white arrow*).

Differential Diagnosis

- ***LV apical infarction; aneurysm with thrombus formation:*** The LV apex is rounded and the wall thickness decreased. Linear enhancement of the subendocardial surface of the myocardium and no enhancement within the crescent-shaped thrombus are typical of this diagnosis.
- *Hypertrophic cardiomyopathy:* Although the apical myocardium appears thickened before gadolinium is given, the wall is clearly markedly thinned once the endocardium is defined. Localized hypertrophic cardiomyopathy usually affects the septal wall.
- *Apical cardiac metastasis:* The appearance of the apex prior to gadolinium administration could suggest an infiltrating metastatic lesion; however, the patient does not have a known malignancy.

Essential Facts

- Most thrombi that form in the LV following myocardial infarction occur within the first 2 weeks, but as early as 48 hours.
- Inflammatory cells infiltrate necrotic myocardium following infarction, inducing platelet and fibrin deposition on the endocardial surface of the myocardium, encouraging thrombus formation.
- Inflammatory markers such as C-reactive protein may help to predict in which patients thrombi are more likely to form.
- Potential embolic complications from LV thrombi portend a poor prognosis.

Other Imaging Findings

- Look for areas of wall motion abnormality, akinesis, marked hypokinesis, or aneurysm as a site of thrombus formation.
- Calcium within or on the surface of the LV thrombus is a sign of chronicity.
- Calcium may be missed on magnetic resonance imaging but should be obvious on computed tomography (CT).

✔ Pearls & ✘ Pitfalls

✔ Describe wall motion abnormalities in a systematic manner:
- If the face of a clock is used for reference, 12:00 is the anterior wall, 3:00 the lateral wall, 6:00 the inferior wall, and 9:00 the septal wall.
- Between these are regions called the *anteroseptal, inferolateral, inferoseptal,* and *anteroseptal segments.*

✘ On CT, the mixing of contrast with non–contrast-enhanced blood is an unusual finding in the LV, but it may be seen in the right side of the heart.

Case 5

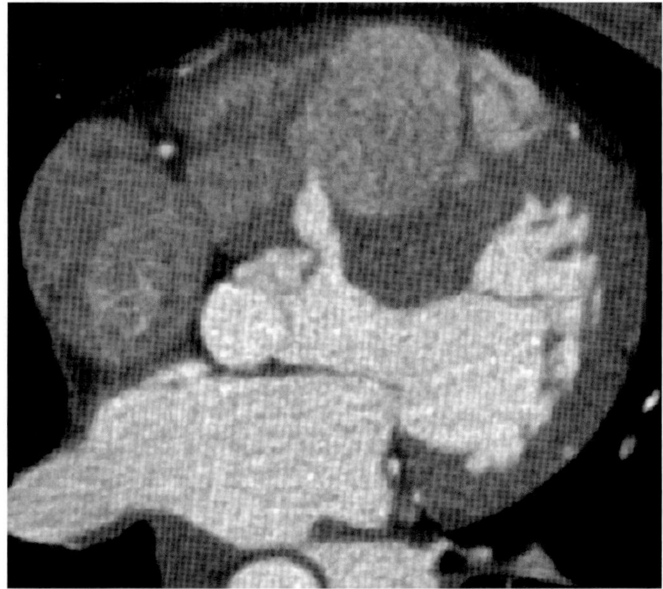
A

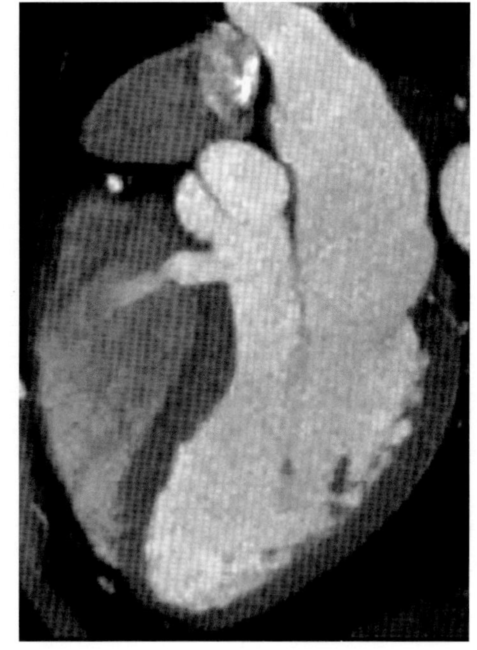
C

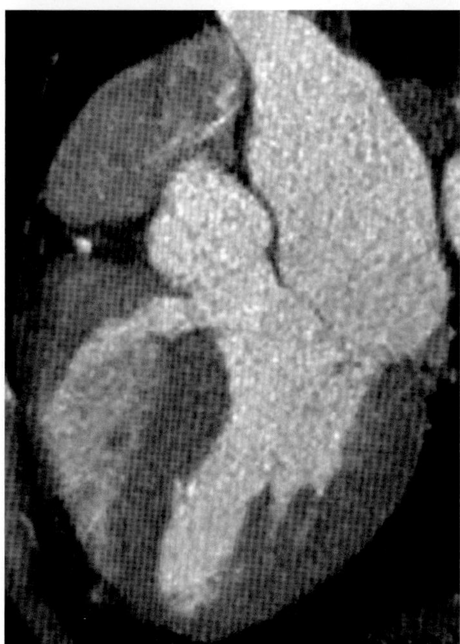
B

Clinical Presentation

A 29-year-old man presents with a murmur. What is the high-signal structure adjacent to the spine, parallel to the aorta? Explain how this structure and the abnormal morphology of the heart (Fig. B) are related.

Imaging Findings

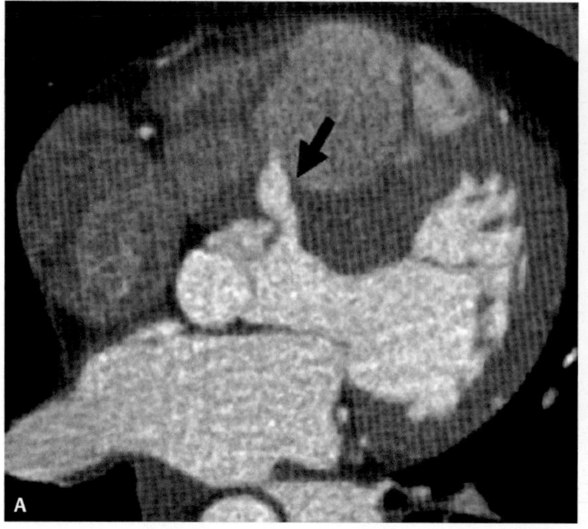
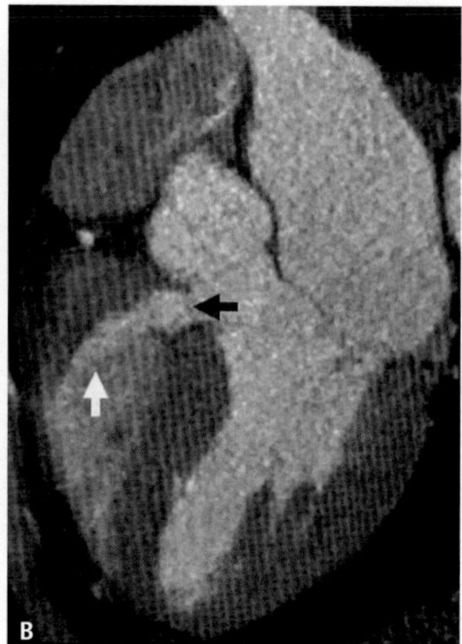
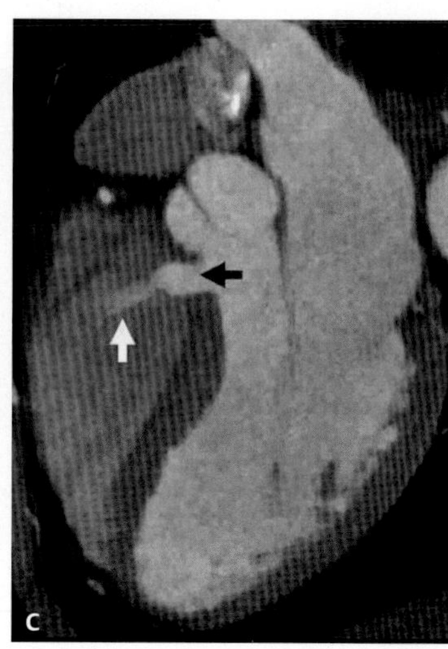

(A) In the axial plane, a defect in the septal wall is seen adjacent to the aortic valve (*black arrow*). In **(B)** systolic and **(C)** diastolic images, the defect in the interventricular septum at the base of the heart (*black arrows*) is seen in a left ventricular (LV) outflow tract view. The more densely enhanced blood in the left side of the heart flows from the left to the right; a jet of contrast-enhanced blood is seen in the right ventricle (*white arrows*).

Differential Diagnosis

- ***Membranous VSD:*** An obvious defect is seen in the interventricular septum, just below the aortic valve, which allows the flow of contrast (blood) from left to right.
- *Muscular VSD:* The muscular interventricular septum is intact and is normal thickness.
- *Aneurysm of the interventricular septum:* An interventricular aneurysm is thought to form during the process of spontaneous closure of membranous defects. Such an aneurysm looks like a windsock, and when completely closed, it does not allow shunting of blood.

Essential Facts

- VSD is the most common congenital heart defect.
- It is one feature of numerous types of congenital heart disease.
- It is the most common symptomatic congenital heart defect in neonates.
- The ventricular septum has four segments: inlet, trabecular, outlet, and membranous.
- Defects of the interventricular septum are classified in different ways:
  - Muscular—entirely surrounded by septal muscle (inlet, outlet, or trabecular)
  - Membranous—lies just below the aortic valve; bordered partially by fibrous tissue inferior to the aortic valve and medial to the mitral valve. The defect may extend to the crista, adjacent to the septal leaflet of the tricuspid valve.
  - Doubly committed, subarterial (combined)—in the outlet septum and bordered partially by fibrous tissue between the aortic and pulmonary valves
  - Inlet—near the mitral valve
  - Outlet—below the aortic valve
  - Supracristal—below the pulmonary valve

✔ Pearls & ✘ Pitfalls

✔ Qp:Qs is a ratio that indicates the degree of shunting, where Qp is the pulmonary resistance and Qs is the systemic resistance.

✔ Restrictive VSD: Qp:Qs < 1.5/1.0
A high-pressure defect exists between the left and right ventricles; the shunt is small, and most children are asymptomatic. A high-frequency holosystolic murmur is noted.

✔ Moderately restrictive VSD: Qp:Qs 1.5/1.0 to 2.5/1.0
This degree of shunting results in a hemodynamic load on the LV. Children present with failure to thrive and congestive heart failure. Holosystolic murmur and apical diastolic rumble are noted.

✔ Nonrestrictive VSD: Qp:Qs > 2.5/1.0
Right ventricle volume overload is seen early, and progressive pulmonary artery overload becomes symptomatic in early life. Holosystolic murmur and apical diastolic rumble are noted.

✔ VSD with Qp:Qs > 2.0/1.0 should be closed before pulmonary hypertension becomes irreversible.

✔ Progressive aortic regurgitation may develop with a restrictive VSD.

✘ View the heart in anatomically correct planes to accurately classify and measure the VSD.

✘ Electrocardiogram-gated computed tomography (CT) or magnetic resonance imaging (MRI) will show the contrast flow or flow void, respectively, through a VSD.

✘ Quantification of the Qp:Qs is possible with MRI and echocardiography but is currently not possible with CT.

Case 6

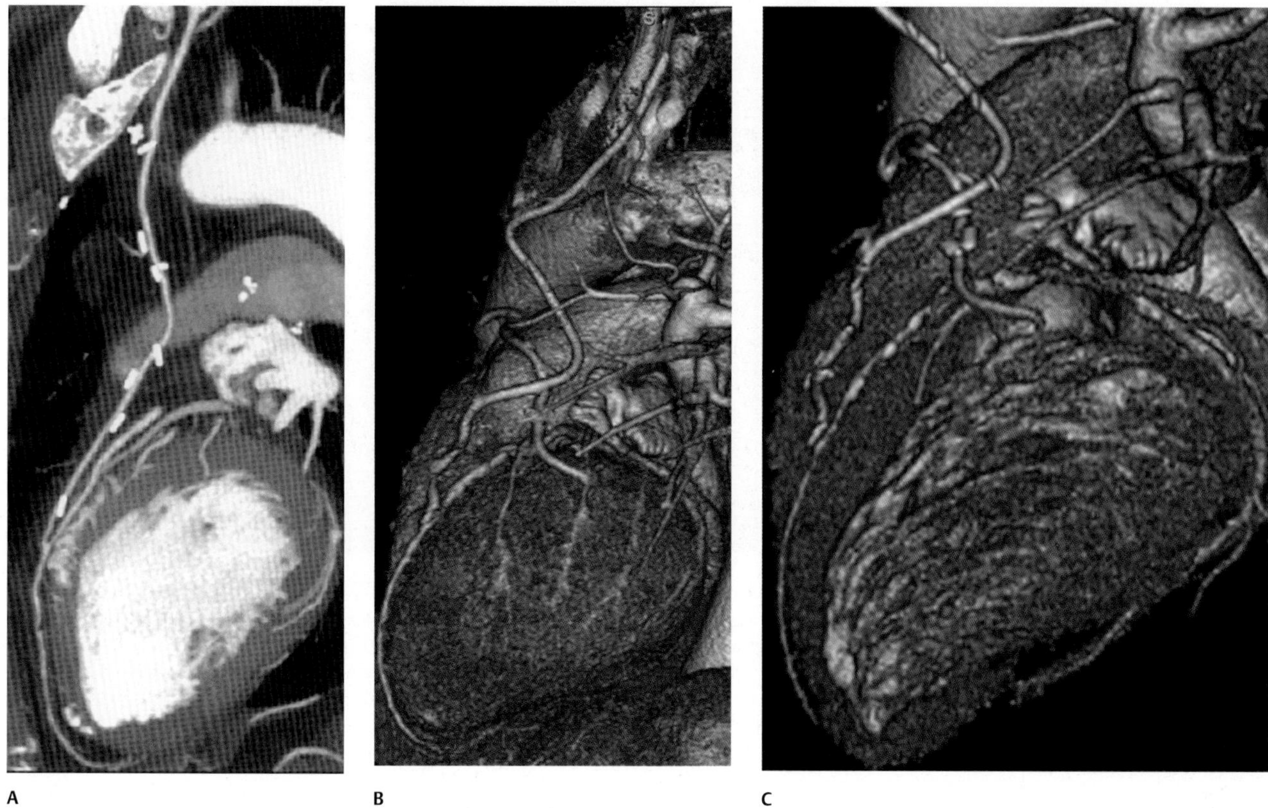

A B C

Clinical Presentation

A 68-year-old man with history of left internal mammary artery (LIMA) coronary artery bypass graft (CABG) to the left anterior descending (LAD) coronary artery after diagnosis of severe proximal LAD stenosis. He now presents with new angina.

Imaging Findings

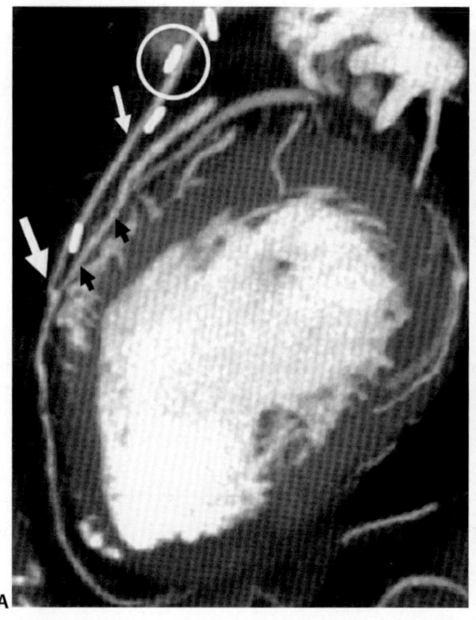
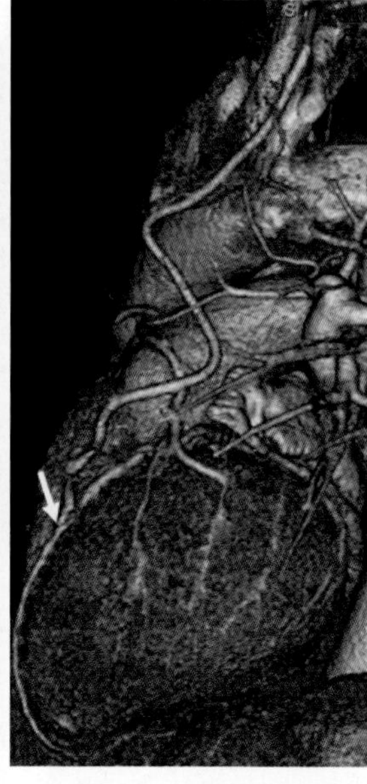
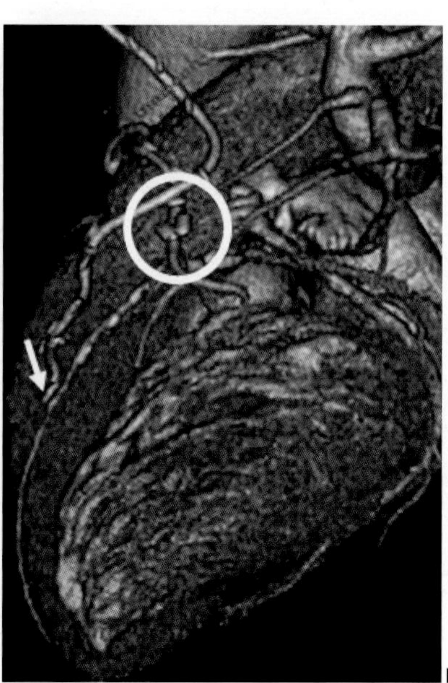

A B, C

(A) In a two-dimensional (2D) planar view, the LIMA bypass graft (*small white arrow*) courses from its origin on the left subclavian artery (not shown) to an end-to-side anastomosis with the mid LAD (*large white arrow*). The proximal LAD is patent (*black arrows*), likely opacified by retrograde flow. The hyperattenuating foci along the course of the LIMA are surgical clips (*white circle*), which are used to close branches of the LIMA.

(B) A three-dimensional surface-rendered view of the heart and the LIMA graft shows the patent anastomosis with the LAD. **(C)** Using a different windowing technique, the surgical clips (*white circle*) are seen. Clips at or near the anastomosis may make it impossible to make a confident diagnosis of patency.

Differential Diagnosis

- ***Patent LIMA–LAD CABG:*** The anastomosis of the LIMA with the LAD is patent, best seen in the 2D view. Retrograde flow into the proximal LAD is a common finding when the stenotic or occlusive lesion is very proximal.
- *Re-established antegrade flow in the LAD:* If a CABG is performed to an epicardial coronary artery that does not have a severe stenosis or occlusion (i.e., the distal myocardium is not ischemic), the CABG will close because blood flow in the native artery is maintained.
- *Saphenous vein–LAD CABG:* Saphenous and other venous grafts are sewn to the ascending aorta, forming an anastomosis with the LAD and other epicardial coronary arteries similar to that shown between the LIMA and LAD.

Essential Facts

- 64 MDCT has been shown to have a sensitivity, specificity, and diagnostic accuracy of 100% for the diagnosis of occlusion of CABG.
- Studies show a slight variation in the sensitivity (100–80%) but agreement in the excellent specificity (91%) and diagnostic accuracy (87%) for determination of flow-limiting stenosis within a graft vessel.
- MDCT allows sensitive and specific determination of CABG patency and stenosis without the risks of an invasive procedure.
- Serial evaluation of CABG patency is essential, especially in patients with multiple grafts, as they may be asymptomatic if only one graft is stenosed or occluded.
- Venous grafts may develop atherosclerotic disease, aneurysms, or pseudoaneurysms.

Other Imaging Findings

- Because of their cephalocaudal course, lesser motion artifacts, and larger luminal caliber, arterial and venous bypass grafts easier to image and follow on multidetector CT imaging than are the native epicardial arteries.
- The metal surgical clips used to close branches of bypass grafts can be beneficial in marking the course of the graft but detrimental if streak artifact obscures the graft–native vessel anastomosis.
- Evaluate native epicardial coronary arteries and myocardium for progressive stenosis and evidence of prior infarction, aneurysm, and thrombus.

✔ Pearls & ✘ Pitfalls

✔ Heart rate control with beta-blockers is recommended to achieve a heart rate between 60 and 65 beats/min.
✔ Use retrospective electrocardiogram (ECG) gating to calculate left and right ventricle function.
✔ Use prospective ECG gating to conserve radiation dose.
✘ Evaluation of CABG vessels may be limited by slowed flow through a graft if there is stenosis and potentially by streak/blooming artifacts from surgical clips and calcium.

Case 7

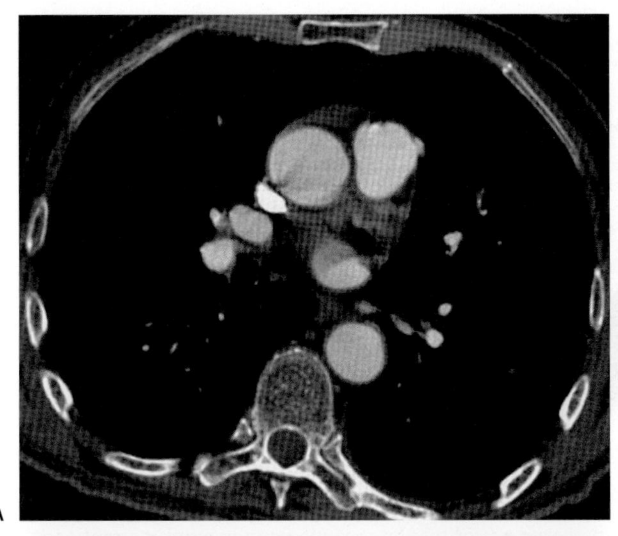
A

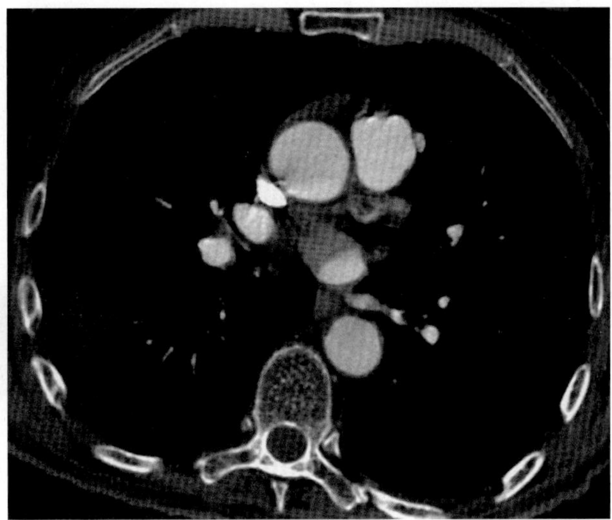
B

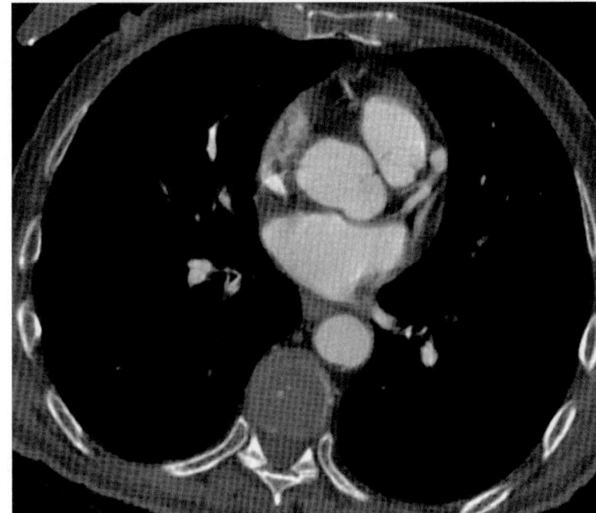
C

Clinical Presentation

Dyspnea on exertion in a 55-year-old man

Imaging Findings

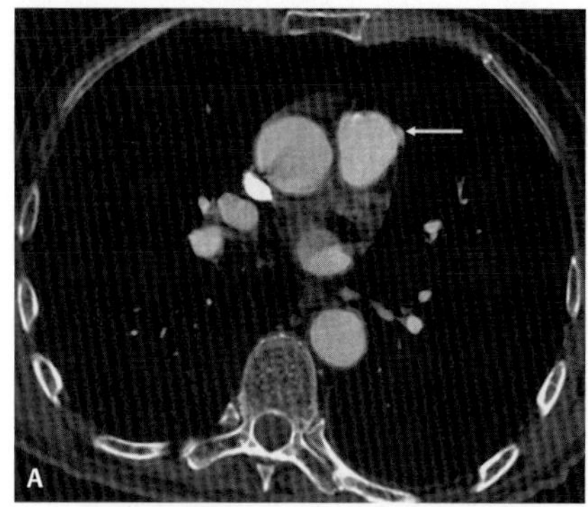

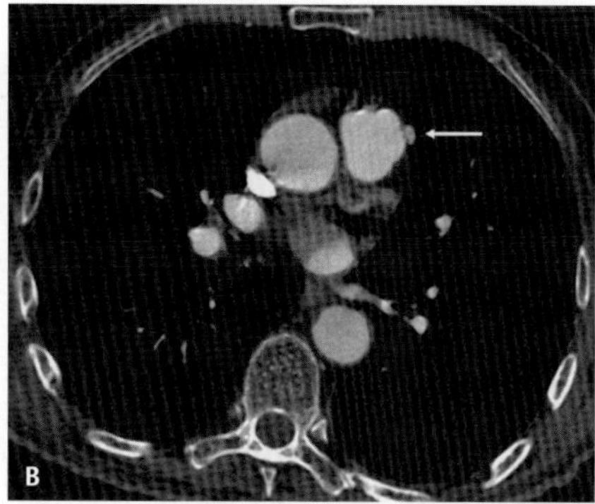

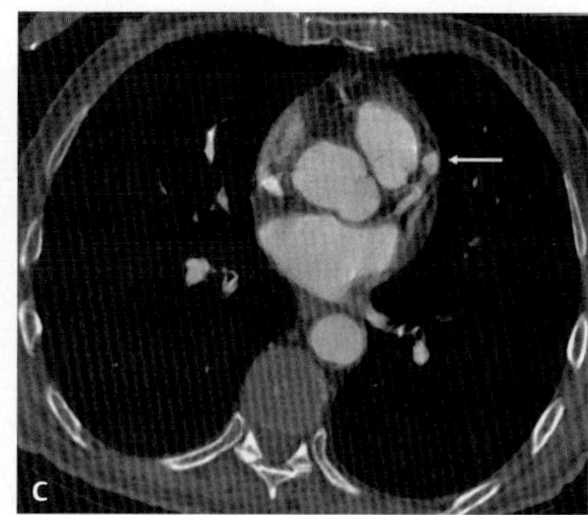

(A–C) Contrast-enhanced computed tomography of the thorax, with axial images at three different levels. An abnormal vessel is seen arising from the trunk of the pulmonary artery and continuing into the position of the left anterior descending coronary artery (LAD).

Differential Diagnosis

- ***Anomalous origin of the left coronary artery from the pulmonary artery (ALCAPA):*** The origin of the left coronary artery from the pulmonary artery, also known as Bland–White–Garland syndrome, is a rare congenital anomaly that induces ischemia and hypoperfused myocardium resulting from "steal" phenomenon, in which blood flow is diverted from the heart to the pulmonary artery.
- *Coronary artery fistula:* A coronary artery fistula may present as an abnormal-caliber vessel in close relation to the main pulmonary artery.

Essential Facts

- ALCAPA is a rare condition seen in 1 in 300,000 live births and accounts for ~0.25% of all cases of congenital heart disease.
  - The flow in the affected coronary artery is reversed and is toward the pulmonary artery.
  - This is one of the most common causes of myocardial ischemia and infarction in children, and if not treated, the mortality rate during the first year of life is ~90%.
  - Occasionally, untreated patients with a lesser degree of ischemia survive until adulthood, and their condition is diagnosed later in life.
  - In the majority of cases, this is an isolated defect, but an association with other anomalies (e.g., atrial and ventricular septal defects and aortic coarctation) has been reported.
  - The goal of surgical correction is to restore two coronary artery systems from the aorta.

Other Imaging Findings

- Untreated patients who survive usually exhibit significant intercoronary collateral circulation with prominent tortuous vessels. The right coronary artery is usually dilated and tortuous as well.

✔ Pearls & ✘ Pitfalls

✔ The landmark case reported by Drs. Bland, White, and Garland (Massachusetts General Hospital) in 1933 was a 3-month-old child with ALCAPA, the son of the prestigious thoracic radiologist Dr. A. O. Hampton.

✔ Other diseases that can present with dilatation of the coronary arteries are vasculitis (Kawasaki disease, polyarteritis nodosa), scleroderma, Ehlers–Danlos syndrome, and fistulas.

Case 8

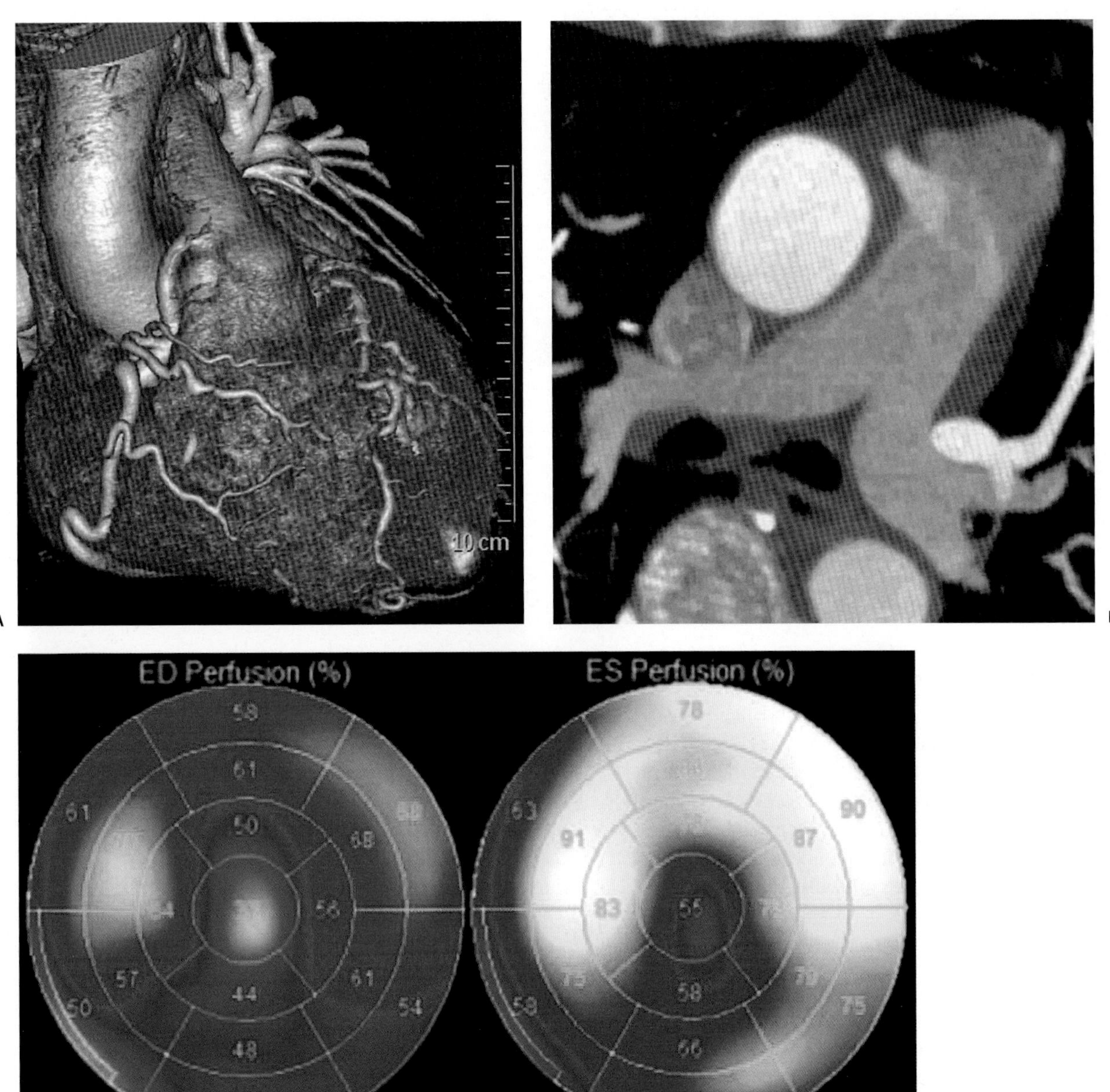

Clinical Presentation

A 74-year-old woman presents with a possible right coronary artery (RCA) anomaly on echocardiogram (ECG).

Imaging Findings

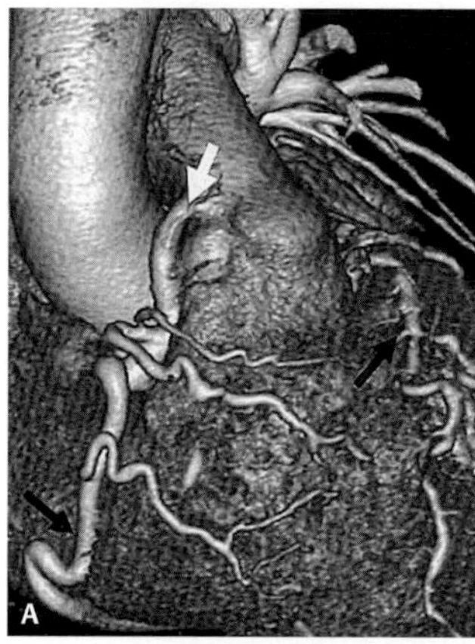

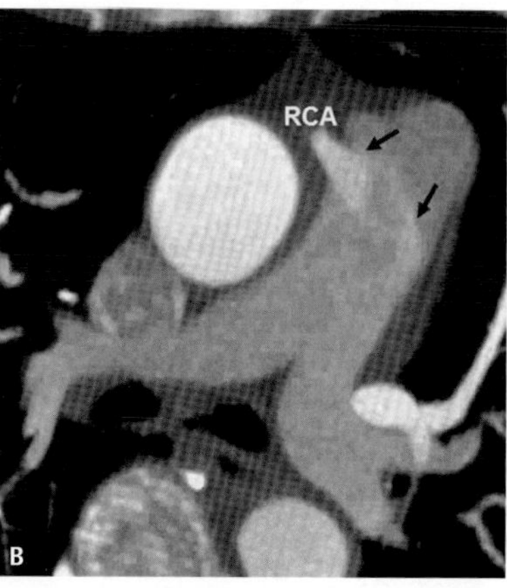

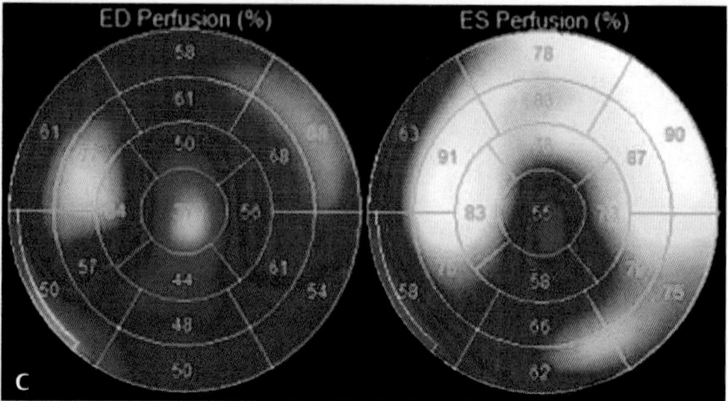

(A) The RCA origin is from the main pulmonary artery (MPA: *white arrow*). The RCA and the left anterior descending (LAD) artery (*black arrows*) are extremely tortuous, but along with their branches, they follow a normal course on the epicardial surface of the heart. **(B)** An oblique view of the main pulmonary artery shows contrast-enhanced blood flowing into the MPA (*arrows*) from the RCA. This MPA steal occurs because of the lower pressure in the MPA than in the RCA. **(C)** Nuclear myocardial perfusion images reveal less blood flow to the inferior wall of the left ventricle (*purple*) than to the anterior and lateral walls (*red* and *yellow*, respectively) in the vascular distribution of the RCA. The defect is larger in diastole than it is in systole.

Differential Diagnosis

- ***Anomalous origin of the right coronary artery from the pulmonary artery (ARCAPA):*** The RCA origin arises from the MPA. An RCA origin is not seen arising from the expected location on the aorta.
- *Coronary vein drainage to the MPA:* Although the abnormal vessel drains into the MPA, its branches are clearly typical of the RCA anatomy. Normal coronary veins drain to the coronary sinus or to the cardiac chambers.
- *Venous coronary artery bypass graft:* Bypass grafts never originate from the pulmonary arteries. There are no other postoperative changes in the chest.

Essential Facts

- ARCAPA is a very rare anomaly, with only 72 cases reported in the literature.
- Embryologically, the truncus arteriosus is the structure from which the ascending aorta and the MPA are formed. Theoretically, the coronary artery origins are displaced from their normal site by abnormal division of the truncus arteriosus. Therefore, the coronary artery may arise from the pulmonary artery instead of the aorta.
- Patients with origin of the RCA from the pulmonary artery may be asymptomatic.
- If the left coronary artery arises from the pulmonary artery, patients present with ischemia in infancy.

Other Imaging Findings

- Nuclear myocardial perfusion imaging as in this patient shows regional deficits.
- Tortuosity of the coronary arteries occurs presumably because of increased flow.
- In the LAD artery, blood flow is antegrade, with a greater volume of blood supplied to the myocardium. Septal and epicardial branches of the left coronary arteries are of large caliber.
- Blood flow in the RCA is retrograde, stealing blood from the myocardium and delivering it to the lower-pressure pulmonary artery.
- Normal coronary blood flow from the epicardial coronary arteries is antegrade during diastole.
- The pulmonic and aortic valves are closed during diastole.
- Myocardial perfusion imaging shows a larger perfusion defect during diastole than in systole because of the steal effect of the ARCAPA.

✔ Pearls & ✘ Pitfalls

✔ Inspect each aortic valve cusp for origins of the coronary arteries.

✔ If the coronary artery origin is not found on the aorta, look elsewhere.

✔ Anomalous coronary artery origins may be from any of the sinuses of Valsalva of the aortic valve, the ascending aorta, or the MPA.

✔ ECG gating is necessary to view the details of the coronary artery anatomy.

✔ The right side of the heart should be nearly empty of contrast-enhanced blood so that the blood flow from the coronary artery into the pulmonary artery can be seen.

Case 9

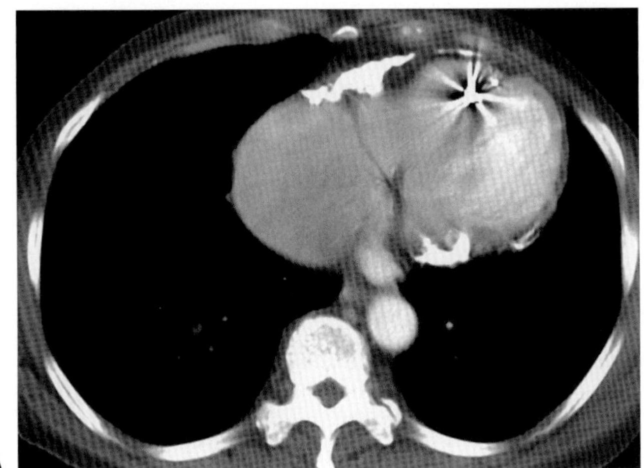

A

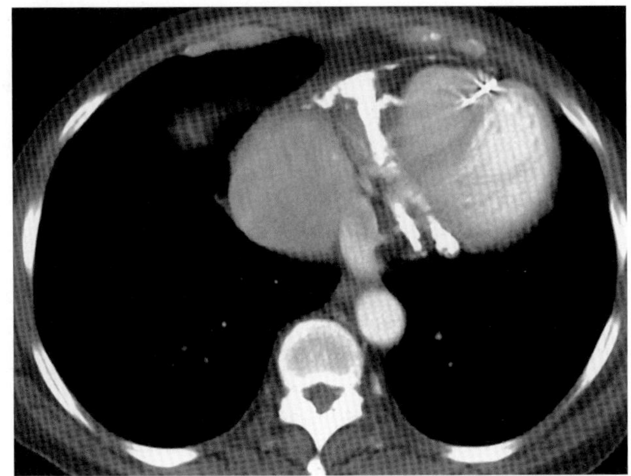

B

Clinical Presentation

Progressive shortness of breath, abdominal swelling, and orthopnea

Imaging Findings

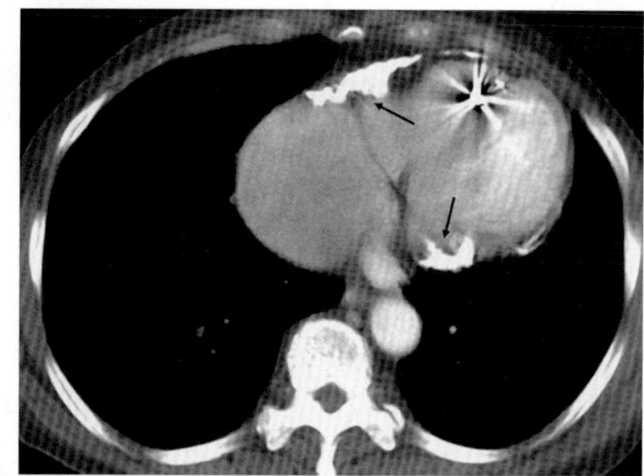

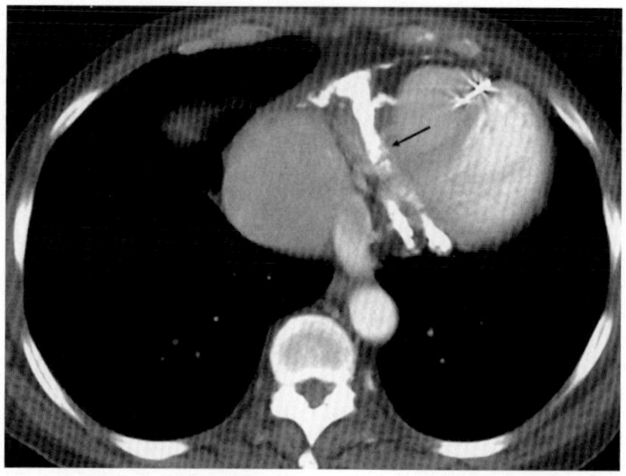

(A,B) Contrast-enhanced computed tomography (CT) of the thorax demonstrates extensive pericardial thickening and calcification (*black arrows*), more prominent on the atrioventricular groove. There is abnormal dilatation of the right atrium and coronary sinus, indicating constrictive physiology.

Differential Diagnosis

- ***Constrictive pericarditis:*** Fibrous or calcified thickening of the pericardium that prevents normal diastolic ventricular filling is characteristic of restrictive pericarditis.
- *Pericarditis without constriction:* Pericardial thickening from diverse acute and chronic inflammatory causes may occur in the absence of a constrictive physiology.
- *Myocardial calcification:* Chronic inflammatory and metabolic disorders may produce myocardial calcification. CT helps differentiate between pericardial and myocardial distribution of calcified plaques.

Essential Facts

- Currently, the most common causes are previous surgery and radiation therapy.
- Other possible causes are infectious pericarditis (tuberculosis, viral), collagen vascular disease, and uremia.
- The physiologic effect and clinical presentation of constrictive pericarditis and restrictive cardiomyopathy are similar.
- Affected pericardium usually exceeds 4 mm in thickness, up to 10 or 12 mm.
- Irregular calcification may occur anywhere over the surface of the heart, but the largest accumulation is usually at the atrioventricular groove.
- Other imaging findings are ventricular deformity with tubular small ventricles and dilated atria.
- After surgery, complete normalization of cardiac hemodynamics is reported in 60% of patients.

Other Imaging Findings

- Signs of impaired diastolic filling include dilatation of the inferior vena cava and hepatic veins, hepatosplenomegaly, and ascites.

✔ Pearls & ✘ Pitfalls

✔ Differentiation between constrictive pericarditis and restrictive cardiomyopathy is crucial, as definitive treatment of restrictive cardiomyopathy is surgical (pericardiectomy or pericardial stripping).

✔ Constrictive pericarditis may be seen in patients with normal pericardial thickness.

✔ Transthoracic echocardiography is limited for evaluating pericardial thickening.

Case 10

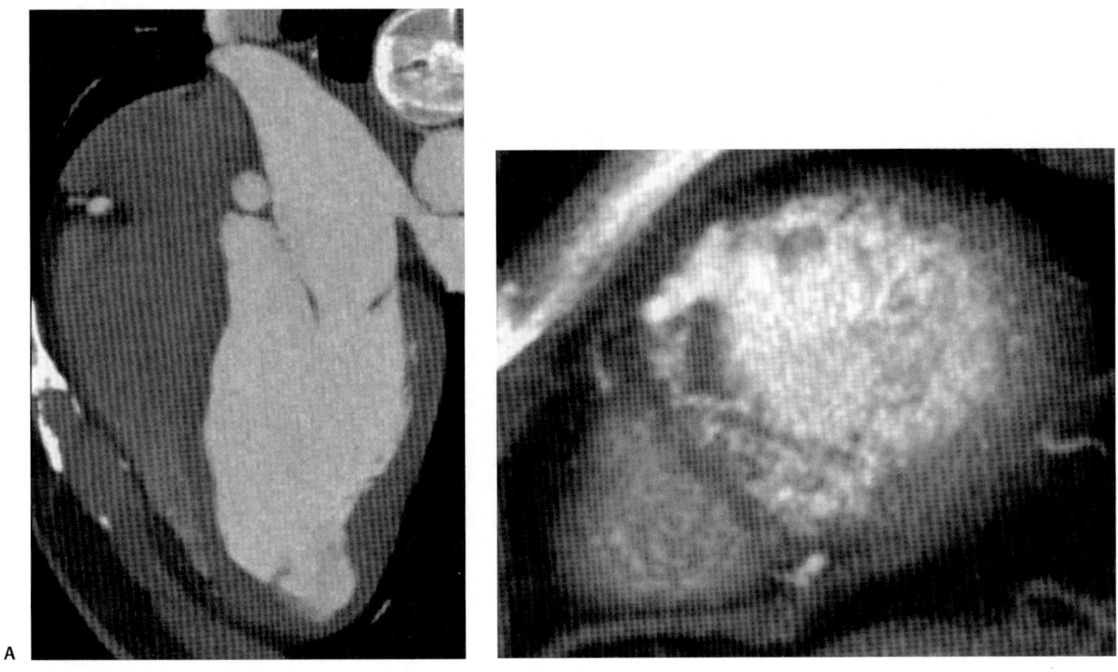

Clinical Presentation

A 63-year-old man presents with ST wave elevation on electrocardiogram (ECG).

Imaging Findings

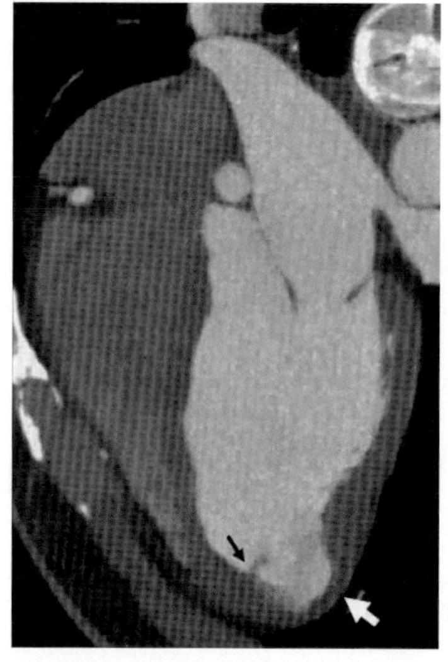

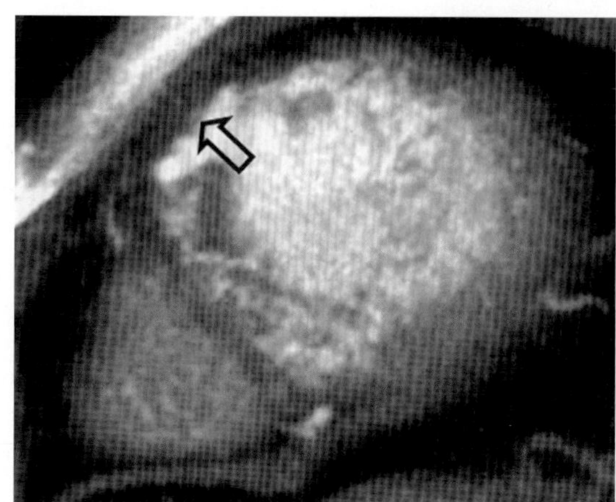

(A) The left ventricular (LV) apex is thin and rounded (*white arrow*). A linear filling defect (*black arrow*) in the apex may represent early thrombus formation. **(B)** In the short axis, focal wall thinning is seen at the apex (*open black arrow*).

Differential Diagnosis

- ***LV apical aneurysm and early thrombus formation secondary to infarction:*** The apex of the LV chamber is thin and aneurysmal, both findings related to remote infarction. A linear filling defect in the aneurysm represents a thrombus that formed in the apex.
- *Dilated cardiomyopathy:* There is only focal myocardial thinning and dilatation at the apex. The remainder of the LV chamber is normal.
- *Ischemic cardiomyopathy:* The computed tomography (CT) findings are classic for focal, completed infarction, not a regional or global LV abnormality, as found with ischemic cardiomyopathy.

Essential Facts

- Normal myocardium has a homogeneous attenuation and uniform thickness on CT.
- Normally, the LV apex is thinner than the adjacent myocardium and has a pointed shape, like the end of a football.
- When one or more of the three principles outlined by Virchow triad are present, such as abnormal blood flow and damage to the endocardial surface in the infarcted myocardium, thrombus is likely to form, as in this patient.

Other Imaging Findings

- An anatomical correlation between calcified and noncalcified coronary artery atherosclerotic disease can be easily distinguished on multidetector CT and should correspond to regions of myocardial infarction.
- Areas of infarcted myocardium show thinning and typically reveal low attenuation, which may represent fat or fibrous tissue replacing or infiltrating the myocardium.
- Wall motion abnormalities may be clearly shown when ECG-gated multidetector CT is performed retrospectively.

✔ Pearls & ✘ Pitfalls

✔ Examine the coronary arteries to diagnose “cutoff” or occlusion of a vessel.

✔ Look for collateralization of coronary artery branches from other epicardial coronary arteries or from transmyocardial collaterals.

✔ The LV myocardium should be imaged in short-axis, vertical, and horizontal long-axis cardiac planes to detect wall thinning, myocardial attenuation abnormalities, and wall motion abnormalities.

✔ Cardiac imaging planes will also allow examination of coronary artery vascular territories.

Case 11

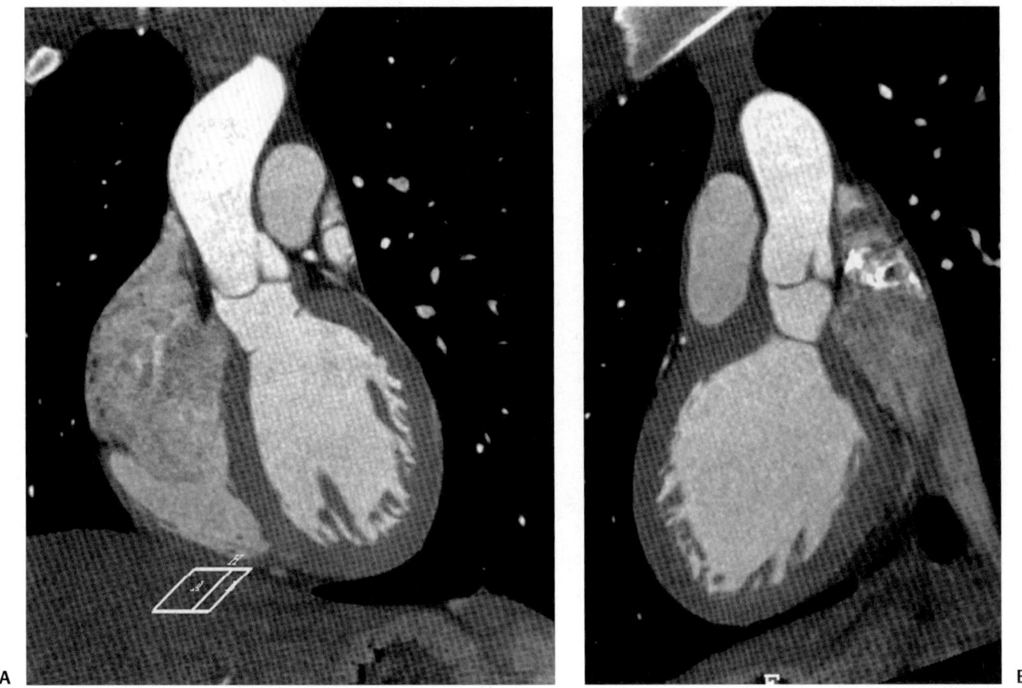

A B

Clinical Presentation

Murmur on a physical examination in a 22-year-old man

Imaging Findings

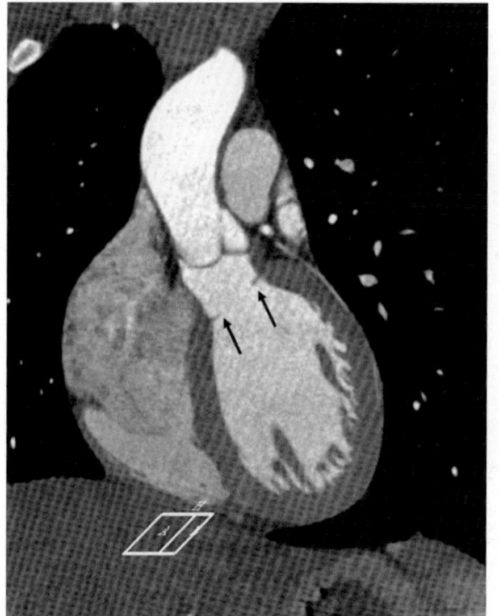

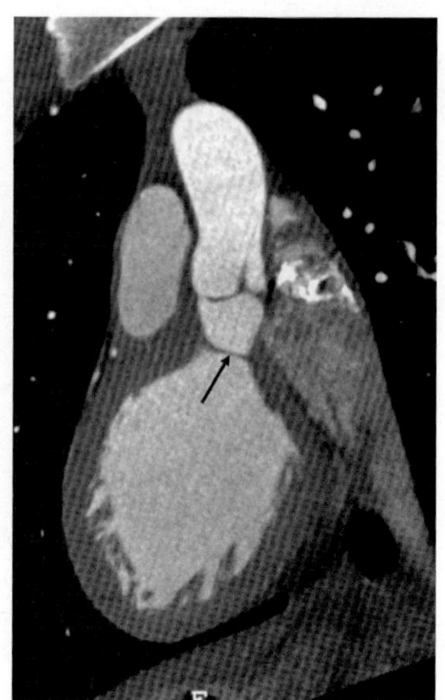

(A,B) Cardiac-gated computed tomography angiogram images with oblique re-formations show a ringlike, thin membrane projecting on the periphery of the outflow tract of the left ventricle (LV).

Differential Diagnosis

- ***Discrete subaortic stenosis (SAS):*** Fixed SAS can be due to a discrete fibrous membrane or diaphragm, muscular narrowing, or both. The discrete membranous type, which is displayed in the images corresponding to this case, is the most common.
- *Muscular subaortic stenosis:* In the muscular form of SAS, the obstruction is more diffuse, resulting in a tunnel-shaped LV outflow tract.

Essential Facts

- The discrete form (membranous type) of SAS is the most common (90%), but the tunnel-type lesion is associated with more significant stenosis of the LV outflow tract.
- Mean age at presentation is 20 years.
- The tunnel type has a distinct female preponderance (7:1).
- The prevalence of discrete fibromuscular SAS is ~6% in adults with congenital heart disease.
- Aortic regurgitation is present in 80% of patients.
- A bicuspid aortic valve is present in one fourth of patients.
- More than one third of patients have a concomitant ventricular septal defect.
- SAS may be part of the Shone's complex (a complex of obstructive lesions including mitral valve stenosis or parachute deformity, bicuspid aortic valve, and coarctation of the aorta).

Other Imaging Findings

- Patients with SAS may present with imaging findings of other congenital heart disease complications: ventricular septal defect, aortic coarctation, atrioventricular septal defect, patent ductus arteriosus, bicuspid aortic valve stenosis, and double-outlet right ventricle.

✔ Pearls & ✘ Pitfalls

✔ *Subaortic stenosis* is a descriptive term that includes a broad spectrum of anomalies, ranging from outlet ventricular stenosis to surgically created long outlet chambers and discrete subaortic membranes.

✔ The degree of SAS may be underestimated by the Doppler-derived pressure gradient in the presence of depressed LV function.

Case 12

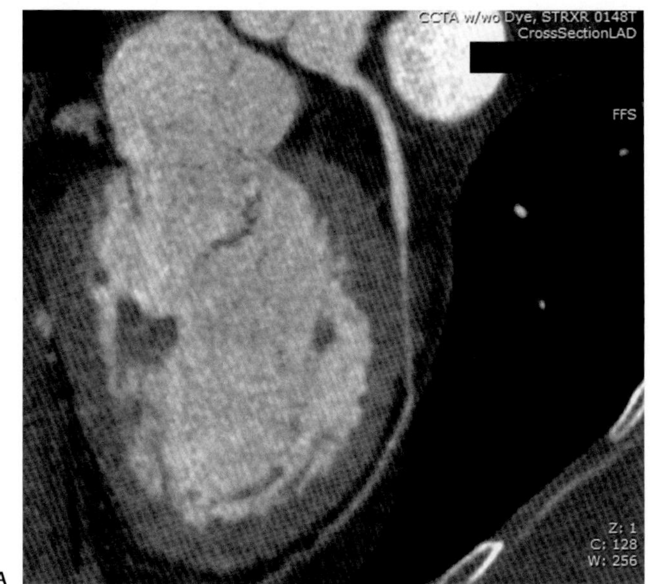

A

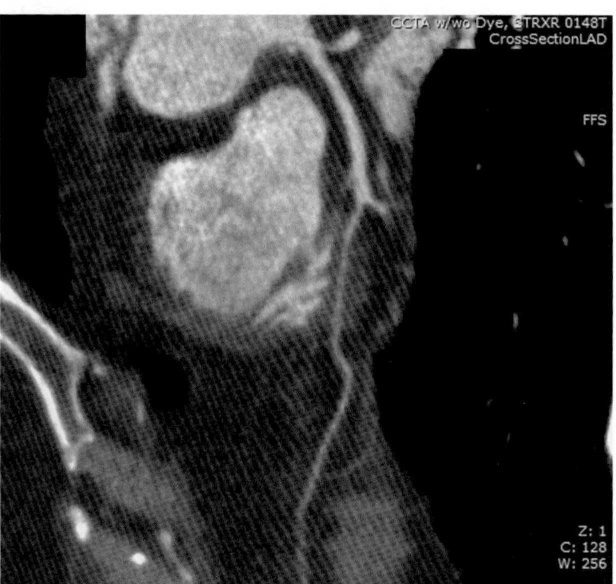

B

Clinical Presentation

A 49-year-old woman presents with atypical chest pain.

Imaging Findings

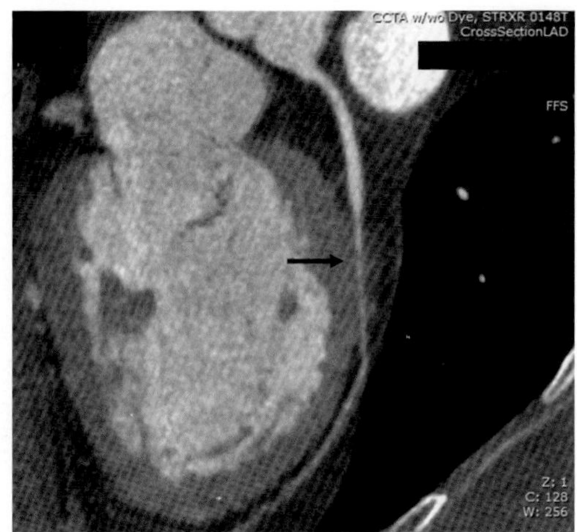

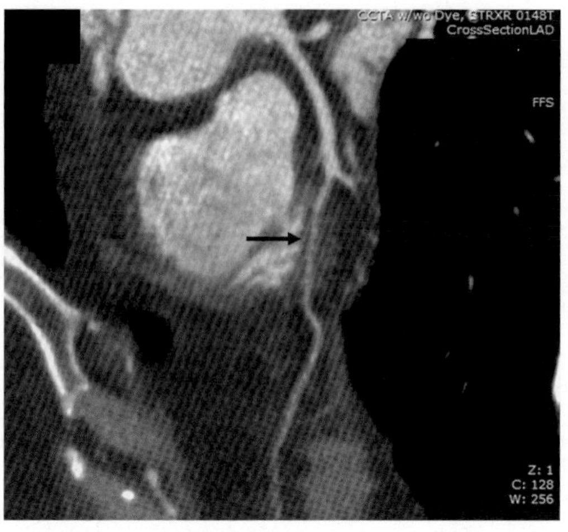

(A,B) Curved multiplanar reconstructions of a computed tomography angiogram (CTA) of the coronary arteries demonstrate mild abnormal narrowing of the middle third of the left anterior descending (LAD) artery (*arrows*) in an intramural segment in which the vessel is covered by ventricular myocardium.

Differential Diagnosis

- ***Myocardial bridge:*** An intramyocardial segment of an epicardial coronary artery, in which the vessel is embedded within the myocardium, is referred to as a *myocardial bridge*.
- *Normal LAD coronary artery:* The curved multiplanar images show a change in caliber as well as myocardium covering the narrow segment, which is not the normal appearance of the LAD coronary artery.

Essential Facts

- The term *myocardial bridge* is defined as a variable-length (4–40 mm), tunneled intramural segment of a coronary artery that normally courses epicardially.
- In an autopsy series, the prevalence of myocardial bridges was between 15 and 85%. In an angiographic series, it was between 0.5 and 16.0%, reflecting the fact that many small, nonconstricting bridges are not visible. A CTA series showed myocardial bridges in 3.5 to 26.0% of patients.
- Most commonly, myocardial bridges occur in the mid-portion of the LAD artery, followed by the diagonal branches, the right coronary artery, and the left circumflex artery.
- In the vast majority of cases, this congenital anomaly is benign and usually asymptomatic.
- The mechanism responsible in symptomatic cases is systolic compression of the tunneled segment by the overlying myocardium.
- Occasionally, this anomaly has been associated with various clinical manifestations. Angina is the most common clinical manifestation (70%). Other manifestations are exercise-induced arrhythmia, myocardial infarction, and sudden death.

Other Imaging Findings

- Angiographic criteria for diagnosis are the "milking effect" and the "step-down/step-up" phenomenon induced by systolic compression of the tunneled vessel.

✔ Pearls & ✘ Pitfalls

✔ Several studies have shown that the tunneled coronary segment is rarely affected by atherosclerosis, but the segment proximal to the myocardial bridge is at increased risk for plaque development.

✔ A dynamic comparison between systole and diastole is important to determine the degree of systolic compression of the intramural segment.

Case 13

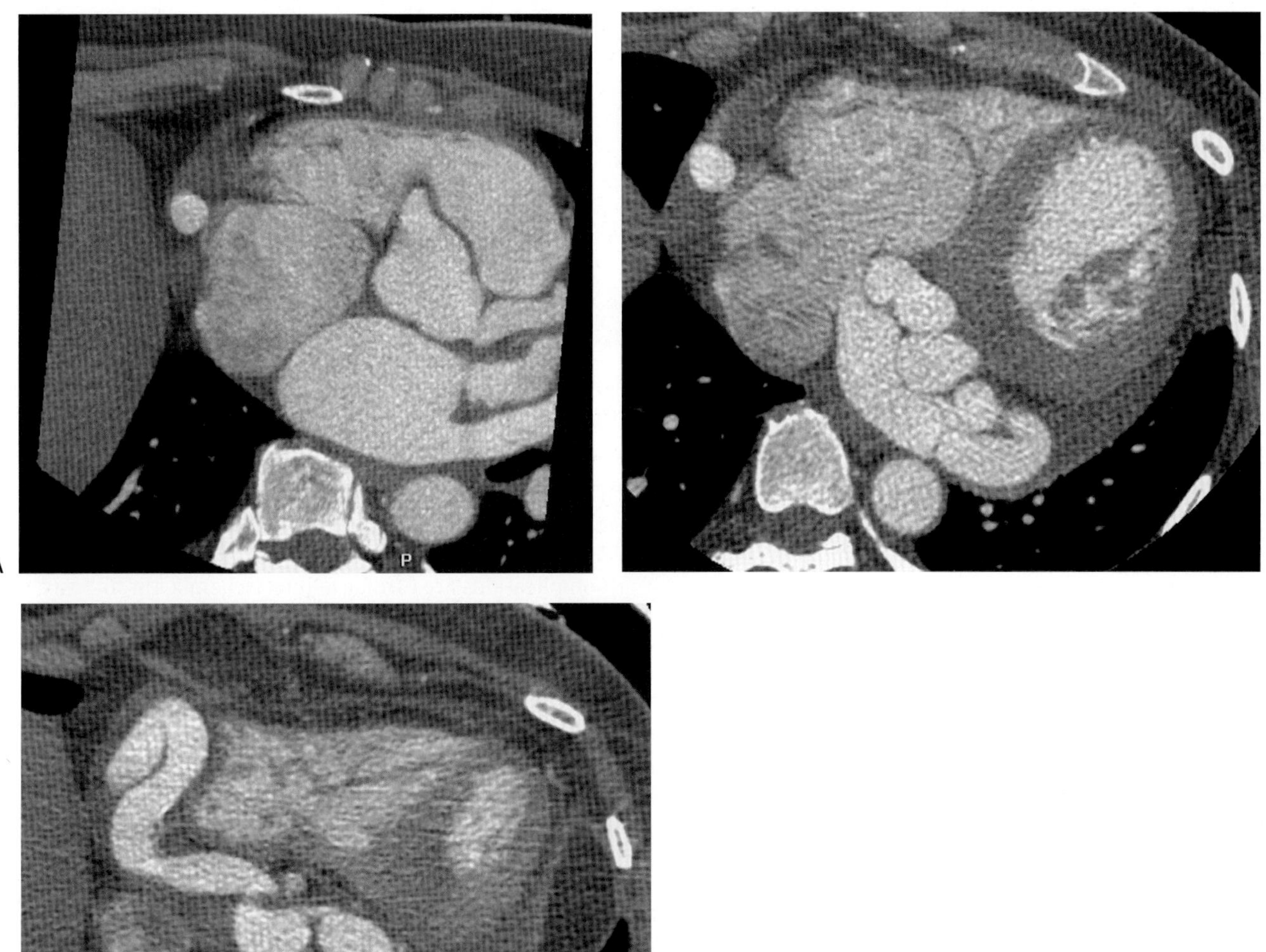

A B C

Clinical Presentation

Dyspnea on exertion and cardiac murmur

Imaging Findings

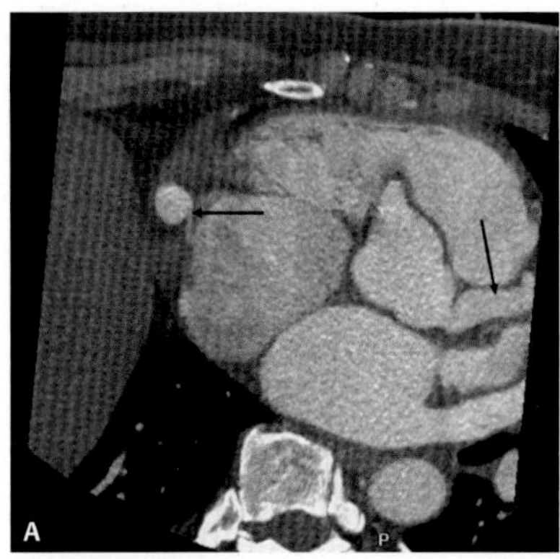

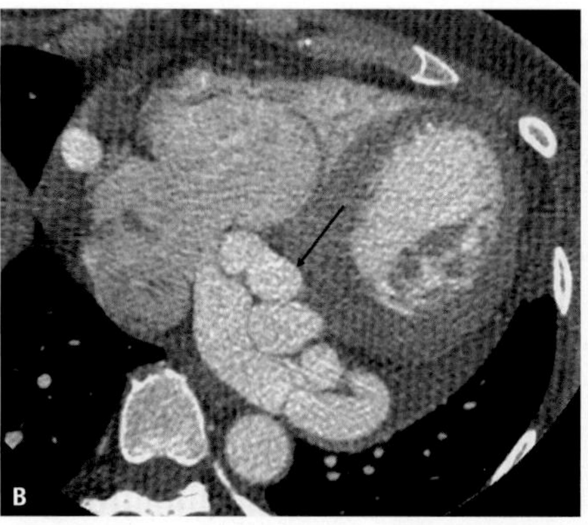

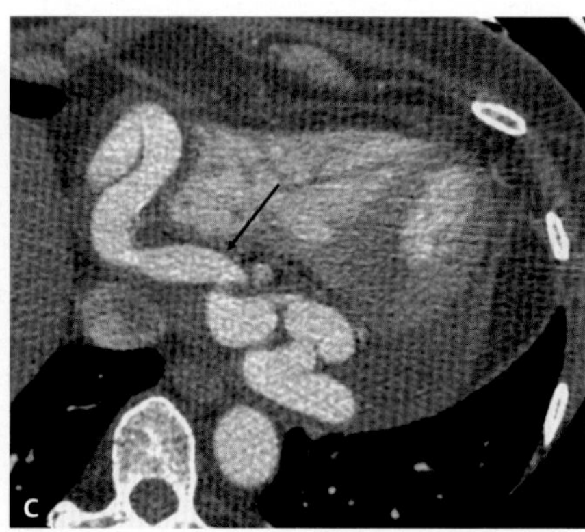

(A–C) Contrast-enhanced cardiac-gated computed tomography angiograms: axial images at multiple levels show abnormal dilatation of both the right and left coronary arteries originating at the ostium and extending distally, as well as abnormal dilatation of the coronary veins and sinus.

Differential Diagnosis

- ***Coronary artery fistula (CAF):*** CAF is a condition in which there is an abnormal communication between the coronary arteries and either the coronary sinus, a cardiac chamber, the pulmonary artery, or the superior vena cava.
- *Coronary artery aneurysm:* Coronary artery aneurysms (from atherosclerosis in adults or Kawasaki disease in children) can present as dilated coronary arteries.
- *Anomalous origin of the left coronary artery from the pulmonary artery (ALCAPA):* In this anomaly, there is also abnormal dilatation and tortuosity of the coronary arteries.

Essential Facts

- CAFs are seen in 0.1% of all cardiac coronary artery catheter angiograms.
- Clinical presentation includes palpitations, chest pain, shortness of breath, and murmur.
- The right coronary artery is more commonly involved (60%) than the left (40%).
- In a small percentage of cases, both coronary arteries are affected.
- The involved coronary artery has increased blood flow and is abnormally dilated and markedly tortuous.
- The most common site of drainage is to the right ventricle, followed by the right atrium (70% to the right side of the heart).
- Complications are cardiac failure, ischemia, thrombosis, arrhythmia, endocarditis, rupture, and death.
- Treatment options are endovascular occlusion and surgical ligation.

Other Imaging Findings

- Focal saccular or fusiform aneurysms may form in the afferent artery, which may calcify.

✔ Pearls & ✘ Pitfalls

✔ CAF creates a shunt in which blood flows from the high-pressure aorta via the coronary artery to the low-pressure cardiac chamber or coronary vein. This may create a steal phenomenon and cause myocardial ischemia.

✔ Acquired CAFs can develop after cardiac surgery or trauma and secondary to inflammatory conditions, such as Kawasaki disease.

Case 14

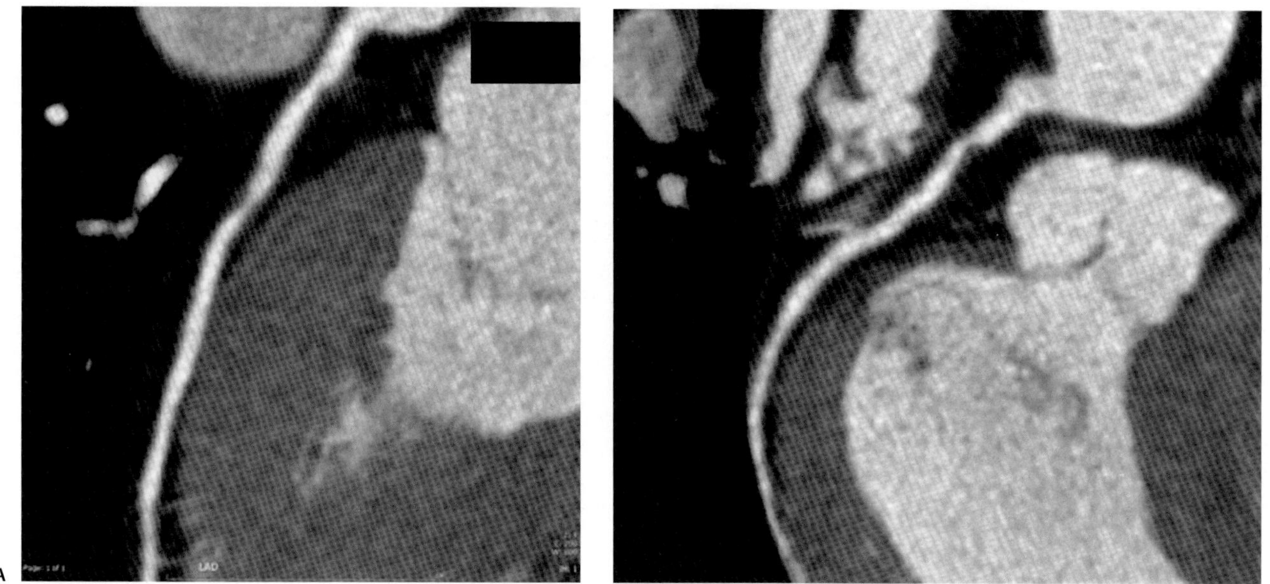

Clinical Presentation

Atypical chest pain and dyspnea on exertion in a 54-year-old man

Imaging Findings

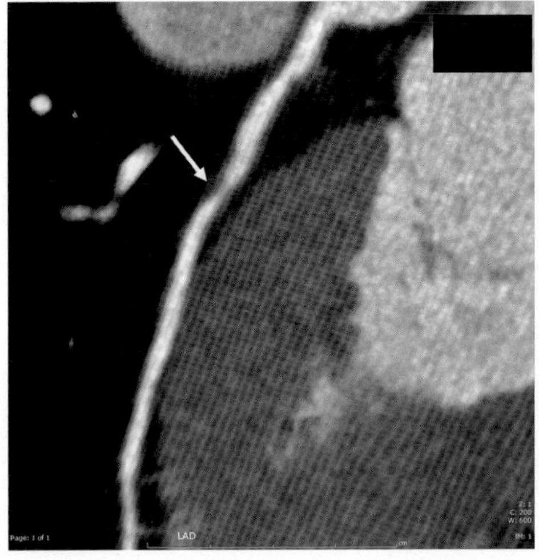
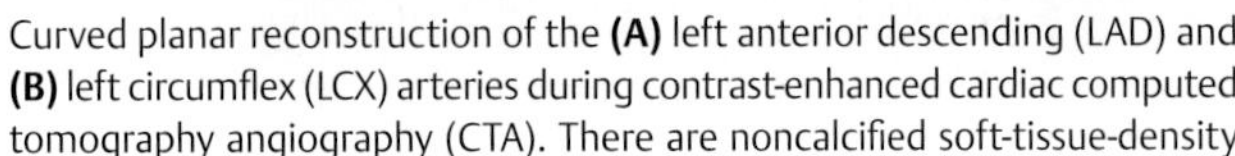
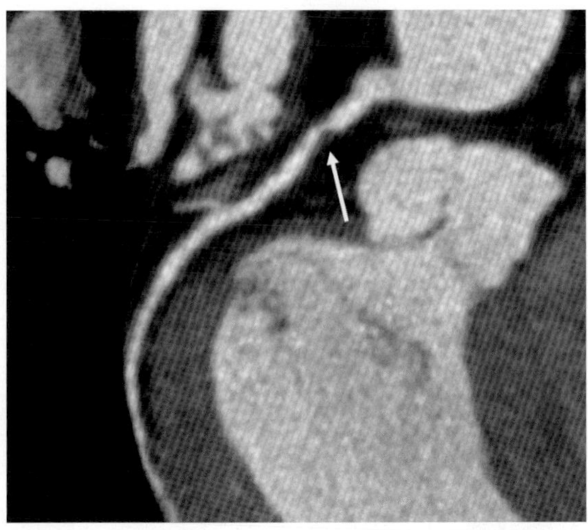

Curved planar reconstruction of the **(A)** left anterior descending (LAD) and **(B)** left circumflex (LCX) arteries during contrast-enhanced cardiac computed tomography angiography (CTA). There are noncalcified soft-tissue-density plaques of both the LAD and proximal LCX coronary arteries, producing mild to moderate luminal narrowing.

Differential Diagnosis

- ***Noncalcified atherosclerotic plaques:*** Noncalcified atherosclerotic plaques can be detected on cardiac CTA. They manifest as areas of abnormal low to intermediate soft-tissue density, depending on the amount of lipid, fibrosis, and thrombus formation.

Essential Facts

- The most common cause of an acute myocardial infarction is the acute formation of a nonobstructive thrombus at the site of preexisting atherosclerotic plaque in a coronary artery that fissures or ruptures.
- Atherosclerotic lesions in arteries are composed primarily of a lipid-rich core and a fibrous cap.
- A large, eccentric lipid core and inflammatory cells (macrophages) are common findings in unstable or ruptured plaques.
- Calcification is generally a marker of plaque stability.
- Nearly two thirds of plaques that rupture have a stenosis of < 50%, with the majority of these being < 70%.
- Coronary artery plaques are commonly eccentric, especially in the early stages.
- Multislice computed tomography has demonstrated the differences in coronary plaque composition between myocardial infarction and stable angina. Noncalcified plaques contribute more to the total plaque burden in myocardial infarction than in angina.

Other Imaging Findings

- As the atherosclerotic plaque progresses, the artery initially enlarges, maintaining a normal- or near-normal-caliber lumen (positive remodeling). Thus, the atherosclerotic lesion may be much larger than suspected from a catheter angiogram.

✔ Pearls & ✘ Pitfalls

✔ One third of all atherosclerotic plaques identified on cardiac-gated CTA are noncalcified.

✔ Between 6 and 50% of patients with a normal calcium score (score = 0) will present with noncalcified atherosclerotic plaques on cardiac CTA. Among them, 4 to 5% will have significant (moderate to severe) luminal narrowing. For that reason and in particular in symptomatic patients (e.g., with chest pain), a normal calcium score is associated with a low risk for a cardiovascular event, but it does not entirely exclude coronary artery disease.

Case 15

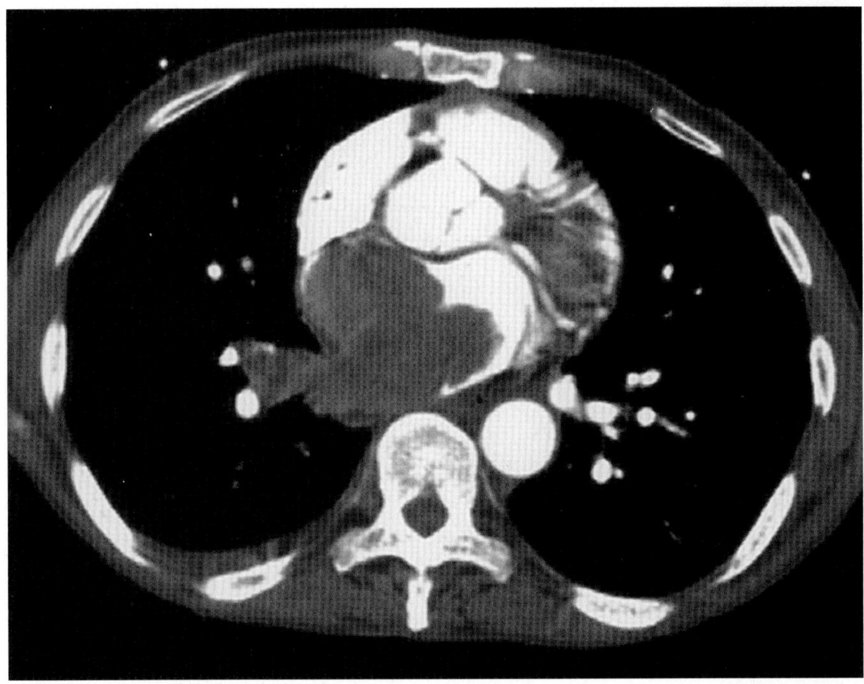

■ Clinical Presentation

Shortness of breath and chest pain in a 65-year-old man with a history of cigarette smoking

Imaging Findings

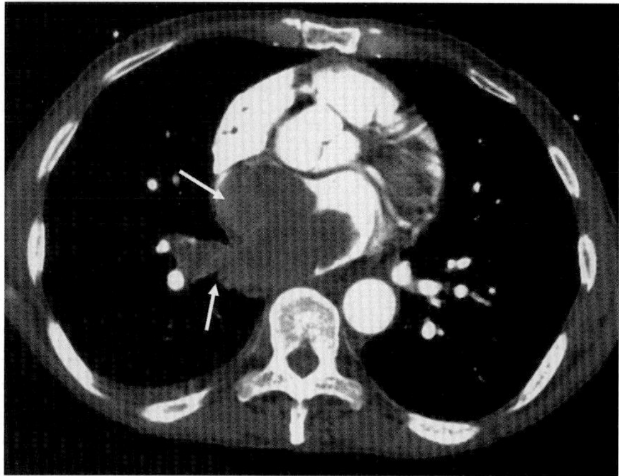

Contrast-enhanced computed tomography of the chest reveals a large soft-tissue mass extending from the right lower lobe pulmonary vein to the left atrium. The mass is lobulated and heterogeneous in density.

Differential Diagnosis

- ***Pulmonary vein extension and left atrial invasion by lung cancer:*** The presence of a tumoral mass within the left atrium with expansion and involvement of a pulmonary vein is characteristic of non–small cell lung cancer.
- *Pulmonary vein sarcoma with extension to the left atrium:* Primary leiomyosarcomas and fibrosarcomas of the pulmonary veins are uncommon but can extend to the left atrium.
- *Angiosarcoma in the left atrium:* Primary sarcomas of the heart can present as intracardiac masses. Primary angiosarcomas more often involve the right atrium than the left, and invasion of a pulmonary vein is not a characteristic finding of this tumor.

Essential Facts

- Pulmonary vein occlusion occurs in up to 6% of patients with lung cancer.
- Sixty to 70% of tumors are squamous cell carcinomas.
- Pulmonary vein occlusion by lung cancer may manifest as segmental veno-occlusive disease, a rare cause of postcapillary pulmonary hypertension.
- The affected lung parenchyma shows congestion and hemosiderosis.
- In a subset of patients, tumor from the involved vein invades the left atrium.
- Non–small cell lung cancer invading the left atrium and the intrapericardial portion of pulmonary veins is classified as T4 and has a poor prognosis.
- Gadolinium-enhanced magnetic resonance angiography has proved useful in the preoperative evaluation of pulmonary veins and left atrial invasion by lung cancer.

Other Imaging Finding

- Transesophageal echocardiography with color Doppler helps to define whether the intracardiac component of the mass is attached to the stalk via the pulmonary vein, with flow around the stalk, or if there is tumoral invasion and infiltration of the vein and cardiac wall.

✔ Pearls & ✘ Pitfalls

✔ The 5-year survival rate after lobectomy or pneumonectomy with partial left atrial resection in the treatment of non–small cell lung cancer is 14%, with a median survival of 25 months.

✔ Benign masses (left atrial thrombi and myxomas) can present as intracavitary masses in the left atrium. Identification of the abnormal appearance of the pulmonary vein and an associated pulmonary lesion is key in distinguishing between these lesions.

Case 16

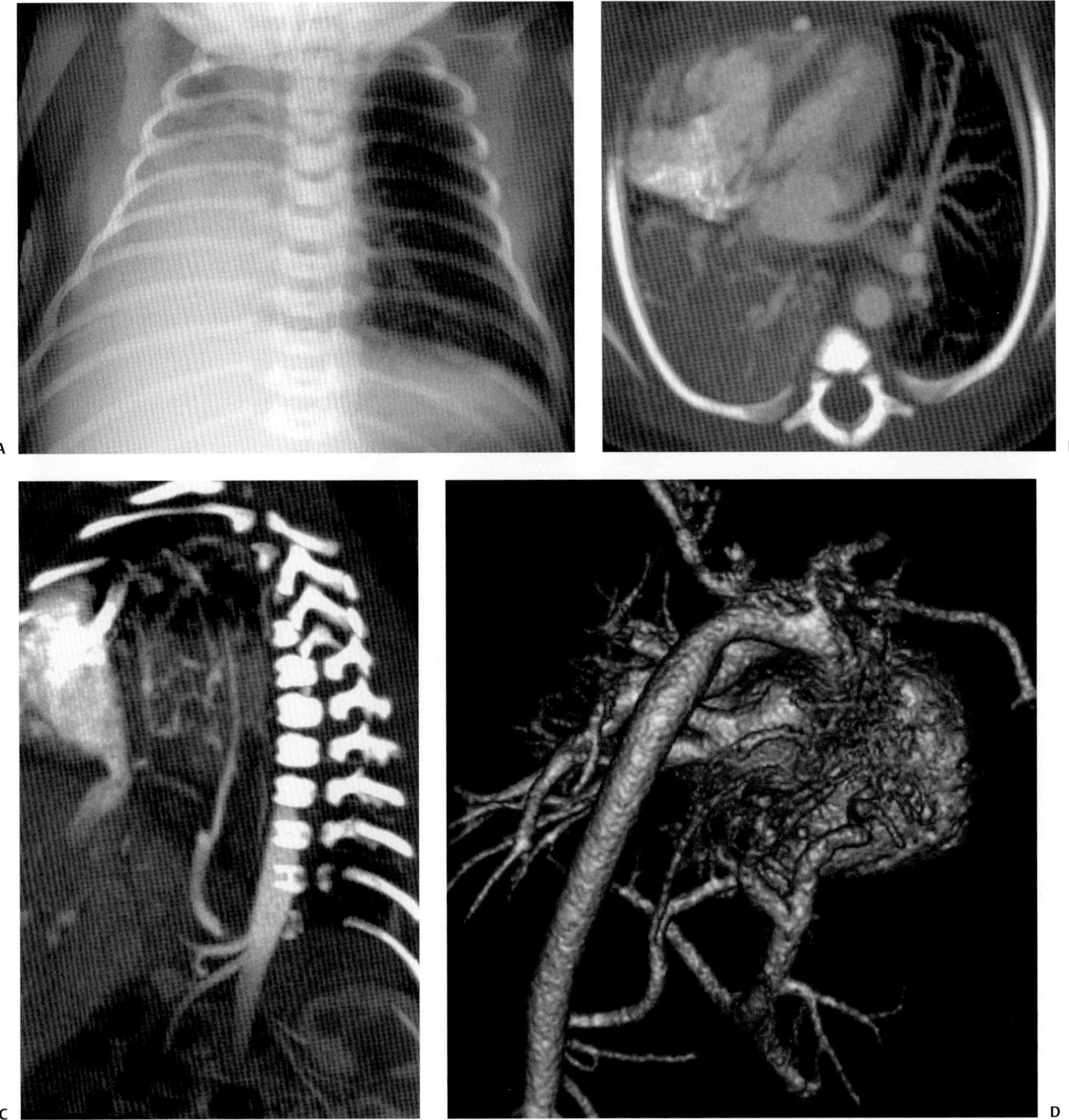

Clinical Presentation

A 6-week-old infant presents with a murmur and presumed dextrocardia based on the initial chest radiograph.

Imaging Findings

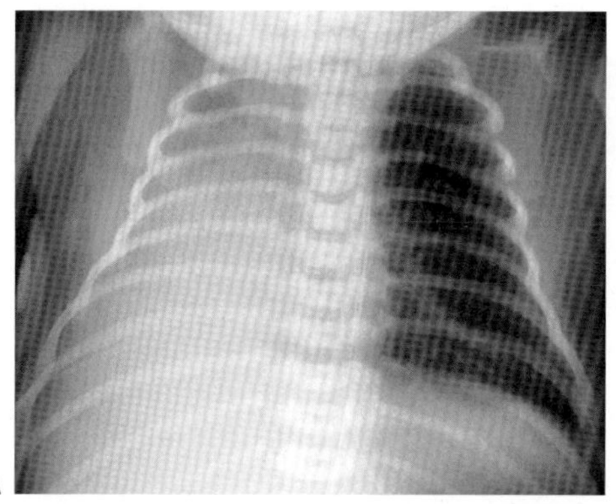
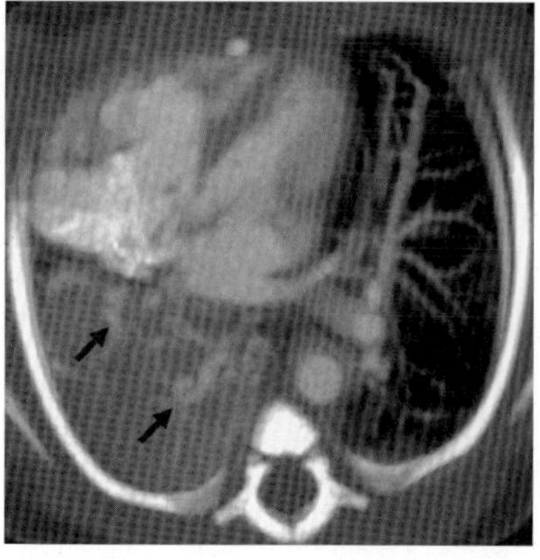
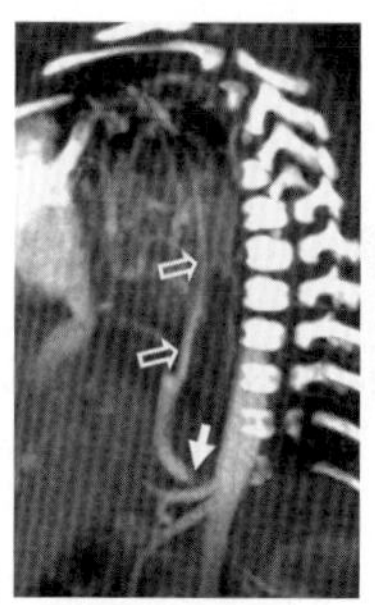
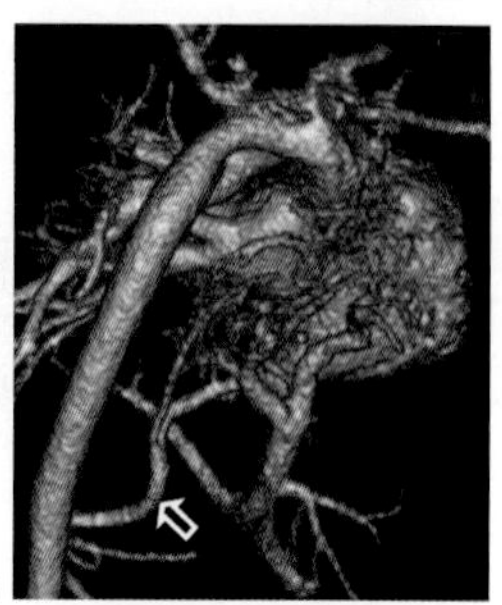

(A) The right hemithorax is completely opacified; the heart is displaced into the right hemithorax (dextroposition). **(B)** This axial computed tomography (CT) image shows the heart in the right hemithorax; in the posterior right hemithorax, a solid mass contains numerous blood vessels (*black arrows*). **(C,D)** Sagittal oblique planar images of the CT data show a large-caliber vessel that arises from the abdominal aorta (*white arrow*) and ascends above the diaphragm into the mass in the right hemithorax (*open arrows*).

Differential Diagnosis

- ***Bronchopulmonary sequestration:*** This abnormal lung parenchyma was enclosed in pleura, a thin layer of tissue. The systemic arterial supply is a clue to the correct diagnosis.
- *Congenital cystic adenomatous malformation (CCAM):* CCAM is a hamartomatous malformation of pulmonary tissue. It may be cystic, solid, or a combination of cystic and solid. The blood supply is from the pulmonary and bronchial arteries, which arise above the diaphragm.
- *Dextrorotation of the heart:* The heart is abnormally positioned in the right hemithorax, but the cardiac apex is on the left. Therefore, the heart is in dextroposition rather than rotated abnormally.

Essential Facts

- Bronchopulmonary sequestration is a malformation or abnormal development of the pulmonary tissue such that the normal communication with the bronchial tree is absent.
- The abnormal lung tissue may be encased by its own visceral pleura (extralobar) or within the normal pulmonary tissue and encased by the normal pleura (intralobar).
- The arterial supply is systemic.
- Venous drainage may be by a pulmonary vein (intralobar) or via a systemic vein (extralobar).
- Cardiac manifestations include congestive heart failure due to left-to-right shunting and murmur from the aberrant systemic artery.
- Noncardiac manifestations include pneumonia, cough, air trapping, and emphysema in the adjacent lung.

Other Imaging Findings

- Dextroposition: The heart is in the right hemithorax, but the cardiac apex is on the left, and intracardiac relationships are normal.
- A cystic or solid mass is seen in the lung base.
- Bronchopulmonary sequestration is extralobar, more often in the lower hemithorax, and subpleural.
- Intralobar sequestration is almost always in the left lower lobe posterobasal segment.

✔ Pearls & ✘ Pitfalls

✔ CT is essential for showing emphysematous changes in the lung.
✔ Multidetector computed tomography angiography shows systemic arterial and venous drainage routes.
✔ Magnetic resonance angiography can clearly reveal the systemic arterial supply and systemic or pulmonary vein drainage without a radiation dose.
✘ Failure to include the upper abdomen in cross-sectional imaging will likely exclude the systemic artery and vein.

Case 17

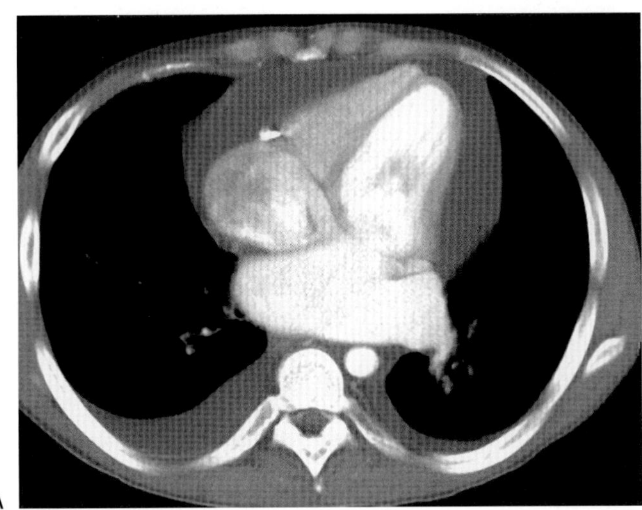
A

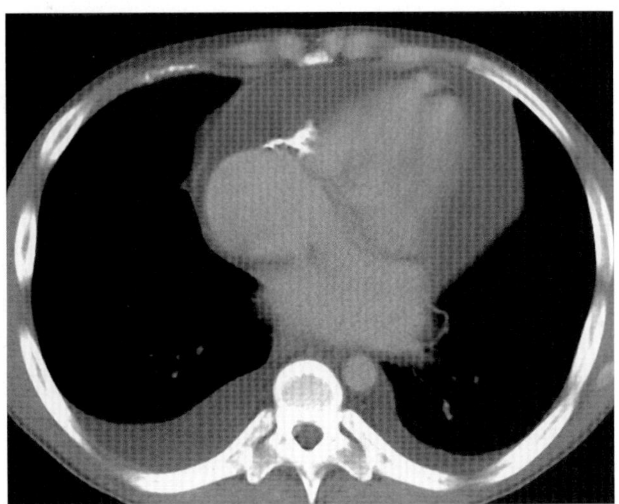
B

Clinical Presentation

Severe dyspnea, orthopnea, and lower extremity edema in a 20-year-old man

Imaging Findings

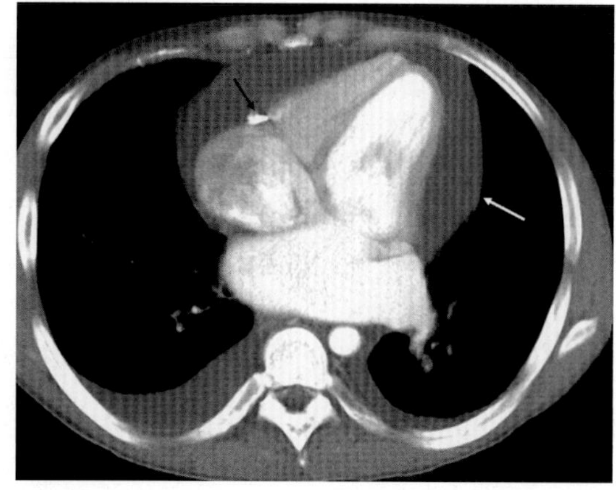
A

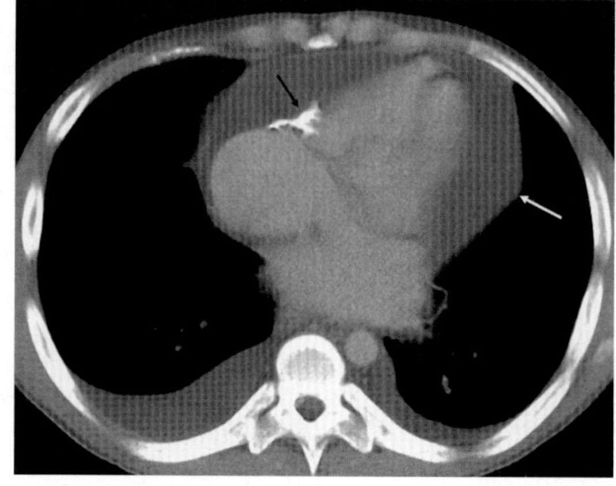
B

Contrast-enhanced computed tomography (CT) of the chest with **(A)** early arterial and **(B)** delayed images. There is an abnormal conical configuration of the heart with significant myocardial thinning of the left ventricle, pericardial fluid, and pericardial calcification (visceral pericardium) at the level of the right atrioventricular groove.

Differential Diagnosis

- ***Effusive constrictive pericarditis (ECP):*** ECP is a syndrome characterized by tamponade physiology, caused by tense pericardial effusion and constriction from a thickened visceral pericardium.
- *Acute pericarditis:* A variable amount of pericardial effusion can be appreciated on CT of patients with acute pericarditis. When large enough or when the accumulation rate is too fast, the cardiac chambers can be compressed. Pericardial calcification of the visceral pericardium and myocardial atrophy are not part of the spectrum of changes expected in an acute process.
- *Constrictive pericarditis:* Constrictive pericarditis is characterized by a constrictive physiology from a chronically inflamed and thickened parietal pericardium that may be calcified.

Essential Facts

- ECP represents 1.3% of all cases of pericardial disease and ~7% of patients presenting with cardiac tamponade.
- The majority of cases of ECP are idiopathic, but this syndrome can develop with any form of pericarditis.
- Other well-documented causes are radiation (postradiation pericarditis), surgery, neoplasia, and tuberculosis.
- A distinctive feature of ECP is the significant role that the visceral layer of the pericardium plays in the pathogenesis of constriction. At surgery or autopsy, affected patients exhibit extensive thickening of both the visceral and parietal pericardium with adhesions between them.
- ECP should be considered when there is focal or global pericardial thickening, tubelike configuration of one or both ventricles, or atrial enlargement associated with pericardial effusion.
- Constrictive pericarditis (including ECP) can be associated with secondary myocardial atrophy, characterized by thinning of the interventricular septum or left ventricular wall (< 1 cm).

Other Imaging Findings

- Unrecognized myocardial atrophy is a frequent cause of intra- and perioperative mortality in patients who undergo pericardiectomy for constrictive pericarditis.

✔ Pearls & ✘ Pitfalls

✔ Cardiac tamponade and constrictive pericarditis have very similar physiologic features. In both conditions, there is a restriction in the filling of the cardiac chambers, as well as an abnormal elevation of the systemic and pulmonary venous pressures.

✔ Drainage of the pericardial fluid or surgical removal of only the parietal pericardium is ineffective when visceral pericardial constriction is also present.

Case 18

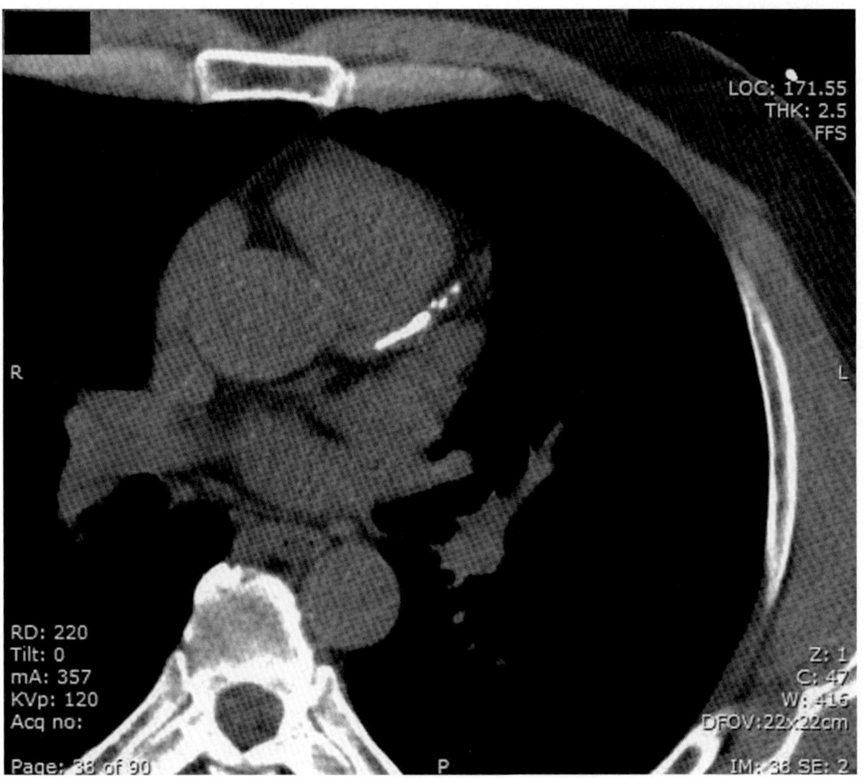

■ Clinical Presentation

A 46-year-old man with atypical chest pain.

Imaging Findings

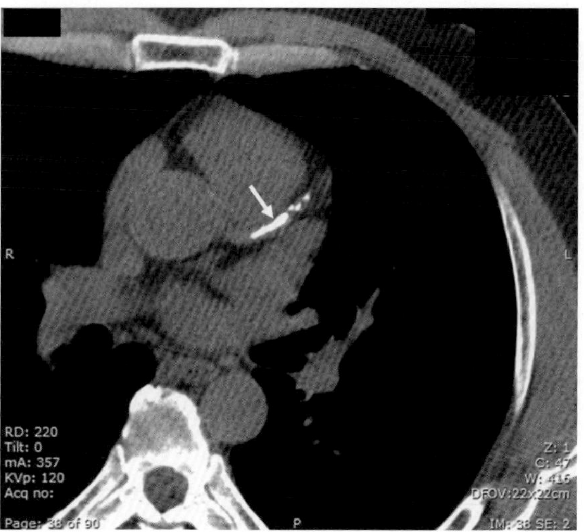

Noncontrast cardiac-gated computed tomography (CT). Axial image demonstrates a linear calcification (*white arrow*) extending from left of the aortic root along the left lateral surface of the heart, following the distribution of the left anterior descending (LAD) coronary artery.

Differential Diagnosis

- ***Coronary artery calcification (CAC):*** Cardiac-gated noncontrast CT shows extensive linear and branching calcium density deposits consistent with CAC.
- *Myocardial calcification:* Calcification can occur in any region of the myocardium, but the most common location is in the anterior left ventricle and apex, in the vascular territory perfused by the LAD artery, secondary to myocardial infarction. The morphology is curvilinear following the myocardial contour.
- *Pericardial calcification:* Pericardial calcification reflects chronic inflammation of the pericardium. Commonly seen calcified deposits are in the atrioventricular groove and interventricular groove.

Essential Facts

- Atherosclerosis is the only vascular disease known to produce CAC.
- CAC is highly prevalent in patients with documented coronary artery disease and is also strongly related to age, particularly after age 50 in men and 60 in women.
- Calcification is only a component of atheroma, so there is a weak correlation between the amount of calcified plaque and the extent of histopathologic stenosis.
- CAC as measured on cardiac CT is defined as a hyperattenuating lesion above a threshold of 130 Hounsfield units (HU) with an area of at least 1 mm^2.
- There are three CT calcium scoring systems: the Agatston score, the volume method score, and the calcium mass score. The most widely used is the Agatston score method, in which the calcium area is multiplied by the CT density number.
- A large meta-analysis (44 studies) has shown that CAC assessment has a high sensitivity (87%), good specificity (75%), and high negative predictive value for the presence of coronary artery disease.
- Measurement of CAC is predictive of death from coronary artery disease or myocardial infarction at 3 and 5 years, and CAC is independently predictive of outcome over and above traditional risk factors.
- The risk for major coronary artery disease events increases 2.1-fold with a calcium score from 1 to 100 and 10-fold with a calcium score > 400 versus risk with a score of 0 (Agatston score).
- With a score ≥ 400, the 10-year coronary artery disease rate is equivalent to that of patients who have diabetes or peripheral arterial disease.

Other Imaging Findings

- Some correlation exists between increased calcium content in the coronary arteries and calcification of the aortic valve.

✔ Pearls & ✘ Pitfalls

✔ Unselected CAC screening is not recommended. The CAC score should be determined in patients judged to be at intermediate risk (10–20% in 10 years) for coronary artery disease.

✔ CAC increases with aging, so an elevated calcium score has less clinical significance and a lower positive predictive value for coronary artery disease in the elderly.

Case 19

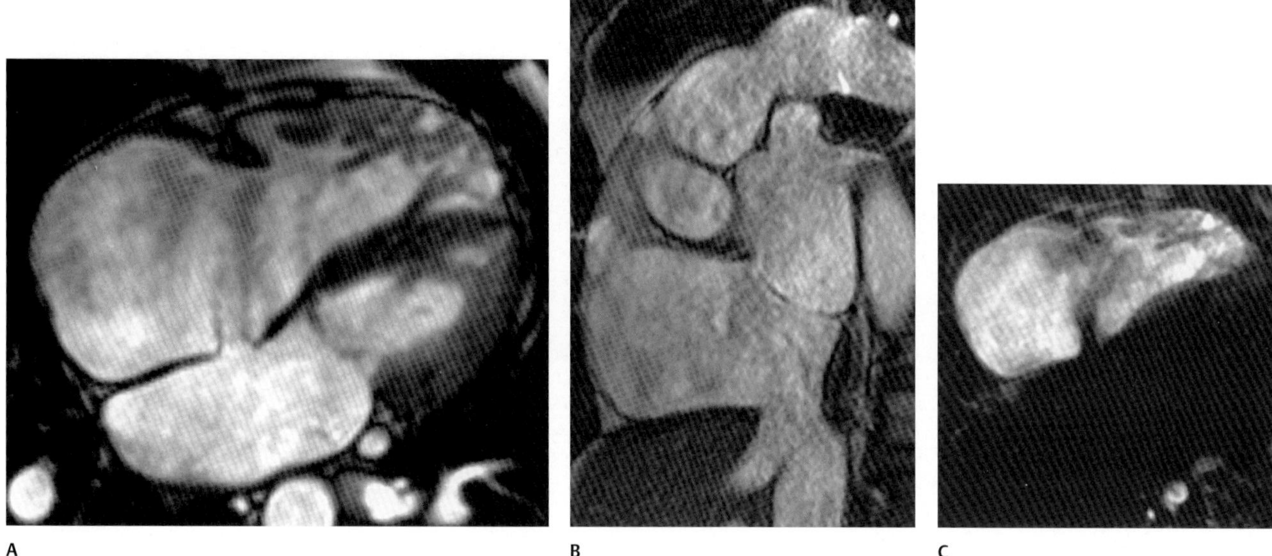

A B C

Clinical Presentation

A 58-year-old man with known congenital heart disease (CHD) and worsening shortness of breath is now unable to maintain activities of daily living. A low-volume murmur is heard on a physical examination.

Imaging Findings

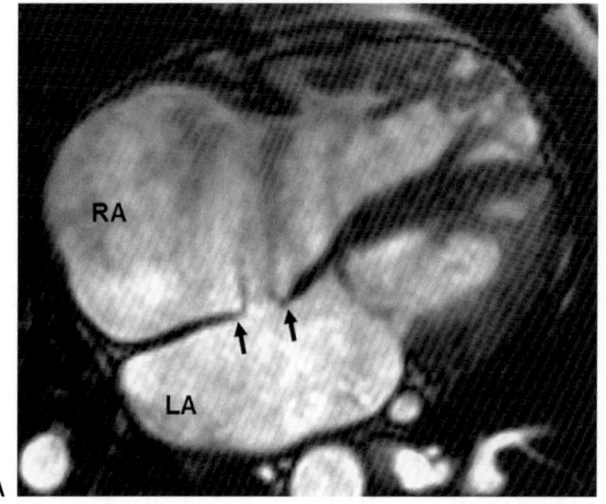

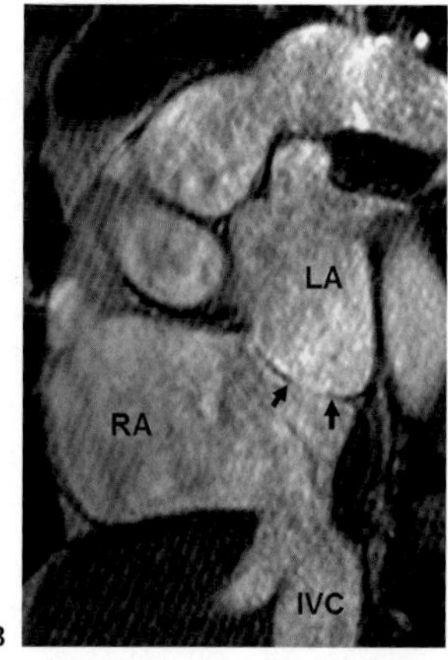

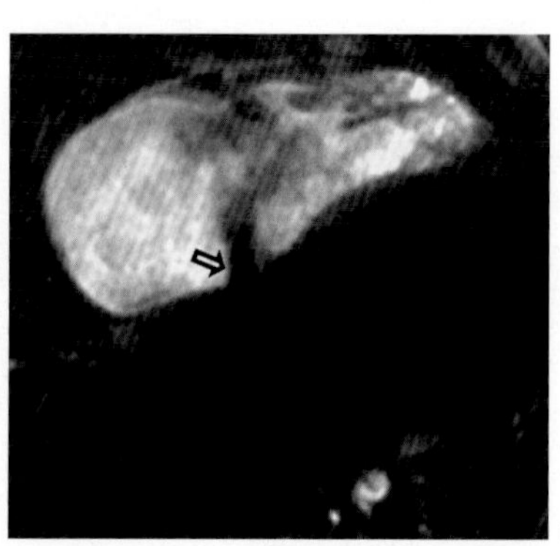

(A) The four-chamber view shows enlargement of the right side of the heart, especially of the right atrium (RA). There is an atrial septal defect (ASD: *arrows*). Note the low signal at the margins of the ASD, due to flow void into the RA. LA, left atrium. **(B)** This short-axis view of the atrial septum shows the superior and posterior rims of the defect. The inferior vena cava (IVC) and a hepatic vein drain into the RA. **(C)** A saturation pulse applied over the left side of the heart saturates protons in the left atrium. The left to right flow of saturated blood protons into the right atrium is now entirely low signal (*open arrow*).

Differential Diagnosis

- ***Secundum atrial septal defect:*** The secundum portion of the atrial septum is partially absent in this adult male patient. He has an audible murmur because blood flow from left to right creates turbulence.
- *Patent foramen ovale (PFO):* The foramen ovale is a small defect in the atrial septum that is normally patent in utero. A PFO usually closes in the postnatal period as pressures on the right side of the heart decrease.
- *Atrioventricular septal defect:* Only the atrial septum is affected in this patient. The ventricular septum is completely intact, and the mitral and tricuspid valves are normally formed.

Essential Facts

- ASD is the second most common form of congenital heart disease, occurring in up to 10% of all patients with congenital heart disease.
- ASD may affect different areas of the interatrial septum (in order of frequency):
  - Ostium secundum: central defect of the fossa ovalis
  - Sinus venosus: superior, adjacent to the superior vena cava (SVC), or inferior, adjacent to the IVC
  - Ostium primum: medial, adjacent to the atrioventricular junction
  - Coronary sinus: involving the coronary sinus
- A large ASD may be a combination of more than one type of ASD.
- Adults with unrepaired ASD become symptomatic because of right-sided heart failure or arrhythmias.
- In pregnancy, women with ASD may present with a louder murmur because of increased circulating blood volume.
- Morbidity and mortality are greater in adults with ASD repair delayed to after age 25 years.

Other Imaging Findings

- Enlargement of the right side of the heart, particularly the RA, is seen on chest radiographs, computed tomography (CT), and magnetic resonance imaging (MRI).
- With a small ASD, a low-signal flow void is usually obvious on MRI because high-velocity blood flow leads to dephasing of the molecular spins in the jet.
- When the ASD is large, the flow across the ASD may be difficult to see on MRI because the velocity of blood flow in the center of the jet is slower; therefore the signal loss is less apparent. As seen in this patient, only the dephasing spins at the edges of the ASD are low signal.
- In cardiac CT, when the left side of the heart is opacified to a greater degree than the right side of the heart, contrast-enhanced blood can be seen passing from the left to the right atrium through a PFO or ASD.

✔ Pearls & ✘ Pitfalls

✔ Measure the anterior, posterior, inferior, and superior remnants of the atrial septum to assist in the evaluation of the potential alternatives for surgical or interventional closure.

✘ The atrial septum is normally quite thin centrally, in the region of the fossa ovalis. Be careful to avoid misdiagnosing ASD when the atrial septum is not well seen on CT and MRI.

Case 20

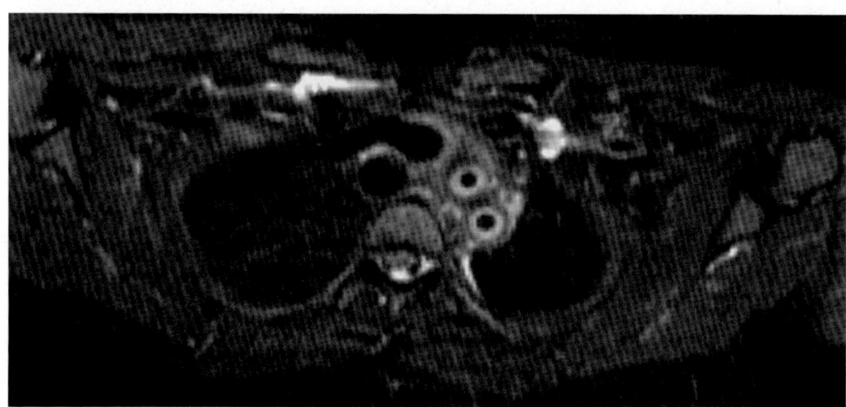

A

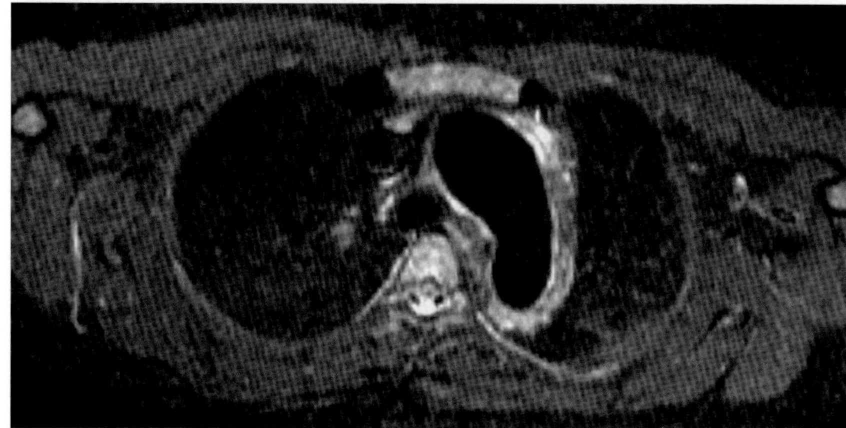

B

Clinical Presentation

A 22 year-old woman presents with chest and left upper extremity pain.

Imaging Findings

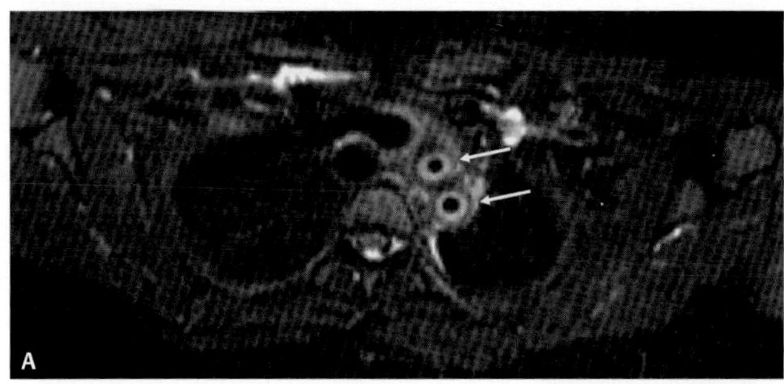

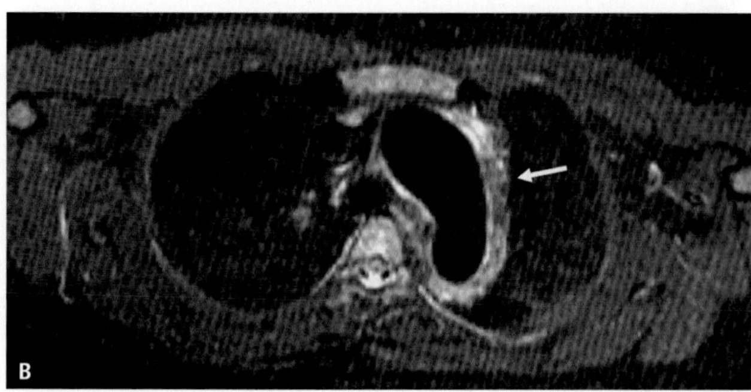

(A,B) Axial T1-weighted fat-suppressed images of the superior mediastinum after gadolinium injection reveal abnormal enhancement and thickening of the aortic arch wall and branches, consistent with an inflammatory process.

Differential Diagnosis

- ***Takayasu's arteritis:*** In a young female patient, the presence of abnormal thickening of the aortic wall associated with abnormal vascular lumen (narrowing, dilatation, or aneurysm) is suggestive of Takayasu's arteritis.
- *Intramural hematoma of the aorta:* Abnormal thickening of the aortic wall can also be seen in intramural hematoma. The presence of a high-density wall in the noncontrast examination is typical of intramural hematoma and helps to differentiate between these two conditions.
- *Giant cell arteritis:* Other forms of large-vessel vasculitis, such as giant cell arteritis, are less common, but they can produce aortic and large artery wall thickening, typically in older women, who have a characteristic clinical presentation that includes temporal artery head pain.

Essential Facts

- Takayasu's arteritis occurs most frequently in young Asian women, although this disorder has been observed worldwide and in all ethnic groups.
- Women are affected 10 times more often than men.
- Most commonly involved vessels are the thoracoabdominal aorta and its branches and the pulmonary arteries.
- Affected vessels exhibit abnormal mural thickening as well as various luminal changes with stenosis, occlusion, dilatation, and aneurysm.
- The acute phase of Takayasu's arteritis, also known as the prepulseless phase, is inflammatory.
- The late (or pulseless) phase of Takayasu's arteritis has been classified as four morphologic types:
  - Type I: involvement of branches of the aortic arch only
  - Type II: a combination of aortic branch obstruction (type I) and atypical coarctation of the aorta (type III). This is the most common type.
  - Type III: atypical coarctation of the aorta
  - Type IV: dilatation of the aorta and its branches

Other Imaging Findings

- Computed tomography angiography (CTA) clearly depicts both luminal and mural changes in the affected vessels, with high accuracy (95% sensitivity and 100% specificity) and is a good imaging modality for the acute phase.
- Magnetic resonance imaging (MRI) is widely used for the diagnosis of this condition and effectively provides excellent anatomical information of the affected vessels and complications. MRI is probably the best imaging modality for the follow-up of these patients, given the significant advantage of not having ionizing radiation.

✔ Pearls & ✘ Pitfalls

✔ Abnormal aortic or pulmonary artery wall thickening with or without luminal abnormality in a young female patient is characteristic of Takayasu's arteritis.

✘ Catheter angiography does not depict arterial wall architecture changes as well as cross-sectional imaging modalities. Additionally, the frequency of ischemic complications secondary to catheter angiography in patients with Takayasu's arteritis is high, so cross-sectional noninvasive imaging techniques are preferred.

Case 21

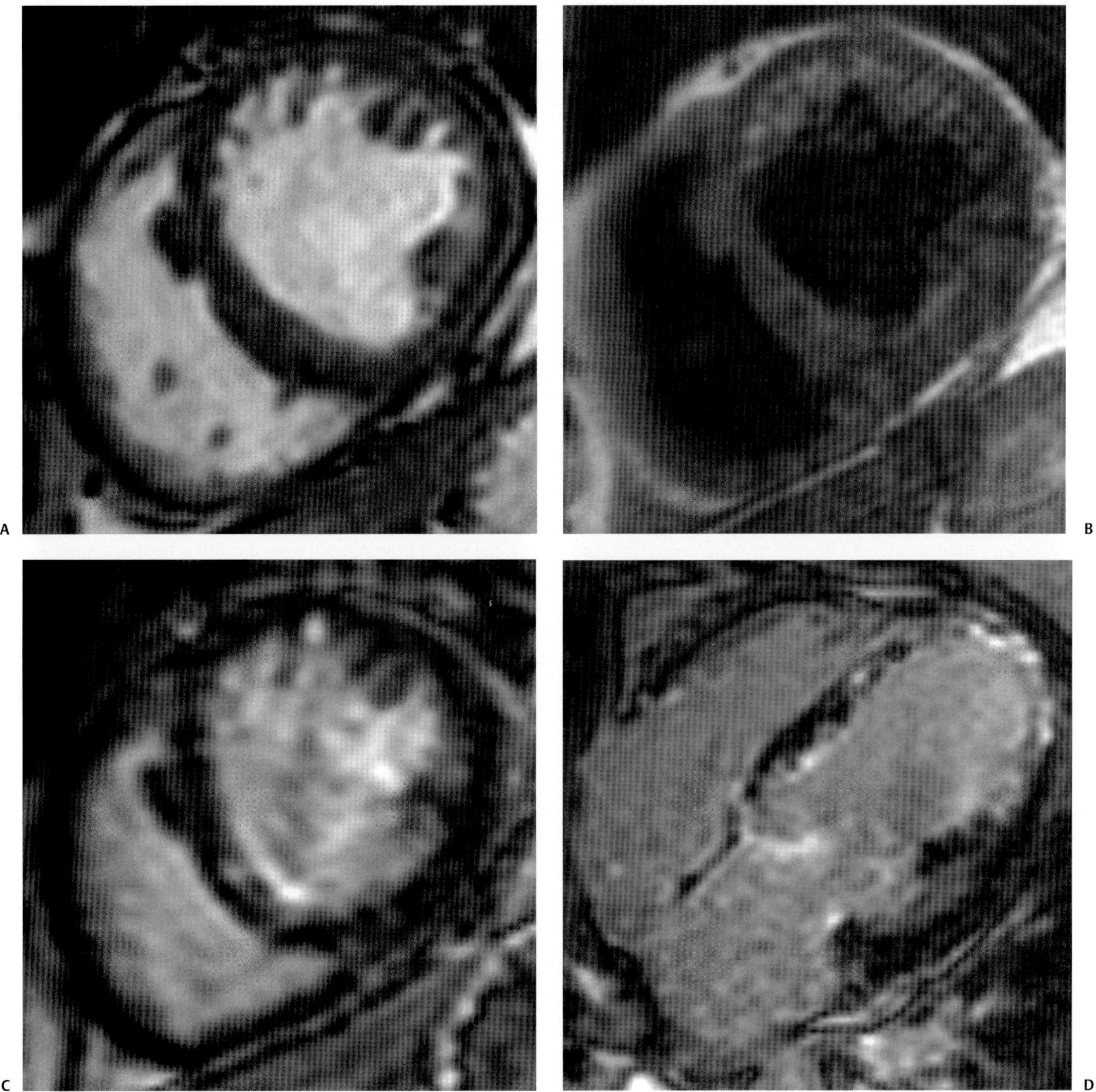

Clinical Presentation

A 62-year-old man with diabetes presents without chest pain but with a troponin leak and ST wave elevation on electrocardiogram (ECG).

Imaging Findings

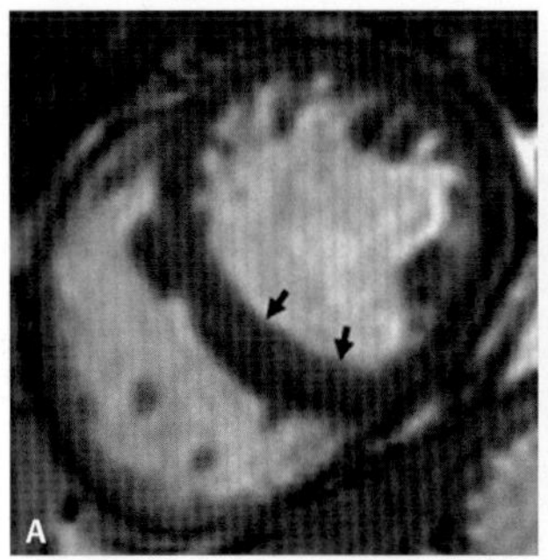

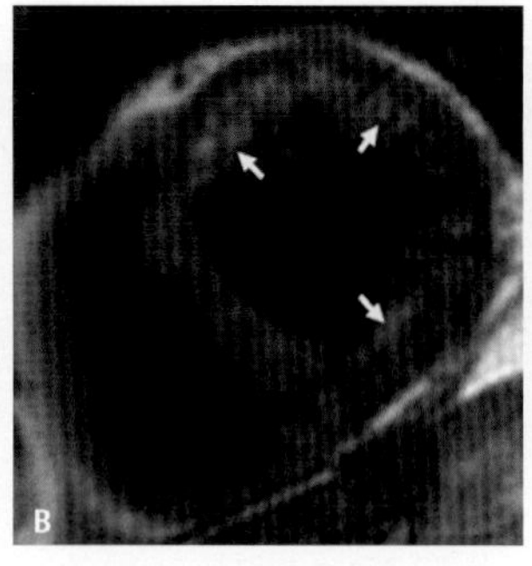

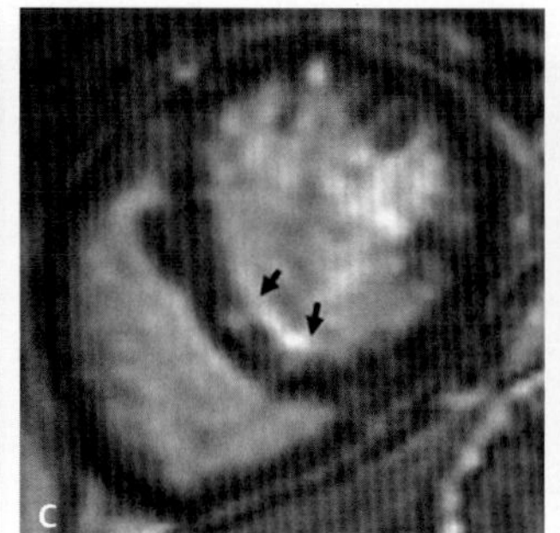

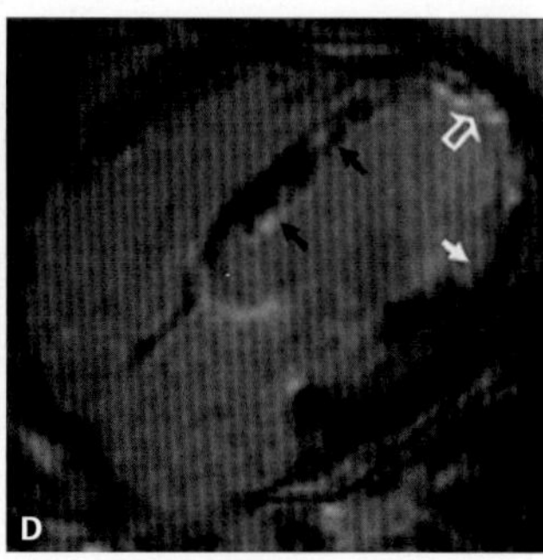

(A) A short-axis image in the midleft ventricle (LV) chamber shows mild thickening of the inferoseptal wall (*black arrows*). **(B)** Closer to the apex, in a short-T2 black blood image, the endocardial myocardium of the anterior, lateral, and inferior walls is thickened and hyperintense (*white arrows*). **(C)** In the same plane as Figure A, following the intravenous administration of gadolinium, the endocardial surface of the inferoseptal wall is hyperintense (*black arrows*), but there is mild motion artifact, and the myocardial signal is not completely suppressed. **(D)** The endocardial enhancement seen in this four-chamber view of the heart involves the septum (*black arrows*), lateral wall (*white arrow*), and rounded apex (*open white arrow*). In this image, the myocardial signal is fully suppressed.

Differential Diagnosis

- ***Multifocal acute and chronic myocardial infarction:*** Segments of the septal and anterior wall of the LV are thickened and edematous, both findings of acute infarction. The apex of the LV is thinned, enhances, and is aneurysmal, findings of chronic infarction.
- *Nonviable myocardium:* The apical myocardium is thinned, but the enhancement is limited to the subendocardial surface, involving < 50% of the wall thickness.
- *Infectious myocarditis:* Multifocal or diffuse myocardial enhancement is often seen with infectious or inflammatory myocarditis, but it is not limited to the endocardial surface.

Essential Facts

- Perfusion defects indicate abnormal blood flow through the myocardium and can be seen in acutely or chronically infarcted or ischemic myocardium.
- Delayed, or late, enhancement refers to enhancement of the subendocardial myocardium and is typical of myocardial infarction.

Other Imaging Findings

- Fibrous tissues such as the tricuspid and mitral valve rings and leaflets also enhance with gadolinium.
- If the signal from normal myocardium is not fully suppressed, foci of infarction can be obscured.
- Motion artifacts can result in signal abnormality that can mimic infarction.

✔ Pearls & ✘ Pitfalls

✔ Following intravenous administration of gadolinium, late enhancement imaging is performed with an inversion recovery turbo fast low-angle shot (FLASH) sequence.

✔ Functional or cine gradient echo sequences are effective in showing wall motion abnormalities.

✘ The magnetic resonance imaging sequence requires adjustment of the inversion time such that signal from normal LV myocardium is suppressed.

✘ Insufficient suppression of the signal from normal myocardium may obscure subtle or small areas of infarction.

Case 22

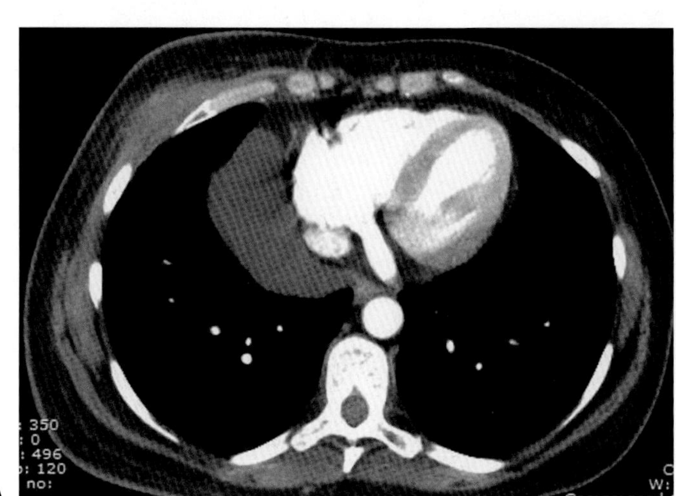

A

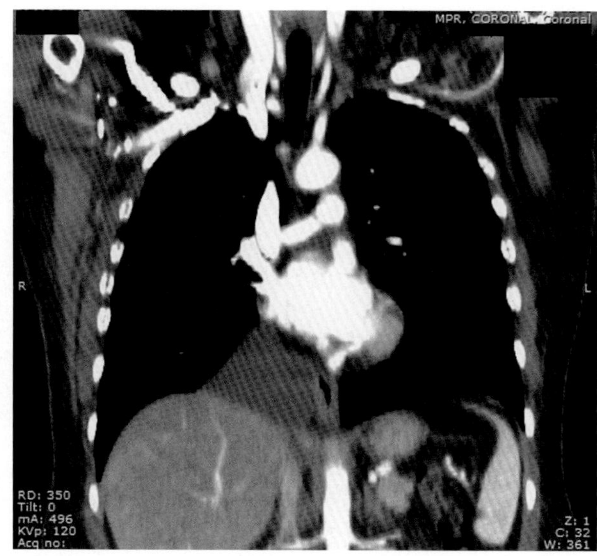

B

Clinical Presentation

Abnormal chest radiograph for respiratory symptoms prompted a computed tomography (CT) scan of the chest.

Imaging Findings

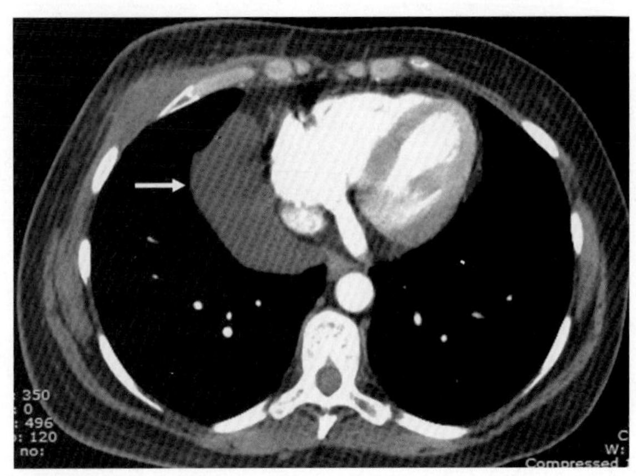

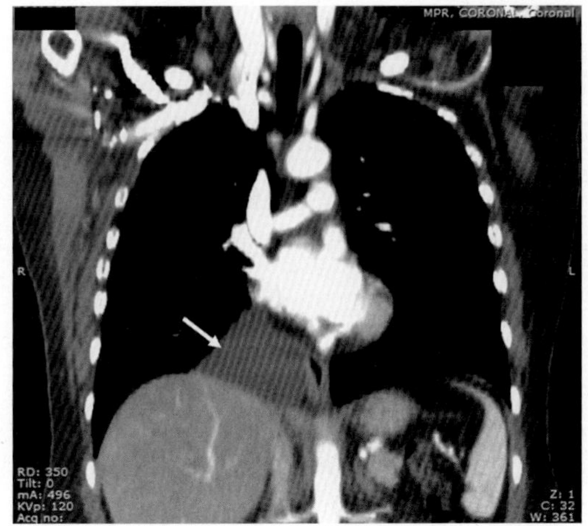

(A,B) Contrast-enhanced CT of the thorax: **(A)** axial image and **(B)** coronal re-formation. There is a nonenhancing round, smoothly marginated fluid-density mass in the right cardiophrenic angle (*white arrow*).

Differential Diagnosis

- ***Pericardial cyst (mesothelial):*** The right cardiophrenic angle is the most common location of a pericardial cyst, but the cysts may be located elsewhere in the mediastinum. It characteristically has water density and a thin wall and exhibits no enhancement after contrast administration.
- *Thymic cyst:* A thymic cyst may be unilocular or multilocular, congenital or acquired, and more often presents in the anterior mediastinum. It occasionally may be associated with thymic tumors, in patients with previous radiation therapy for mediastinal lymphomas, or with infectious or inflammatory conditions.
- *Hydatid disease:* In a case of pericardial involvement from hydatid disease, the pericardial cyst will likely exhibit additional features, such as a thick wall, septation, multiloculation, and calcification, which are rarely seen in a mesothelial pericardial cyst.

Essential Facts

- Pericardial mesothelial cysts are usually asymptomatic, but they occasionally may manifest with chest pain, dyspnea, or cough.
- They result from an abnormal development of the coelomic somatic cavities in the embryo.
- The cyst wall is composed of a single layer of mesothelial cells covering a connective tissue membrane.
- The estimated prevalence of pericardial cysts is 1 per 100,000 persons.
- Ninety percent of cysts are located in the cardiophrenic angles, with the right more commonly involved.
- When in an atypical location, pericardial cysts may be similar in appearance to bronchogenic, thymic, and duplication cysts.

Other Imaging Findings

- On magnetic resonance imaging, pericardial cysts typically have low or intermediate signal intensity on T1, homogeneously high signal intensity on T2 and fluid-sensitive sequences, and no enhancement after gadolinium injection. Cysts with hemorrhagic content or highly proteinaceous fluid may exhibit high signal intensity on T1.

✔ Pearls & ✘ Pitfalls

✔ Pericardial cysts are contiguous and connected to the pericardium, and they are inseparable from the pericardium and cardiac border.

✘ In conventional radiography, epicardial fat or a Morgagni hernia may present as a round soft-tissue density in the cardiophrenic angle, similar to a pericardial cyst. Cross-sectional imaging is required to confirm the cystic nature of the lesion and to differentiate it from other mediastinal abnormalities.

Case 23

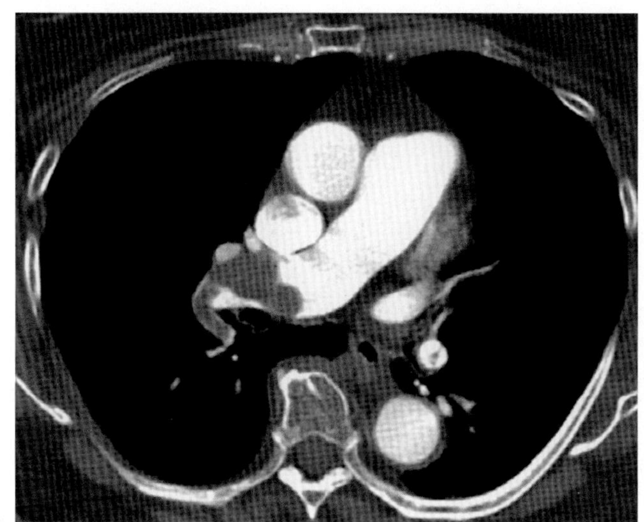
A

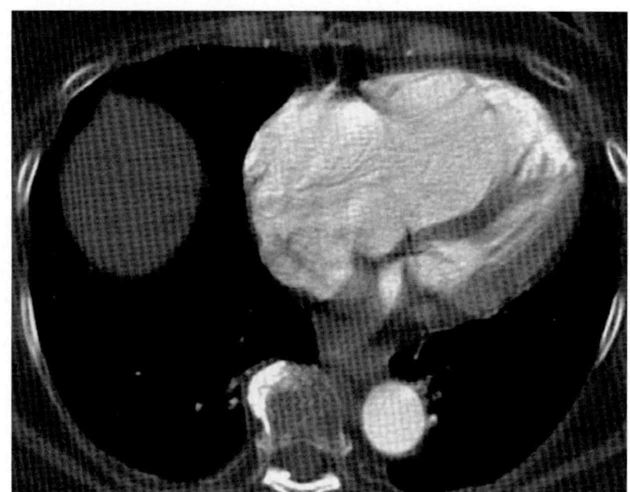
B

Clinical Presentation

A 75 year-old woman presents with acute chest pain and shortness of breath.

Imaging Findings

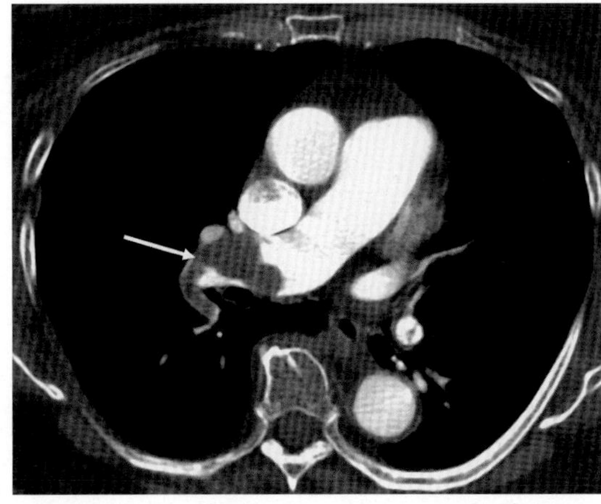

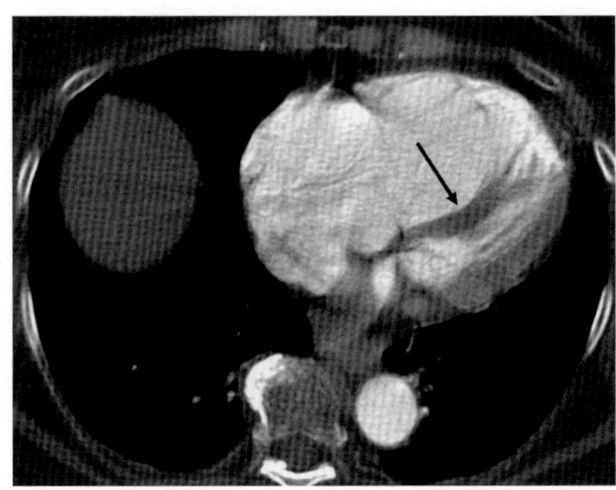

(A) Contrast-enhanced computed tomography (CT) of the chest reveals a large filling defect in the right pulmonary artery and a smaller one in the left lower lobe. **(B)** Contrast-enhanced chest CT at a lower level shows significant enlargement of the right atrium and ventricle and abnormal bowing of the interventricular septum to the left (*black arrow*). Note the significant reduction in the size of the left ventricle (LV).

Differential Diagnosis

- ***Acute right ventricular (RV) dysfunction secondary to pulmonary embolism***
- *Pulmonary embolism:* A massive pulmonary embolism, which occludes a significant portion of the pulmonary vascular bed, can induce acute pulmonary hypertension and dysfunction of the RV.
- *Pulmonary embolism and dilated cardiomyopathy:* Pulmonary emboli can be seen in patients with dilated cardiomyopathy, but dilated cardiomyopathy typically causes dilatation of both the right and left ventricles. The LV is usually more significantly enlarged and presents with more significant hypokinesis than the RV.

Essential Facts

- Severe acute pulmonary embolism, usually with obstruction of > 30% of the pulmonary vasculature, can induce acute right heart failure with circulatory collapse and death (> 50%).
- Pulmonary vasculature obstruction produces elevation of the pulmonary vascular resistance, which is worsened by the release of vasoactive agents from tissue, platelets, and plasma, as well as reflex vasoconstriction and hypoxemia.
- This entire process induces significant pulmonary hypertension.
- The physiologic and clinical impact of the embolic event depends not only on the magnitude of the embolic process but also on the patient's underlying cardiopulmonary reserve.
- Qualitative and quantitative assessment of right heart dysfunction on multidetector computed tomography angiography in patients with acute pulmonary emboli is possible by identifying dilatation of the RV and deviation of the interventricular septum toward the LV.
- The presence of a ratio of the RV to the LV diameter > 1 and left septal bowing has high sensitivity (78–92%), specificity (100%), and positive predictive value (100%) compared with echocardiography for identifying RV dysfunction and is associated with increased morbidity and 30-day mortality.

Other Imaging Findings

- RV dysfunction produces increased volume and pressure in the right atrium, which may reflect upstream increased pressure with dilation of the inferior and superior venae cavae and azygos vein.

✔ Pearls & ✘ Pitfalls

✔ Computed tomography (CT) has higher sensitivity and specificity than echocardiography for the detection of right heart dysfunction in patients with acute pulmonary emboli. Ventricular CT measurements obtained from four-chamber views are superior to those from axial views for this assessment.

✘ Pulmonary artery (PA) diameter > 30 mm indicates precapillary pulmonary hypertension, but this measurement has a better correlation with chronic pulmonary hypertension than with acute events. The diameter of the PA or the ratio of the diameter of the PA to that of the aorta is not a good indicator of the severity of acute pulmonary embolism or a predictor of mortality.

Case 24

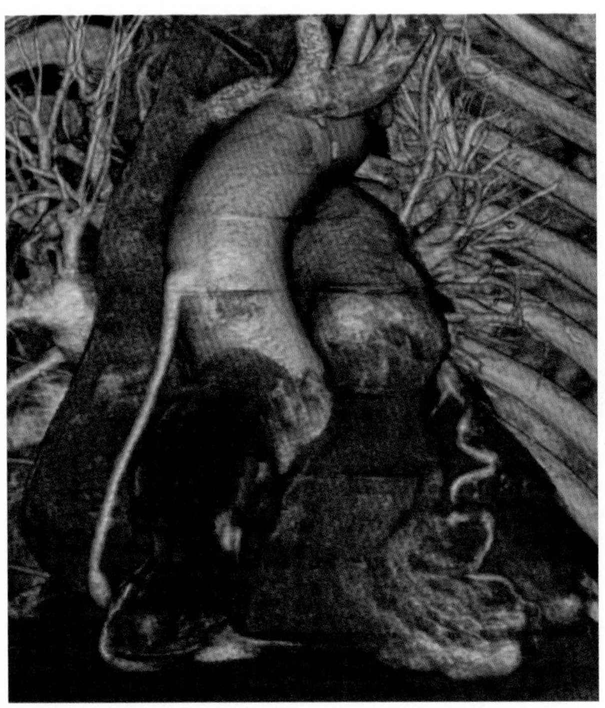

A

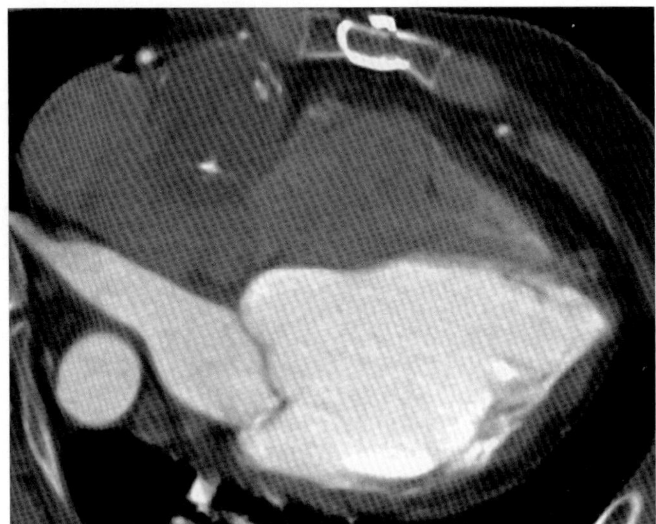

B

Clinical Presentation

A 32-year-old man presents with a history of congenital heart disease that was treated in infancy. The patient is slightly cyanotic.

Imaging Findings

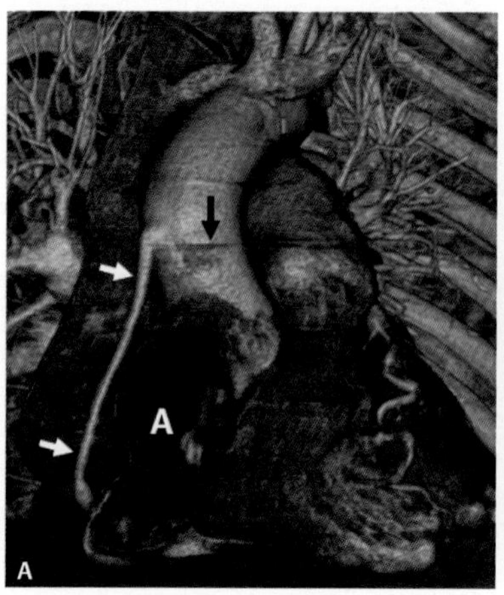

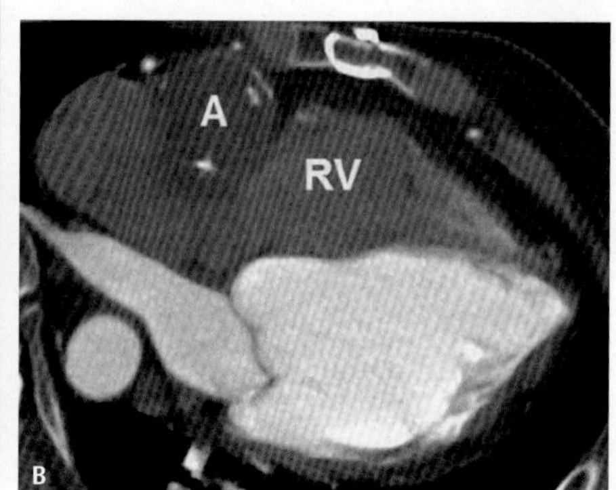

(A) In a coronal three-dimensional view of the heart, a mass is in the expected position in the right coronary artery (RCA) (A). A venous coronary artery bypass graft (CABG) extends from the ascending aorta to the distal RCA (*white arrows*), bypassing the thrombosed vessel. Linear artifact (*black arrow*) is due to sternal wires. **(B)** In a four-chamber view of the heart, the round low-attenuation thrombus (A) also contains curvilinear calcium. It causes a mass effect on the right ventricle (RV) and atrium.

Differential Diagnosis

- ***Giant thrombosed aneurysm of the RCA:*** The RCA is occluded by thrombus, which contains calcium, a feature of a chronic process.
- *Postoperative thrombus in the pericardial sac:* The myocardium is not thickened. The left ventricle (LV) is usually small in hypertrophic cardiomyopathy.
- *Lymphoma:* Dilatation of the LV can be seen in patients with ischemic cardiomyopathy, but the myocardial signal should remain normal on nonenhanced images.

Essential Facts

- The incidence of coronary artery aneurysms during angiography is < 1%.
- Coronary artery aneurysms are diagnosed when the diameter of the vessel lumen is 150% that of the normal vessel.
- RCA aneurysms account for ~50% of coronary artery aneurysms, with the remainder divided between the left anterior descending and left circumflex arteries.
- Atherosclerosis is the most likely etiology.
- Other important causes are Kawasaki disease and collagen vascular disorders such as Ehlers–Danlos and Marfan syndromes.
- Thrombosis is a well-known complication.

Other Imaging Findings

- Diffuse coronary artery ectasia
- Atherosclerotic disease
- Myocardial infarction
- Tricuspid valve dysfunction

✔ Pearls & ✘ Pitfalls

✔ Multidetector computed tomography is increasingly used to diagnose CABG patency.

✘ Iatrogenic coronary artery aneurysm formation following cardiac catheterization is a rare event and usually involves the ostia.

Case 25

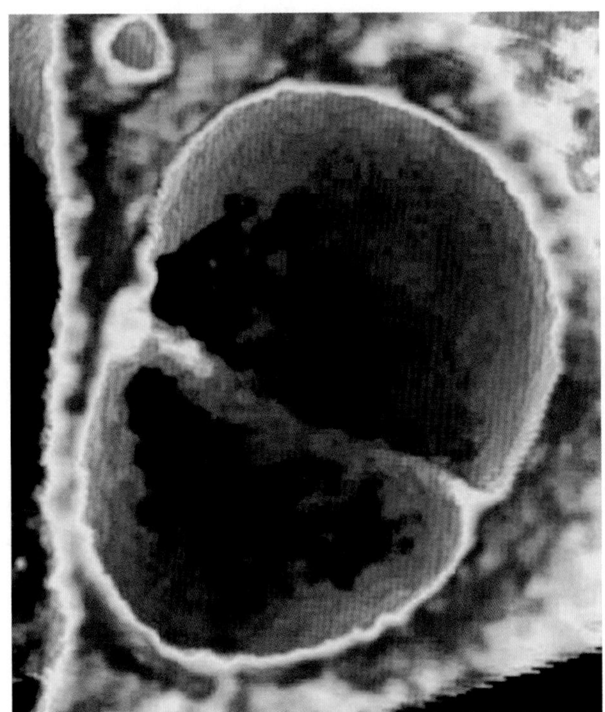

A

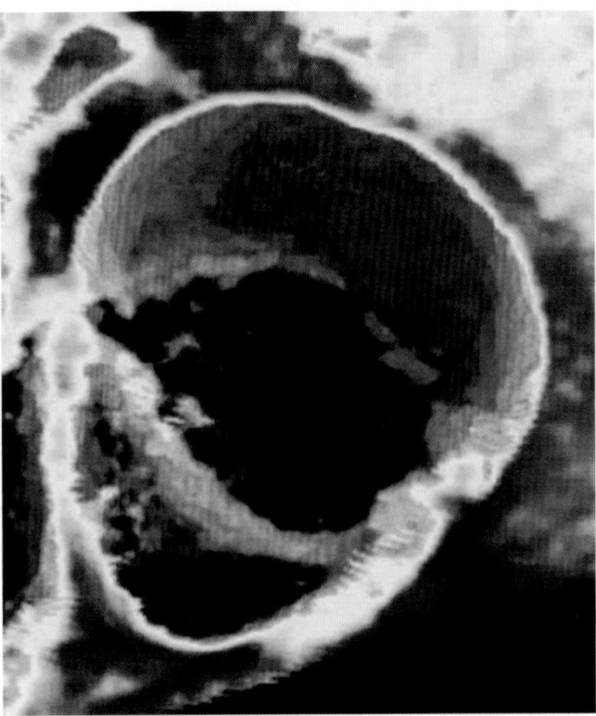

B

Clinical Presentation

A 35-year-old male presents with atypical chest pain and has had an abnormality detected on echo. The aortic valve usually has 3 cusps. What is the nature of malformation of this aortic valve? What are the typical formations of aortic valve malformation?

Imaging Findings

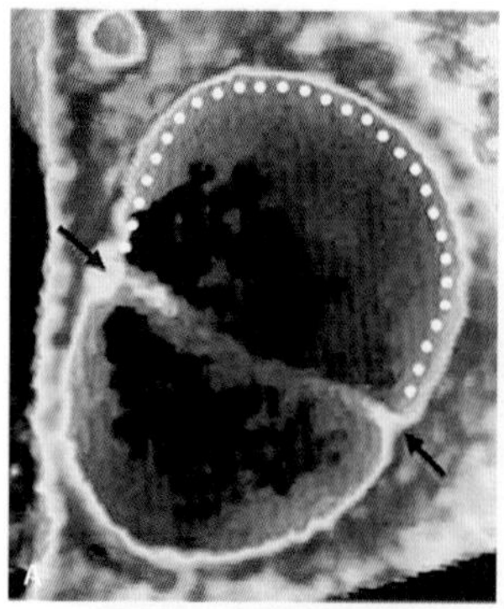

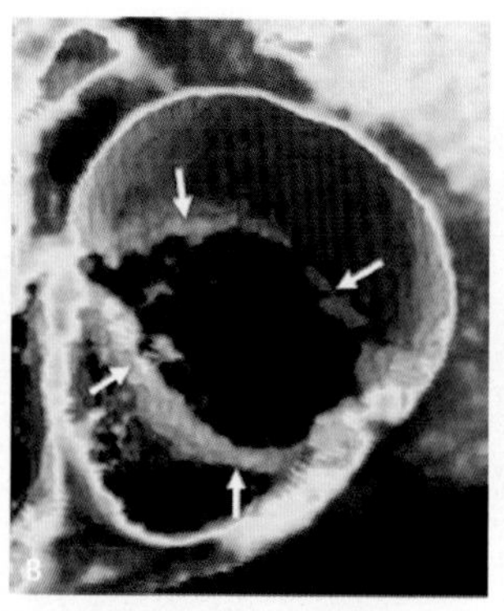

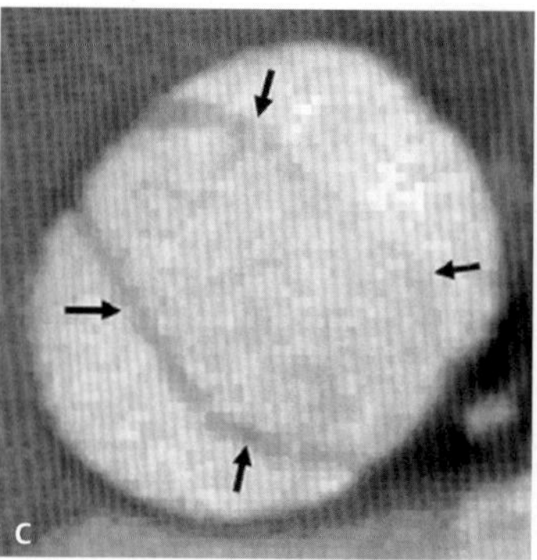

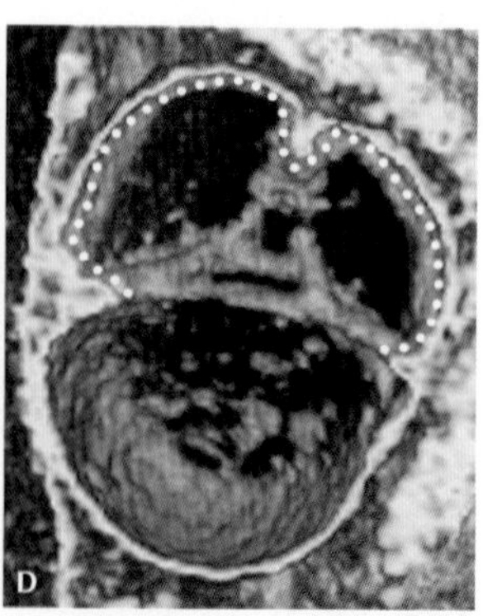

(A,B) Three-dimensional images of the aortic valve show a bicuspid aortic valve in a closed (diastolic) and open (systolic) position. The valve cusps are slightly asymmetric, as there is probably fusion of the right and left cusps (*dotted line*). The open valve is shaped like the mouth of a fish (*white arrows*). **(C)** In another patient, a two-dimensional image of the bicuspid aortic valve shows the fish mouth configuration as the nearly equal-size leaflets open (*black arrows*). **(D)** In a third patient, a three-dimensional image of the aortic valve shows fusion of the right and left coronary cusps (*dotted white line*).

Differential Diagnosis

- ***Bicuspid aortic valve:*** There are two nearly symmetric leaflets of the aortic valve, one of the many ways in which the aortic valve can have a bicuspid configuration.
- *Aortic valve stenosis:* Although bicuspid valves may be stenotic, this patient did not have a dilated ascending aorta, a finding that commonly accompanies stenosis of the aortic valve, no matter the cause.
- *Biological (tissue) prosthetic valve:* Prosthetic biological valves are used in the aortic position, but they are constructed to have three valve cusps, similar to the normal native aortic valve. Biological valves are made of pericardial tissue from pigs (porcine), cows (bovine), or other species.

Essential Facts

- Bicuspid aortic valves occur in ~2% of the population.
- Bicuspid aortic valves may function normally for many years without treatment.
- The risk for aortic root dissection in patients with bicuspid aortic valves is 5%.
- In 25% of patients, the aortic valve annulus may enlarge, potentially leading to incompetence of the valve and/or dissection.
- Aortic valve stenosis is due to the accelerated aging process in bicuspid valves and results in sclerosis and calcification of the valve leaflets.
- Obstruction to left ventricular outflow is usually at the level of the aortic valve.
- In addition to narrowing of the aortic valve orifice by sclerotic, thickened, and calcified leaflets, the mobility of the leaflets is reduced, further contributing to stenosis.
- The aortic valve area index is helpful for determining the severity of aortic valve stenosis of any cause:
  - Mild: 1.5 to 2.0 cm^2 (indexed: 0.9–1.1 cm^2/m^2)
  - Moderate: 1.0 to 1.5 cm^2 (indexed: 0.6–0.9 cm^2/m^2)
  - Severe: < 1.0 cm^2 (indexed: < 0.6 cm^2/m^2)
  - Critical: < 0.75 cm^2 (indexed: < 0.45 cm^2/m^2)

Other Imaging Findings

- Aortic valve leaflets may be partially fused, or there may be two nearly symmetric valve leaflets.
- If the aortic valve is stenotic, post-stenotic dilatation of the ascending aorta is likely to be present.
- Bicuspid aortic valve is not uncommon in patients with coarctation of the aorta.
- When bicuspid aortic valve is associated with coarctation of the aorta, premature atherosclerotic disease is found in the coronary arteries.

✔ Pearls & ✘ Pitfalls

✔ Retrospectively, electrocardiography-gated computed tomography scans are needed to show the open and closed positions of the valve.

✔ Reconstructed en face views of the aortic valve are the most valuable for evaluating the structure of a bicuspid aortic valve.

✘ Valve leaflets thickened by an infectious or inflammatory process such as bacterial or rheumatic fever may be fused and function as a bicuspid valve.

Case 26

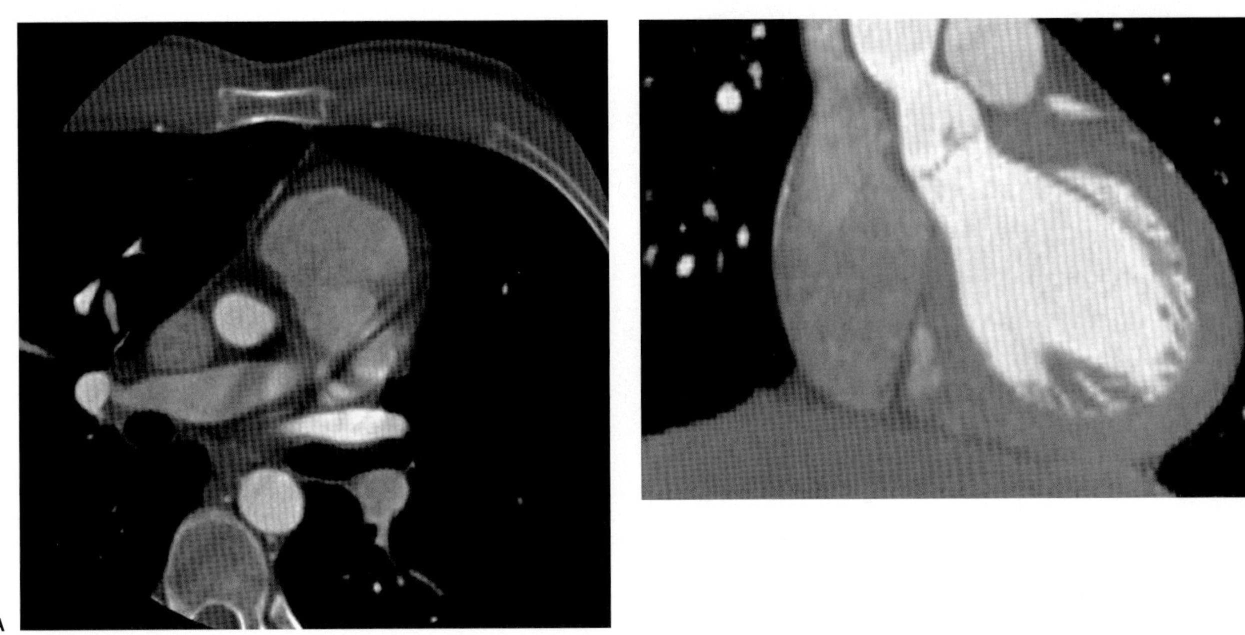

Clinical Presentation

A 22-year-old woman presents with dyspnea, chest pain, and systolic murmur.

Imaging Findings

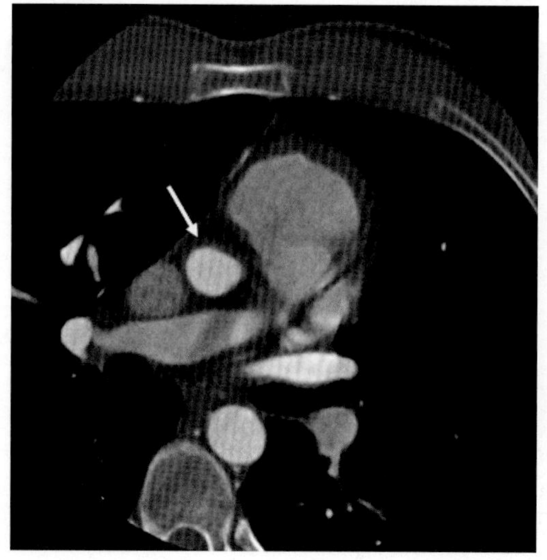

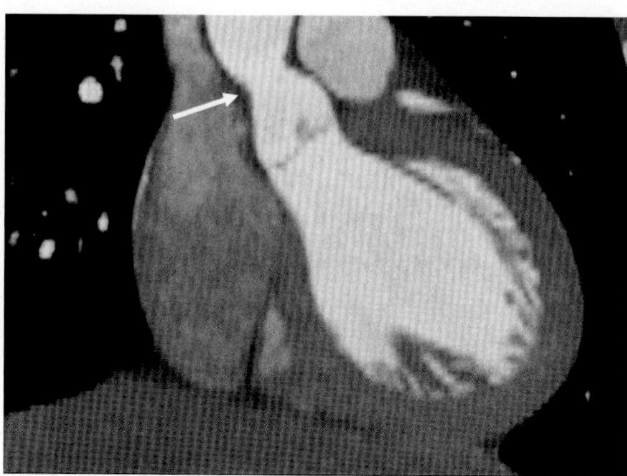

Contrast-enhanced cardiac-gated computed tomography angiography: **(A)** Axial and **(B)** coronal images demonstrate abnormal narrowing and an hourglass deformity of the proximal ascending aorta (*white arrows*).

Differential Diagnosis

- ***Supravalvular aortic stenosis (SVAS):*** SVAS is a rare condition in which there is abnormal narrowing of the aorta above the level of the aortic valve, resulting in left ventricular (LV) outflow obstruction.
- *Hypoplastic ascending aorta:* The hypoplastic ascending aorta is the diffuse type of SVAS.
- *Aortic coarctation:* The typical location of the aortic narrowing in coarctation is distal to the origin of the left subclavian artery.

Essential Facts

- The prevalence of SVAS is not known. In an autopsy series of patients with congenital heart disease, the prevalence rate was 0.67%.
- Underlying abnormality is a disruption of the elastin gene (*ELN*) on chromosome 7 (7q11.23), which can be familial (autosomal-dominant) or sporadic. This produces a reduced number and a disorganized pattern of elastic fibers in the aortic media.
- SVAS can be associated with Williams–Beuren syndrome, which, besides SAVS (71%), includes elfinlike facies, hypercalcemia, pulmonary artery stenosis, and mitral valve prolapse.
- SVAS can present as a focal hourglass deformity or as diffuse hypoplasia of the ascending aorta just above the level of the coronary arteries.
- Several other arteries may be narrowed, in particular the peripheral pulmonary arteries (83%), followed by the coronary, renal, carotid, innominate, and mesenteric arteries.
- Aortic, pulmonary, and/or mitral valve cusps may be thickened, resulting in stenosis or insufficiency.
- More than 50% of patients with SVAS present with an associated aortic valve abnormality, especially bicuspid aortic valve.
- Patients with SVAS may present with concomitant aortic coarctation or congenital heart disease (e.g., tetralogy of Fallot, ventricular septal defect).
- Complications include LV hypertrophy, myocardial ischemia, infarction, sudden death, and stroke.

Other Imaging Findings

- Coronary arteries show dilatation, tortuosity, and accelerated atherosclerosis, changes probably related to the elevated systolic pressure seen in SVAS.

✔ Pearls & ✘ Pitfalls

✔ Surgery, with enlargement of the narrow sinotubular region, including the ascending aorta, is recommended in symptomatic cases (angina, chest pain, and syncope) or when the pressure gradient across the stricture is ≥ 50 mm Hg. Balloon angioplasty has not proved useful.

✘ SVAS is not a condition restricted to the ascending aorta. A significant number of patients have changes involving other vessels, such as the pulmonary arteries, arch vessels, abdominal aorta, renal arteries, and iliac arteries.

Case 27

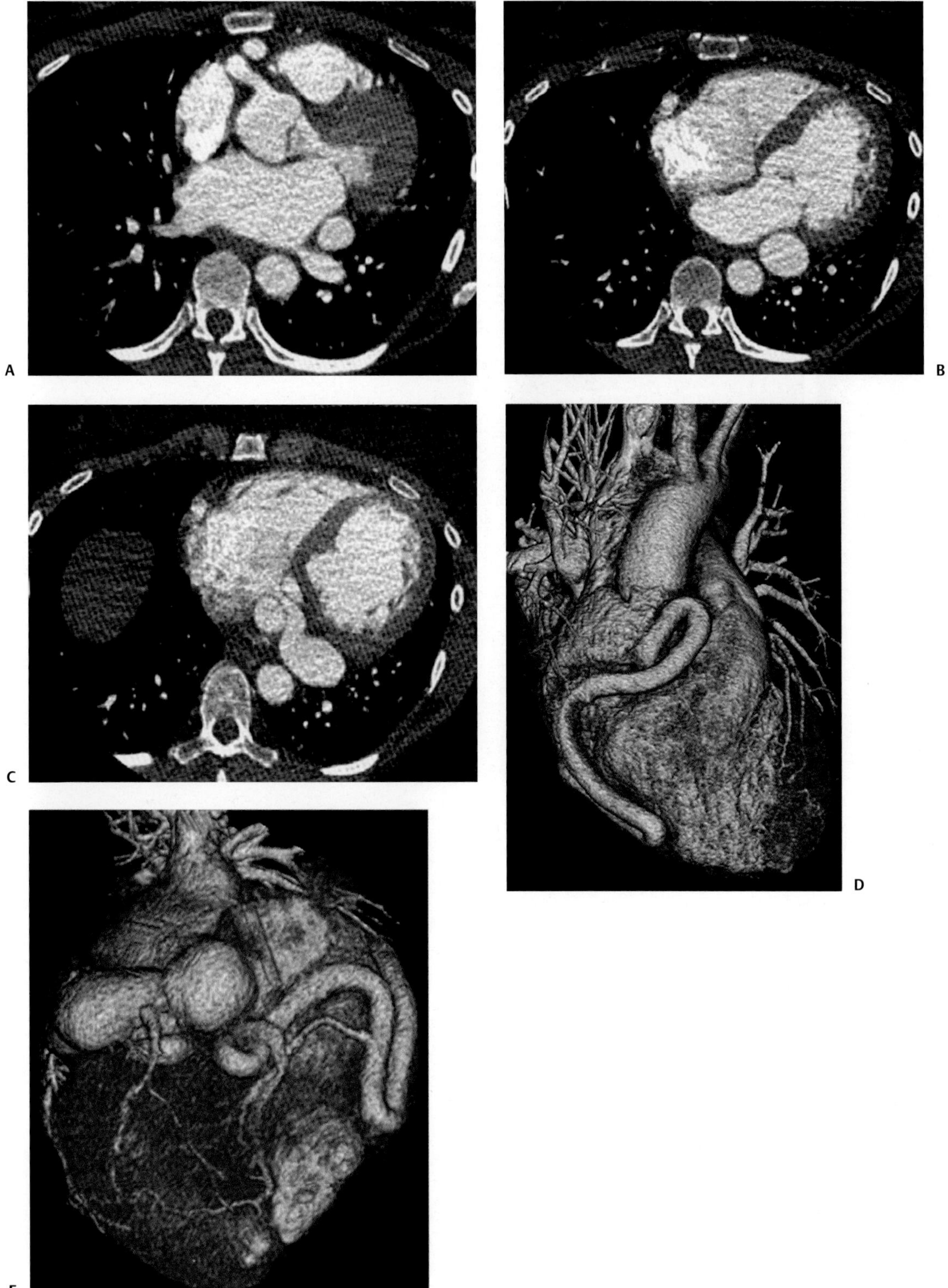

Clinical Presentation

A 43-year-old woman presents with a right coronary artery (RCA) anomaly discovered on an echocardiogram. Computed tomography (CT) was requested to define the anatomy before surgical repair.

Imaging Findings

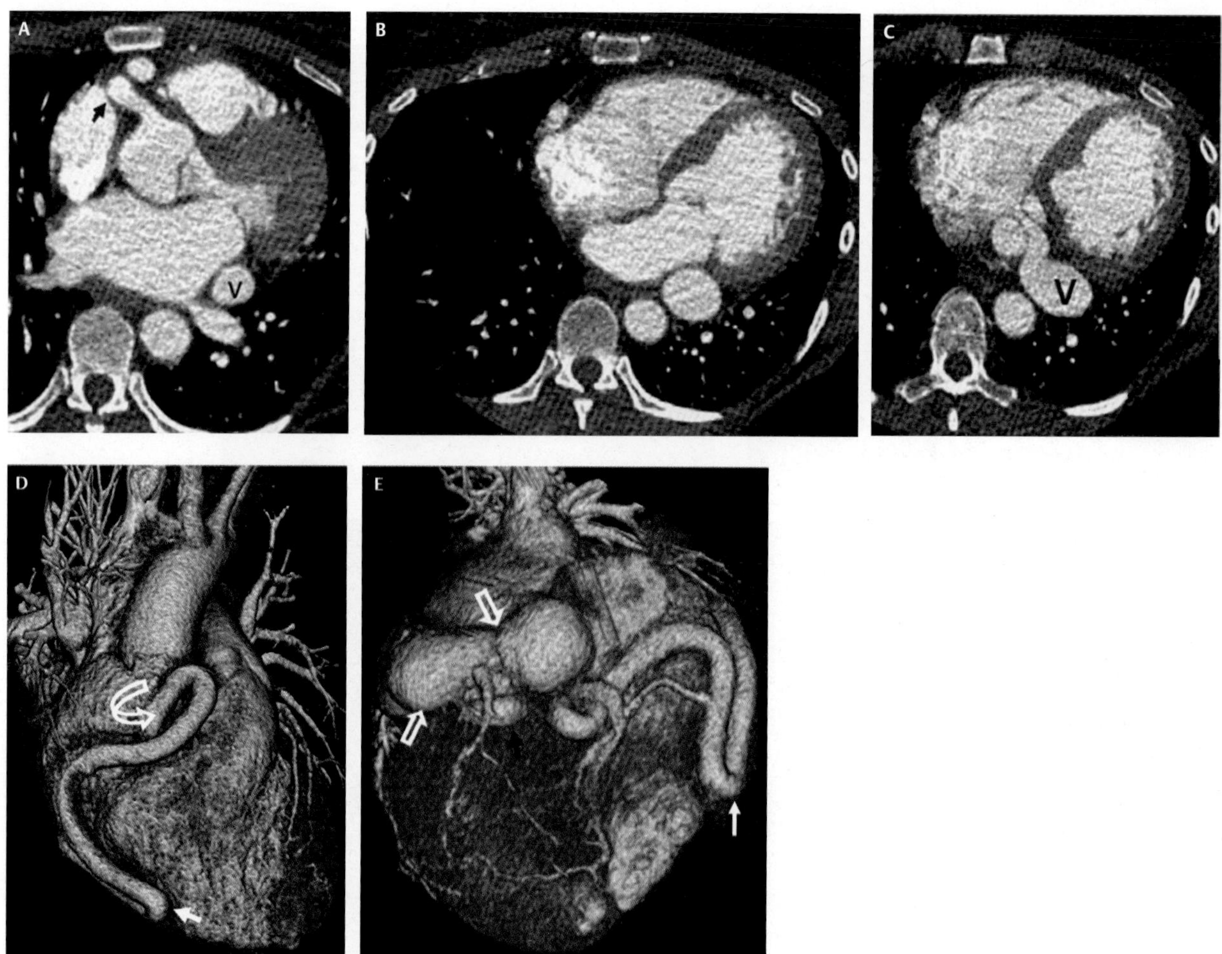

(A) In the axial plane, the RCA origin is enlarged (*black arrow*). On the left cardiac border is an abnormal vascular structure (V). **(B)** Adjacent to the left arterial border, a vascular structure (V) is larger caliber than the descending thoracic aorta. **(C)** Inferiorly, a larger vessel (V), the coronary sinus, drains toward the right atrium. **(D)** In this three-dimensional reconstruction, the RCA is enlarged and tortuous. The vessel arises normally from the aorta and makes two 180-degree turns (*curved open arrow*) and continues to the right posterolateral surface of the right side of the heart (*white arrow*). **(E)** On the inferolateral surface of the heart, the RCA (*white arrow*) continues to the crux of the heart, where there is an aneurysm (*black arrow*). A communicating but separate vascular structure, the coronary sinus (*open white arrows*) is markedly dilated.

Differential Diagnosis

- ***RCA-to-coronary sinus fistula:*** The RCA is markedly enlarged and very tortuous. It connects inappropriately to the coronary sinus, another hallmark of a coronary artery fistula.
- *Anomalous origin of the RCA from the pulmonary artery:* Anomalous origin of a coronary artery from the pulmonary artery is a rare anomaly. The coronary artery is typically mildly enlarged.
- *Fusiform aneurysm of the RCA:* Coronary artery aneurysm is defined as an increase in the diameter of the vessel to 150% of the normal diameter.

Essential Facts

- Fifty-five to 65% of congenital coronary artery fistulas involve the RCA; 7% of these drain to the coronary sinus.
- Clinical symptoms include cardiac failure, ischemia, thrombosis, arrhythmia, and rupture, which may lead to pericardial tamponade.
- Transcatheter occlusion and surgical transection have both been shown to be successful treatment options.

✔ Pearls & ✘ Pitfalls

✔ Magnetic resonance imaging and multidetector CT are capable of providing excellent diagnostic imaging of coronary artery fistulas.

✔ Three-dimensional reconstructed images from these studies are essential before transcatheter or surgical treatment is attempted.

✘ Tortuosity and wide fistulous connections will make a transcatheter approach less successful.

Case 28

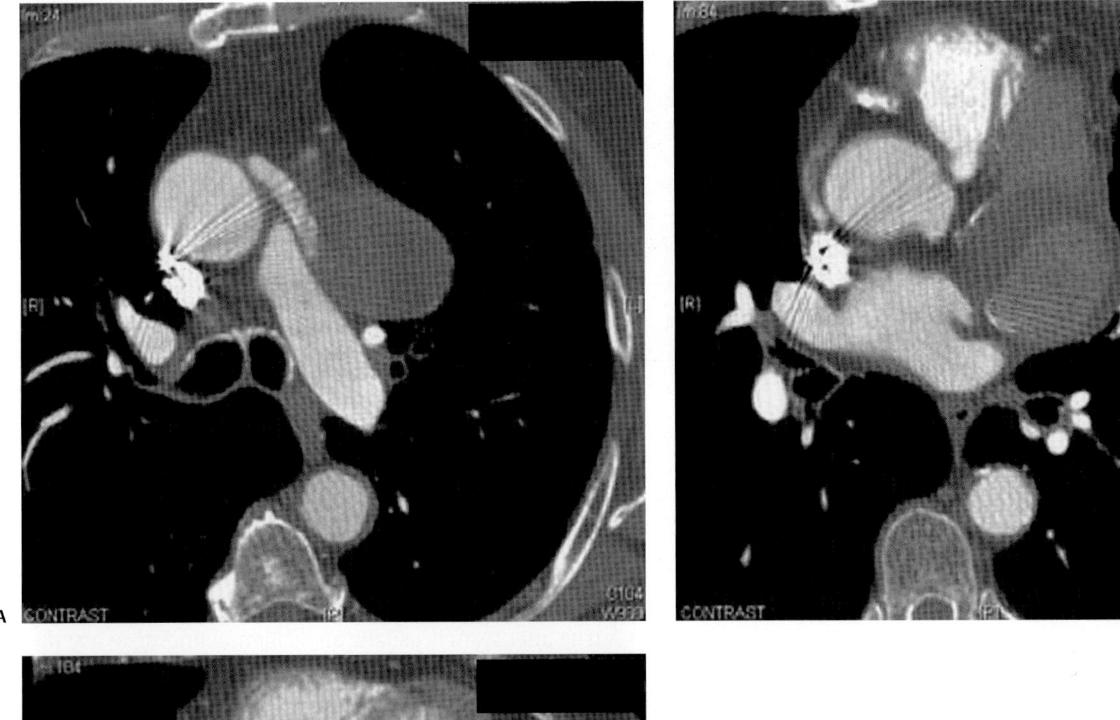

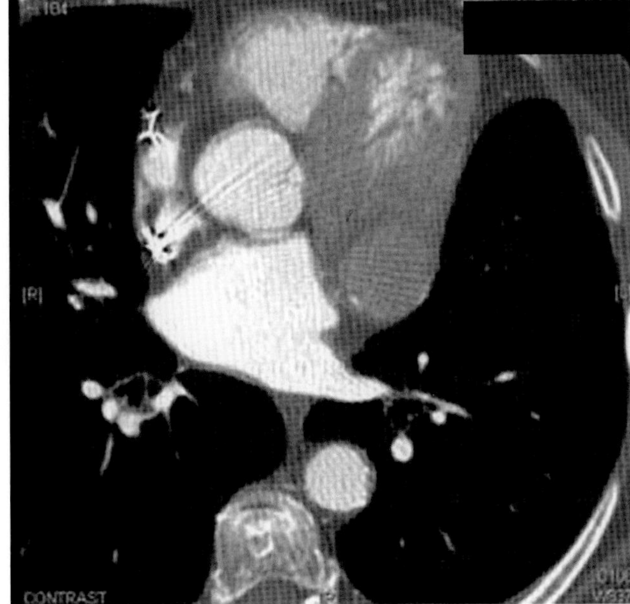

■ Clinical Presentation

Abnormal chest radiograph in a patient with a history of revascularization surgery 7 years before

Imaging Findings

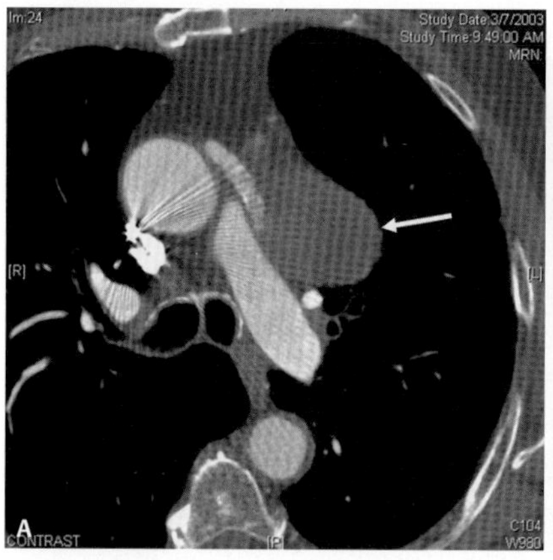

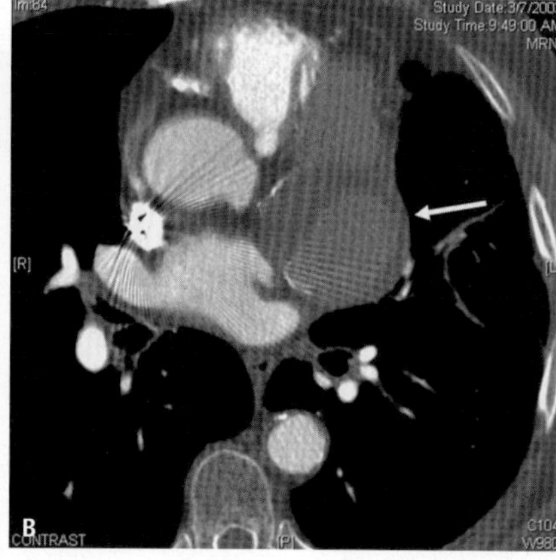

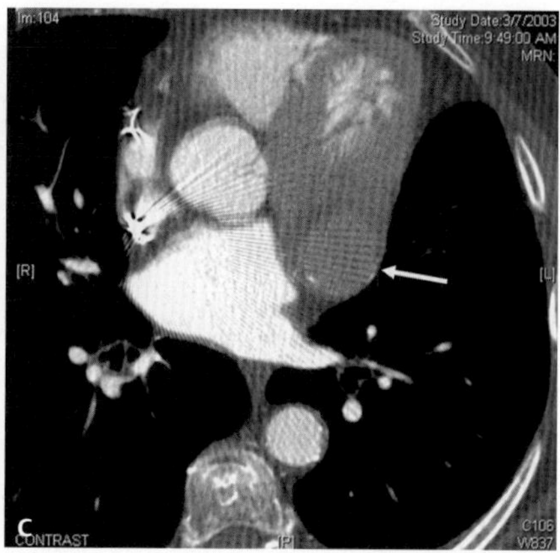

(A–C) Contrast-enhanced cardiac-gated computed tomography angiography: Axial images at three different levels demonstrate a left-sided venous graft and an aneurysmal vascular structure with mural thrombus on the left aspect of the cardiac silhouette along the left atrioventricular groove (*white arrows*).

Differential Diagnosis

- ***Saphenous vein graft aneurysm (SVGA):*** In patients with a medical history of coronary artery disease and bypass graft surgery, the presence of a vascularized mediastinal mass should raise the possibility of an SVGA.
- *Coronary artery aneurysm:* In adult patients, native coronary artery aneurysms are secondary to atherosclerotic disease, are relatively small, and follow the anatomical distribution of the native coronary artery tree. The affected wall shows atherosclerotic disease.
- *Mediastinal tumor:* A mediastinal tumor can present as a soft-tissue density or as an enhancing mass. The patient's age and past medical history, the morphology, and the relation of the tumor to the adjacent structures are key elements for narrowing the differential diagnosis.

Essential Facts

- SVGA is defined as dilation of the graft to 1.5 times the expected diameter of the vessel.
- SVGAs are classified as true aneurysms when all layers of the vessel wall are involved and as pseudoaneurysms or false aneurysms when there is abnormal disruption of one or more layers of the vessel wall. False aneurysms are more common, develop earlier, and typically arise at suture lines. True aneurysms are rare and develop later in the postoperative period (> 1 year).
- More commonly affected vessels are an SVG graft to the left anterior descending artery, followed by an SVG graft to the right coronary artery. An SVG graft to the circumflex or obtuse marginal artery is less commonly involved.
- True aneurysms usually result from intimal hyperplasia and atherosclerotic involvement of the graft with atheroma formation and plaque rupture. A small proportion of true aneurysms are infectious (mycotic) or related to dehiscent surgical sutures.
- Most true aneurysms are fusiform and symmetric, whereas false aneurysms are more commonly saccular and asymmetric.
- A true aneurysm is usually an incidental finding in asymptomatic patients, presenting as a mediastinal or hilar mass on a chest radiograph, whereas a false aneurysm is more commonly symptomatic (chest pain, angina, and bleeding).
- Contrast-enhanced computed tomography shows a vascular tubular or fusiform structure in continuity with the vein graft, with variable degrees of intramural thrombus.
- Complications include rupture, mass effect and compression of mediastinal structures, thrombus formation, distal embolization, ischemia, and infarction.

Other Imaging Findings

- On magnetic resonance imaging, an SVGA appears as a mixed-density tubular or vascular mass along the heart border. Contrast-enhanced images show the lesion to enhance simultaneously with the descending aorta and later to the pulmonary arteries.

✔ Pearls & ✘ Pitfalls

✔ The best treatment option for SVGA is controversial depending on the clinical presentation, size, expansion rate, comorbidity, and life expectancy. Some experts advocate observation for small asymptomatic true aneurysms. Larger, symptomatic true aneurysms and all false aneurysms should be more aggressively treated with either surgery or endovascular intervention.

✘ Selective catheter coronary angiography can underestimate the true diameter of a partially thrombosed SVGA.

Case 29

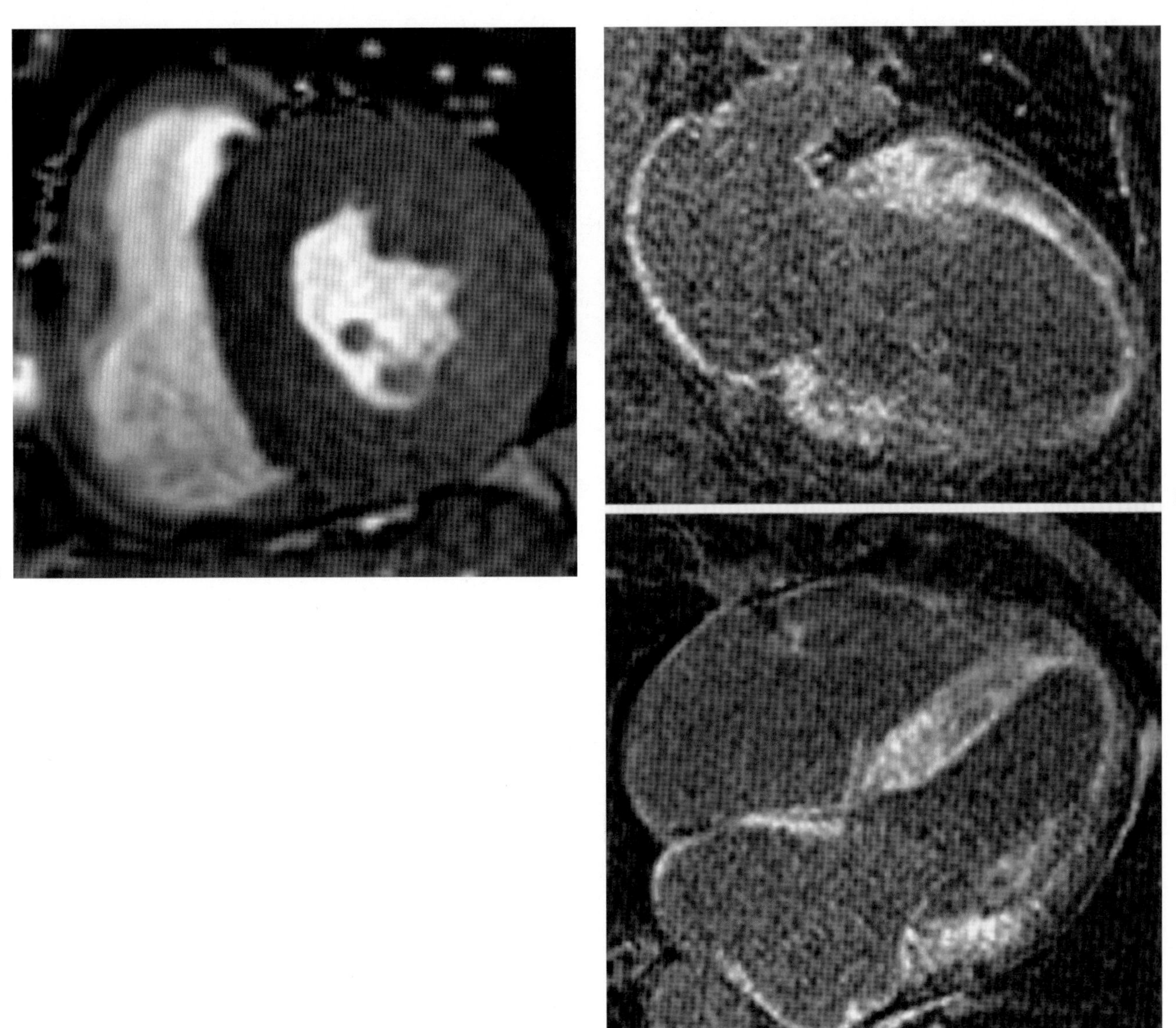

Clinical Presentation

A 73-year-old man presents with shortness of breath, low ejection fraction, and other abnormalities found on a transesophageal echocardiogram.

Imaging Findings

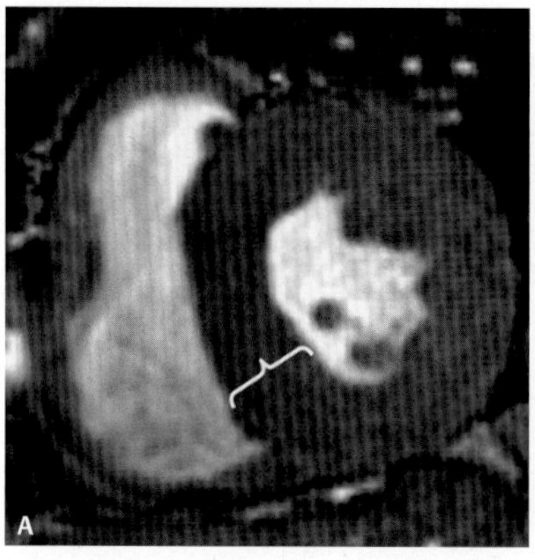
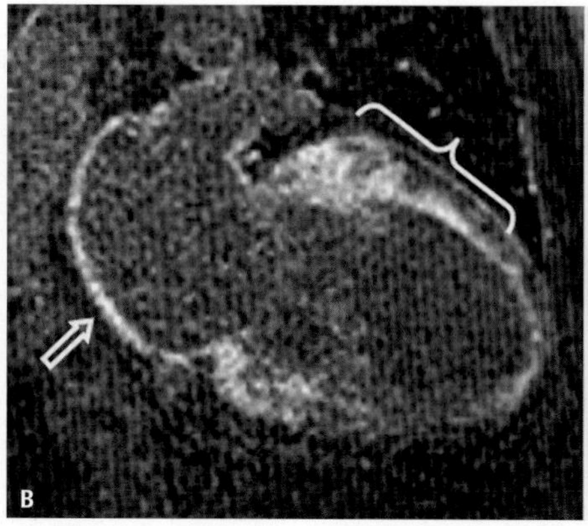
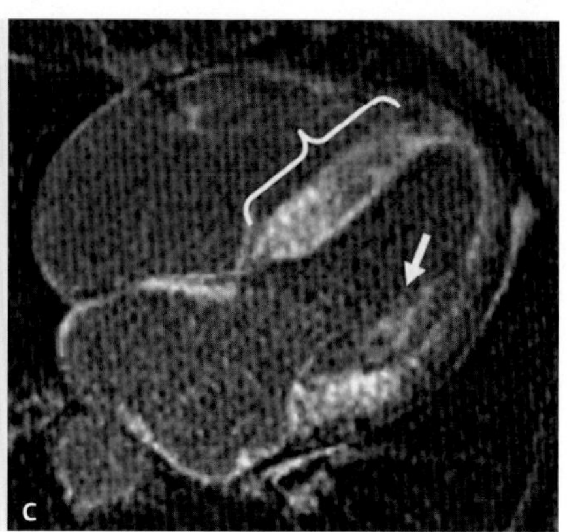

(A) The left ventricle (LV) myocardium is hypertrophic, or thickened, in a concentric manner (*white bracket*). The right ventricle (RV) myocardium is also diffusely thickened. **(B,C)** Vertical long-axis (VLA) and horizontal long-axis (HLA) inversion recovery images of the heart were performed 10 minutes after the intravenous administration of gadolinium. The inversion time (TI) required for suppression of the myocardial signal was 350 milliseconds, which results in suppression of the blood pool. The pattern of enhancement is patchy throughout the LV myocardium (*brackets*) and the atrial wall (*open arrow*). The posterior papillary muscle also enhances (*white arrow*).

Differential Diagnosis

- ***Cardiac amyloidosis:*** Deposition of amyloid protein in the myocardium results in hypertrophy of the myocardium by expanding the extracellular space, increasing the volume of the myocardium. The volume of the LV remains normal.
- *Cardiac sarcoidosis:* Sarcoid cardiomyopathy results in hypertrophy of the myocardium, as in this case. Although myocardial enhancement is typical, the pattern of enhancement is not as extensive, allowing myocardial suppression at typical TI values of 200 to 250 milliseconds.
- *Idiopathic cardiomyopathy:* Cardiomyopathy without a known cause is classified as idiopathic. Typically, in this group of diseases, hypertrophy of the LV is asymmetric, with greater involvement of the interventricular septum.

Essential Facts

- Insoluble fibrillary protein (amyloid) is deposited in the interstitial space of the myocardium.
- Amyloid protein is also deposited in other visceral organs.
- Primary amyloidosis (AL type): cardiac amyloidosis is usually found with primary amyloid disease.
- Secondary amyloidosis (AA type) rarely affects the heart.
- The AA type of amyloid protein can replace normal myocardium. When this happens, the muscle becomes stiff (wall motion is restricted), resulting in restrictive cardiomyopathy.
- Primary amyloidosis is often seen in patients with multiple myeloma.

Other Imaging Findings

- Typical findings of restrictive cardiomyopathy are seen with magnetic resonance functional analysis:
- LV wall thickness is increased.
- Gadolinium enhancement is patchy and heterogeneous, and it is seen throughout the myocardium.
- It can be very difficult to suppress the signal of the normal myocardium on delayed gadolinium images.
- When a long TI is selected, the blood pool may become hypointense to the hyperintense signal of the myocardium.

✔ Pearls & ✘ Pitfalls

✔ Myocardial enhancement may be so intense that it is difficult or nearly impossible to determine if the myocardial signal is suppressed adequately when typical TIs of 200 to 250 milliseconds are used.

✔ Suppression of the myocardial signal on the delayed gadolinium sequences may be incomplete.

✘ Gadolinium enhancement that is limited to the endocardial surface is much more likely to indicate myocardial infarction.

✘ If it is difficult to suppress the signal of the myocardium on delayed gadolinium enhanced images, the diagnosis of cardiac amyloidosis should be strongly considered.

Case 30

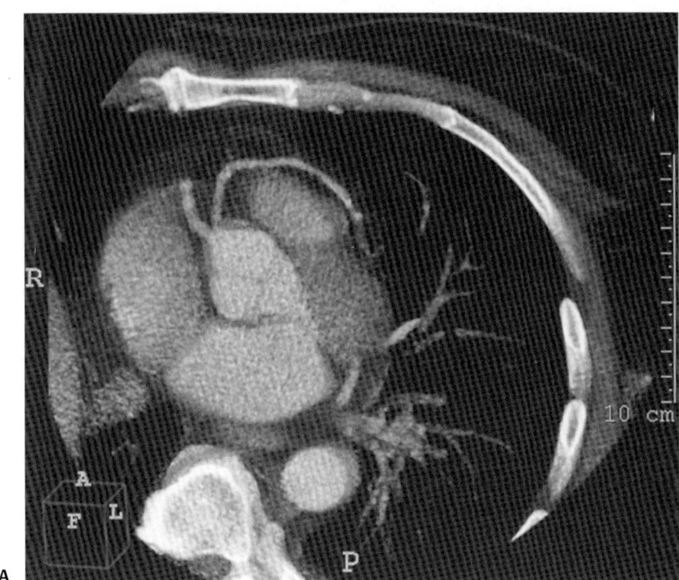

A

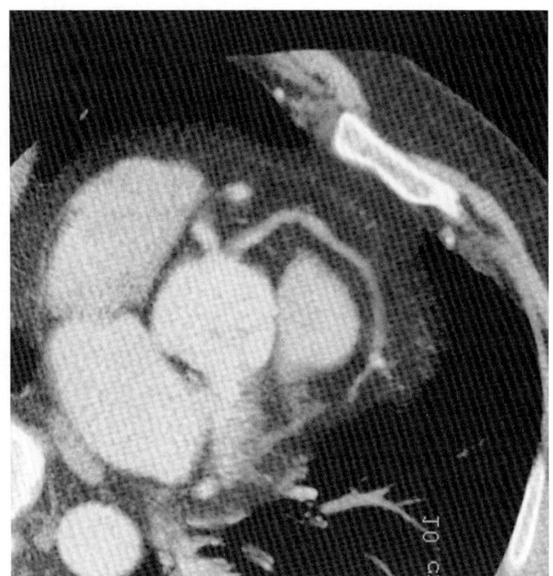
B

■ Clinical Presentation

Atypical chest pain in a 49-year-old man

Imaging Findings

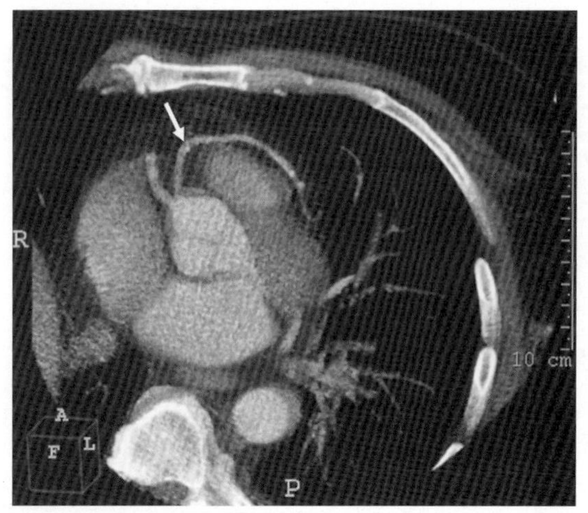

A

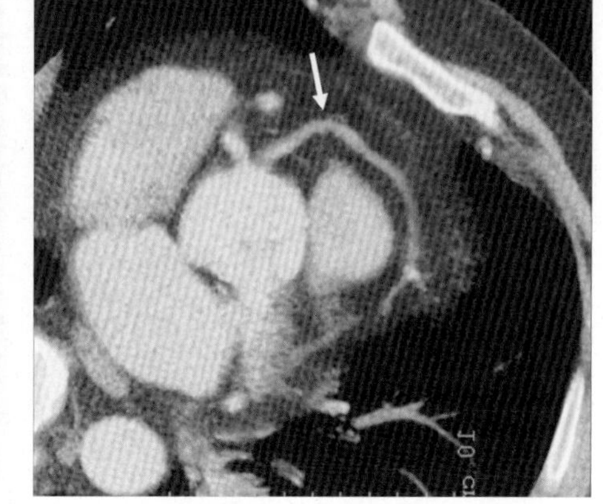
B

(A,B) Contrast-enhanced cardiac-gated computed tomography angiography: **(A)** Axial and **(B)** oblique axial maximum-intensity projection images show an abnormal pattern and origin of the coronary arteries. Both the right and left coronary arteries are identified arising from the right coronary sinus (*white arrows*).

Differential Diagnosis

- ***Anomalous origin of the left coronary artery (LCA) from the right coronary sinus:*** Aberrant LCA from the right coronary sinus can originate from the same ostium as the right or independently. In this case, it arises from a separate ostium. The anomalous vessel runs anteriorly and to the left in a prepulmonic course (benign type).
- *Normal origin of the LCA and its branches:* The normal anatomy of the coronary artery system consists of independent origins of the right and left coronary arteries, each from its corresponding coronary sinus. The vessels in the images shown do not follow this pattern.

Essential Facts

- The LCA may arise from the right sinus of Valsalva either as an independent vessel or as a branch of a single coronary artery.
- In 75% of cases, the LCA follows an interarterial course (between the right pulmonary artery and the aorta) to reach the left side of the heart; this pattern (malignant type) is associated with a high risk for sudden cardiac death (27%).
- Other possible paths are prepulmonic (as in this case), retroaortic, and septal.

Other Imaging Findings

- Besides the correct identification of the course of the abnormal vessel, proper identification of the shape of the ostium is important. An anomalous artery may have an acute kinking with a slitlike ostium.

✔ Pearls & ✘ Pitfalls

✔ Coronary artery anomalies should be considered in athletes and young adults who present with chest pain, exertional dyspnea, and syncope. These types of anomalies account for 13% of cases of sudden cardiac death in competitive athletes, second only to hypertrophic cardiomyopathy.

✘ Unlike the interarterial course of an anomalous LCA, an anomalous origin of the left circumflex artery from the right coronary artery is generally of no clinical significance.

Case 31

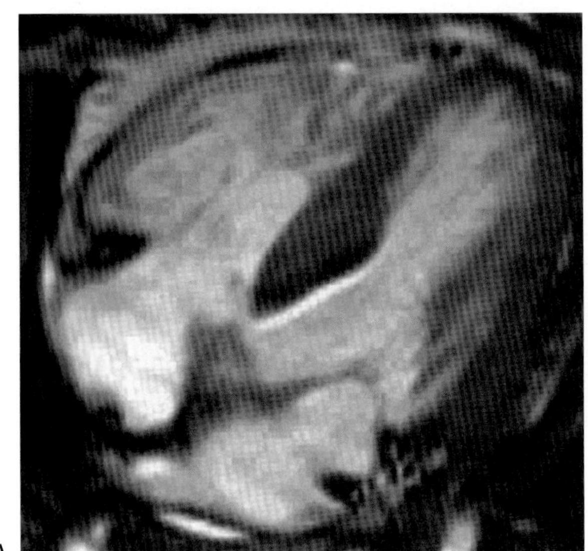
A

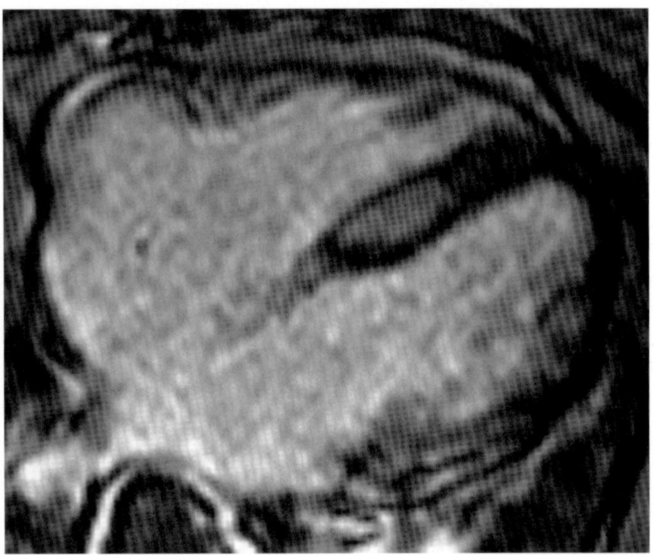
B

Clinical Presentation

A 35-year-old man presents with chronic pulmonary disease and arrhythmia.

Imaging Findings

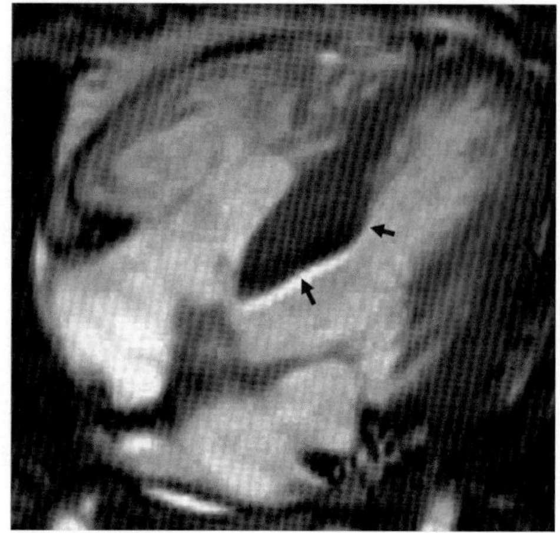
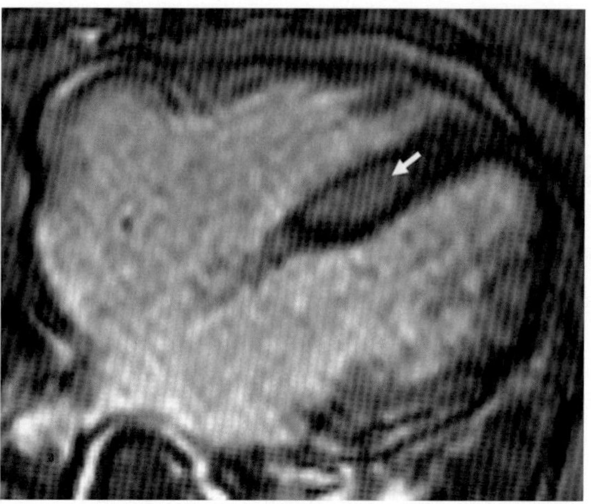
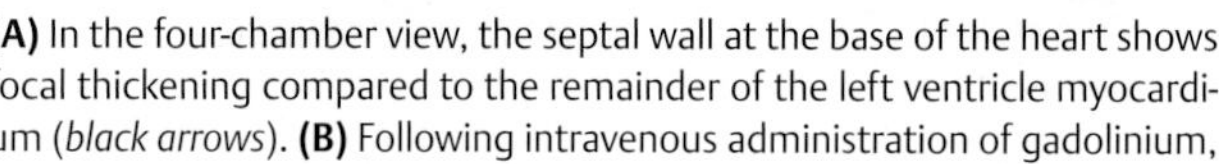

(A) In the four-chamber view, the septal wall at the base of the heart shows focal thickening compared to the remainder of the left ventricle myocardium (*black arrows*). **(B)** Following intravenous administration of gadolinium, a delayed image in a slightly foreshortened four-chamber plane reveals enhancement of the mid myocardium of the basal septal wall, in the region of myocardial thickening (*white arrow*).

Differential Diagnosis

- ***Cardiac sarcoidosis:*** The LV chamber is dilated, and the wall thickness is normal. The gradient echo T2* images show decreasing myocardial signal as the echo time is increased, a property of increased conspicuity of iron deposits in the myocardium.
- *Acute septal infarction:* The myocardium is not thickened. The LV chamber is usually small in hypertrophic cardiomyopathy.
- *Expected findings following septal ablation:* Dilatation of the LV chamber can be seen in patients with ischemic cardiomyopathy, but myocardial signal should remain normal on nonenhanced images.

Essential Facts

- Only 5% of patients with systemic sarcoid disease have cardiac sarcoid disease.
- Cardiac sarcoid disease is the most common cause of sudden cardiac death.
- Heart block is the most common arrhythmia.
- Histologic findings of cardiac sarcoidosis have been found at autopsy in 20 to 50% of patients with pulmonary sarcoidosis.
- Cardiac involvement may be clinically silent.
- The clinical sequelae of sarcoid granulomas within the myocardium range from asymptomatic conduction abnormalities to fatal ventricular arrhythmias.
- Chronic sarcoid infiltration may demonstrate primarily middle myocardial and epicardial delayed enhancement in a noncoronary distribution.
- Myocardial inflammation in sarcoidosis often involves the septum and sometimes the LV wall, whereas papillary muscle and the right ventricular wall are rarely affected.

Other Imaging Findings

- Sarcoid infiltrates are visible on magnetic resonance imaging (MRI) as intramyocardial focal zones with increased signal intensity on both black blood and early enhanced images because of edema associated with inflammation.
- In the acute phase, first-pass perfusion studies do not show segmental ischemic defects but range from normal to early increased segmental enhancement.
- Cine MRI functional images in patients with cardiac sarcoidosis may exhibit segmental contraction abnormalities.
- With severe cardiac involvement, massive infiltration may sometimes lead to diffuse myocardial thickening and marked contraction abnormalities.
- In severe disease, congestive cardiomyopathy and heart failure develop secondary to conduction and contraction abnormalities.
- Advanced cardiac sarcoidosis is characterized by septal wall thinning, systolic and diastolic LV dysfunction, regional wall motion abnormalities, and pericardial effusion.
- Early cardiac sarcoidosis is difficult to diagnose; enhancement diminishes after steroid therapy.
- With thallium 201, segmental defects are seen in areas of myocardial deposits.

✔ Pearls & ✘ Pitfalls

✔ Correlate cardiac findings with chest radiograph and computed tomography (CT) imaging.

✔ Mediastinal and hilar lymphadenopathy, pulmonary fibrosis and nodules, and pleural disease are primary findings on CT.

✘ Imaging findings are not specific for the diagnosis of cardiac sarcoidosis.

✘ Myocardial biopsy is the only known method for definitive diagnosis.

Case 32

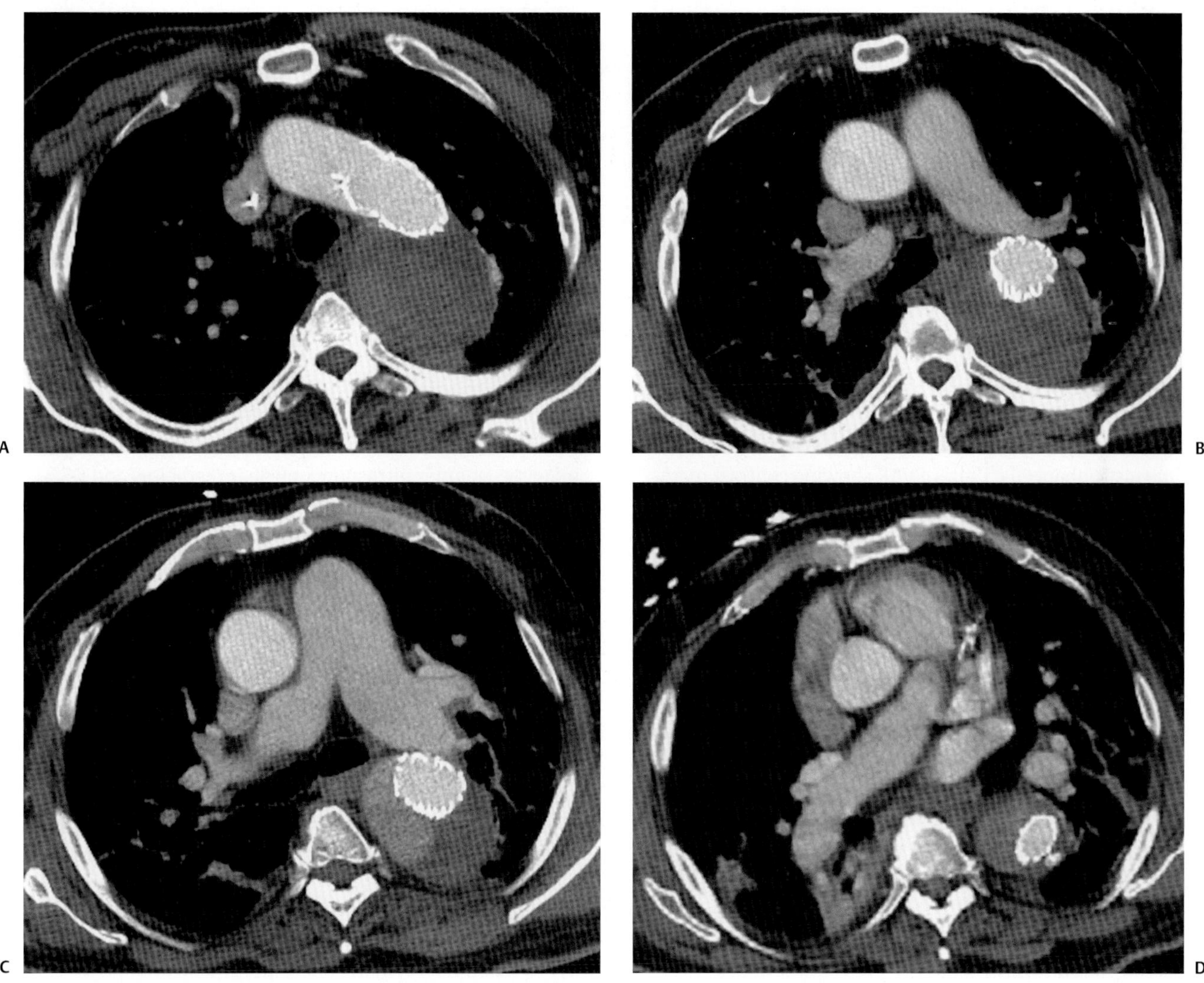

Clinical Presentation

Follow-up computed tomography (CT) scans in a patient with a history of treated aortic aneurysm

Imaging Findings

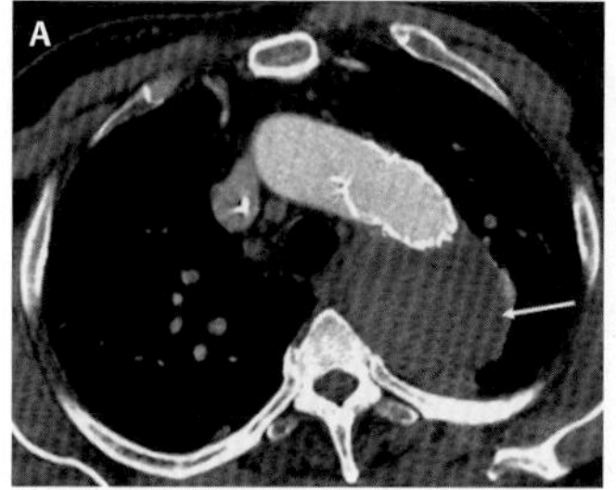

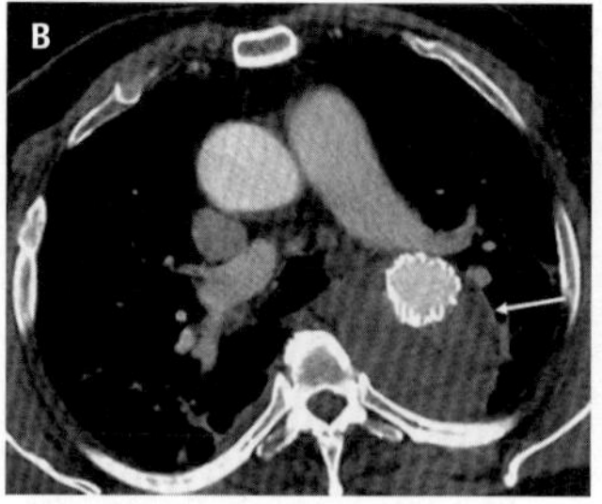

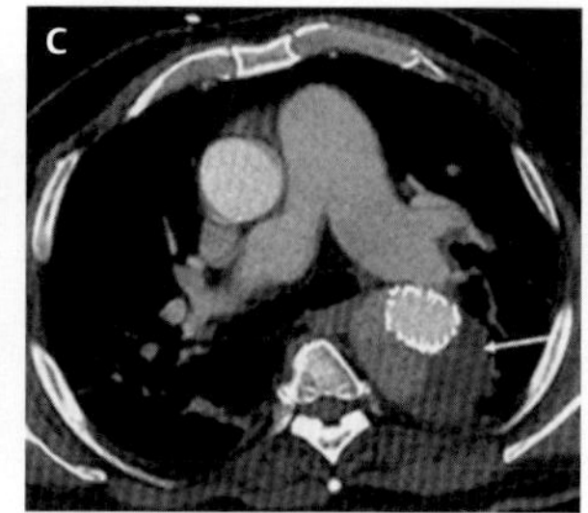

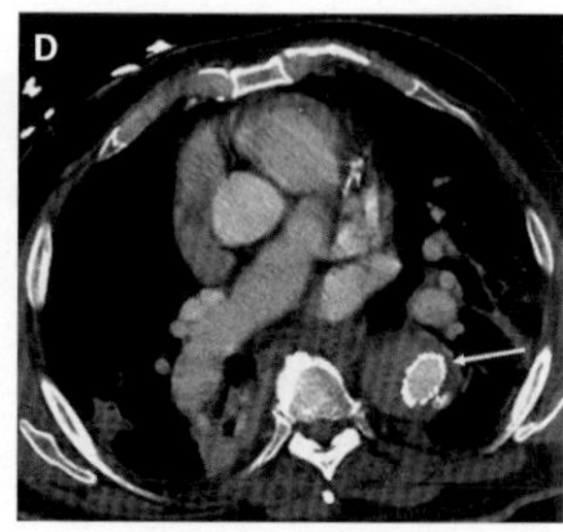

(A–D) Contrast-enhanced computed tomography angiography (CTA) of the aorta: axial images at four different levels are shown. An endovascular aortic stent-graft is seen extending from the mid aortic arch to the descending aorta. There is residual extraluminal contrast opacification of the aneurysm sac in the dilated and stented segment.

Differential Diagnosis

- ***Endoleak after endovascular aneurysm repair (EVAR):*** Contrast-enhanced CT after EVAR showing contrast material flowing outside the stent-graft and inside the aneurysm sac is consistent with an endoleak

Essential Facts

- Stent graft placement is an alternative to surgery for the treatment of descending thoracic aortic aneurysms, aortic ulcers, fistulas, mycotic aneurysms, traumatic aortic injury, and thoracic descending aortic dissections.
- Incidence of endoleak after stent-graft placement for endovascular repair of aortic condition varies from 0 to 33% (average ~12%).
- Endoleaks are classified into five categories based on the source of the blood flow:
  - In type I endoleak, the blood flow originates from the stent-graft attachment site.
  - In type II, there is retrograde flow into the aneurysm through aortic branch vessels.
  - In type III, there is structural failure of the stent-graft from fracture, perforation, or junctional separation in modular devices.
  - Type IV endoleaks result from stent-graft fabric porosity.
  - Type V endoleaks result from expansion of the aneurysm without an obvious endoleak (referred to as *endotension*), likely from an occult endoleak or ultrafiltration of blood across the stent-graft wall.
- Although CTA is excellent for endoleak detection, it has limited ability to determine blood flow direction and appropriate classification.
- Digital subtraction angiography (DSA) is required for precise classification and treatment decisions.
- Lifelong imaging surveillance is needed for patients with EVAR.
- CTA, typically every 6 to 12 months, is currently the most commonly used imaging technique for this purpose.

Other Imaging Findings

- Besides CTA, gadolinium-enhanced magnetic resonance imaging, Doppler ultrasound, nuclear medicine, and DSA play a role in the surveillance, detection, and treatment of patients with EVAR and endoleaks.

✔ Pearls & ✘ Pitfalls

✔ Treatment options for endoleaks vary depending on the cause and source of the abnormal flow. Type I (attachment site) and type III (graft defect or failure) are repaired immediately. Type II (collateral vessel) can be embolized. A subset of type II (40%) and most type IV (graft wall porosity) spontaneously become thrombosed. Type V (endotension) may require conversion to open surgery.

✘ Endoleaks have variable flow rates, so a triphasic CT protocol is needed for their detection, including a noncontrast examination followed by an early arterial phase and a delayed phase.

Case 33

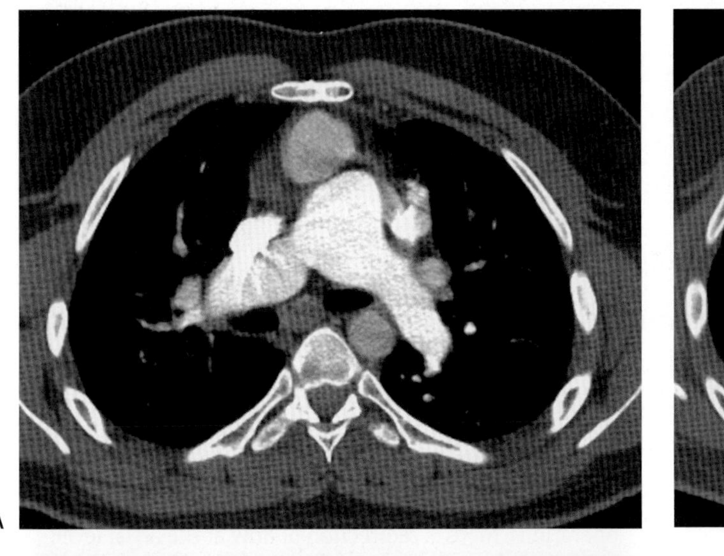
A

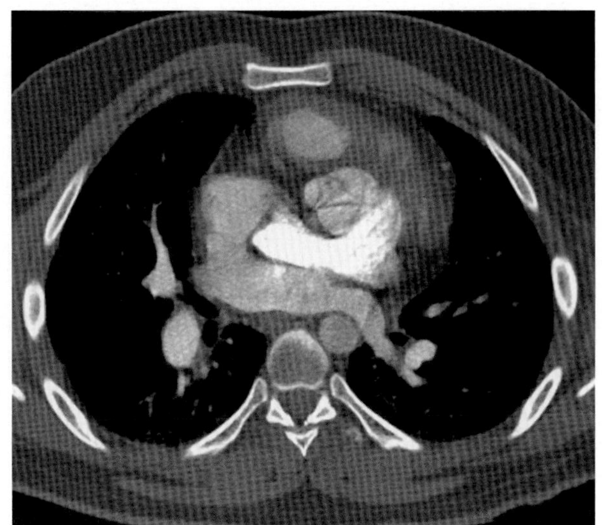
B

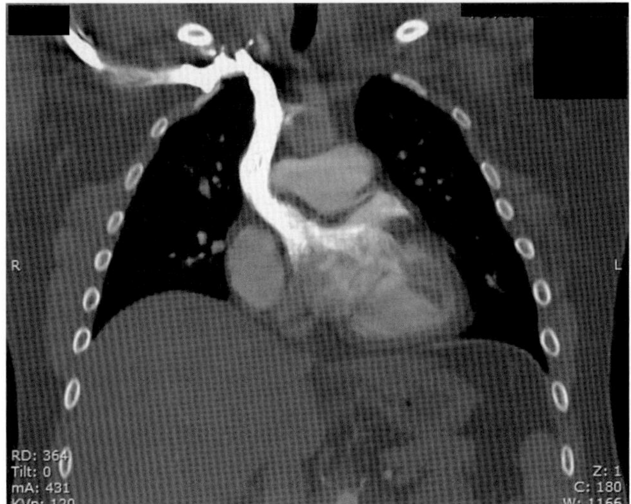

C

Clinical Presentation

Shortness of breath in a 22-year-old man with a past medical history of cardiac disease

Imaging Findings

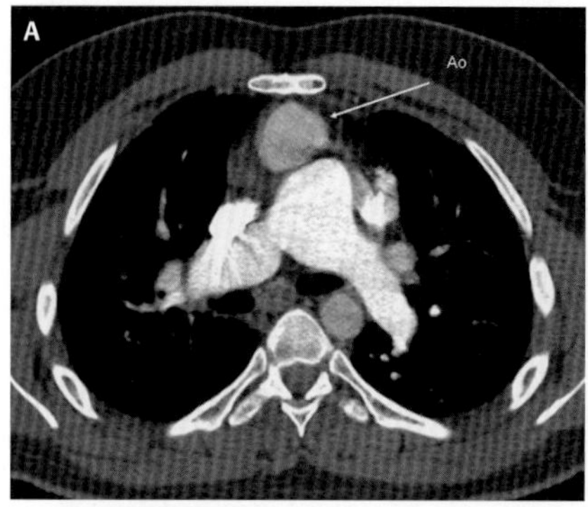

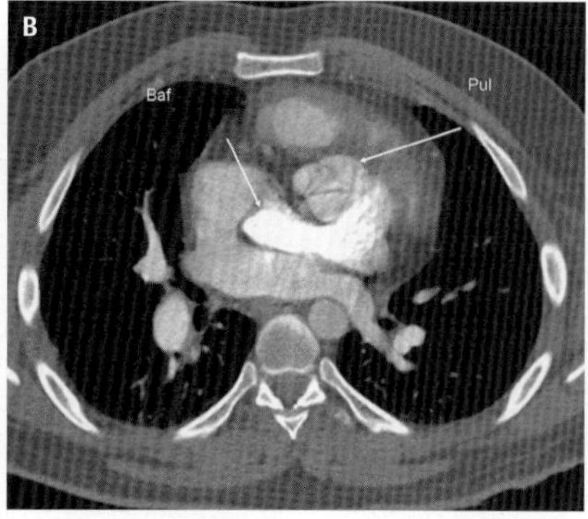

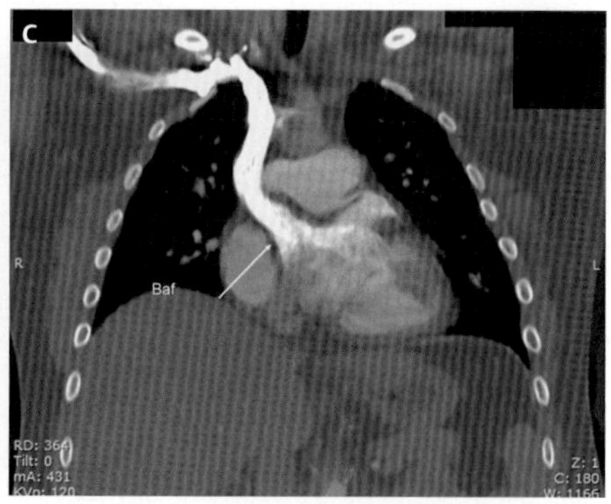

(A–C) Contrast-enhanced cardiac computed tomography (CT) images show the aorta arising in an anterior position from the right ventricle (RV) and the pulmonary artery arising to the left from the left ventricle (LV). The blood returning from the systemic venous system is directed into the LV and then into the pulmonary artery by a surgically created pericardial baffle.

Differential Diagnosis

- ***Dextro-transposition of the great arteries (D-TGA):*** The presence of an anterior position of the aorta in contiguity with the RV and to the right of the pulmonary artery, along with the pulmonary artery arising from the LV, is consistent with a D-TGA.
- *Levo-transposition of the great arteries:* In this so-called congenitally corrected transposition, there is both atrioventricular and ventriculoarterial discordance. The aorta arises from the RV, the pulmonary artery is connected to the RV, the right atrium connects with the LV, and the left atrium connects with the RV.

Essential Facts

- In D-TGA, also known as *complete transposition*, the aorta arises in an anterior position from the RV and the pulmonary artery arises from the LV. Because the transposed aorta is also to the right, this is considered a dextro-transposition.
- This type of transposition creates a complete separation of the pulmonary and systemic circulation, which is incompatible with life.
- For infants with this condition to be able to survive, there must be communication between the two circuits, usually though the ductus arteriosus or patent foramen ovale.
- Affected infants present with cyanosis from birth, tachypnea, and not uncommonly, heart failure.
- Without early intervention, the prognosis is very poor, with a 90% mortality rate in the first 6 months.
- Immediate management includes infusion of prostaglandin E to maintain patency of the ductus arteriosus and creation of an atrial septal defect by means of a balloon (Rashkind procedure).
- In the "atrial switch" operation (Mustard or Senning operation), there is redirection of flow at the atrial level. The atrial septum is excised, and a baffle within the atria is constructed to direct systemic venous flow into the LV (which is connected to the pulmonary artery) and the pulmonary venous flow into the RV (which is connected to the aorta), as in this case, restoring the physiologic pattern of circulation.
- The "arterial switch" operation (Jatene operation), which is more commonly done, is a more anatomical correction. The proximal pulmonary artery and ascending aorta are transected above the semilunar valves and coronary arteries, then switched so that the aorta is connected to the valve arising from the LV, and the pulmonary artery is connected to the valve arising from the RV. The coronary arteries are also relocated to the neo-aorta.
- Surgical techniques have dramatically changed the prognosis of patients, and affected children are reaching adulthood and living almost normal lives.

Other Imaging Findings

- In D-TGA, the aorta and the pulmonary arteries lie parallel and almost in the same sagittal plane, with the aorta slightly more anterior and to the right of the pulmonary artery.

✔ Pearls & ✘ Pitfalls

✔ Almost all patients with L-TGA have associated congenital heart anomalies, in particular ventricular septal defect (70%) and pulmonic stenosis (50%).

✔ Most often, D-TGA occurs without associated cardiac anomalies, and without early intervention it is not compatible with postnatal life.

Case 34

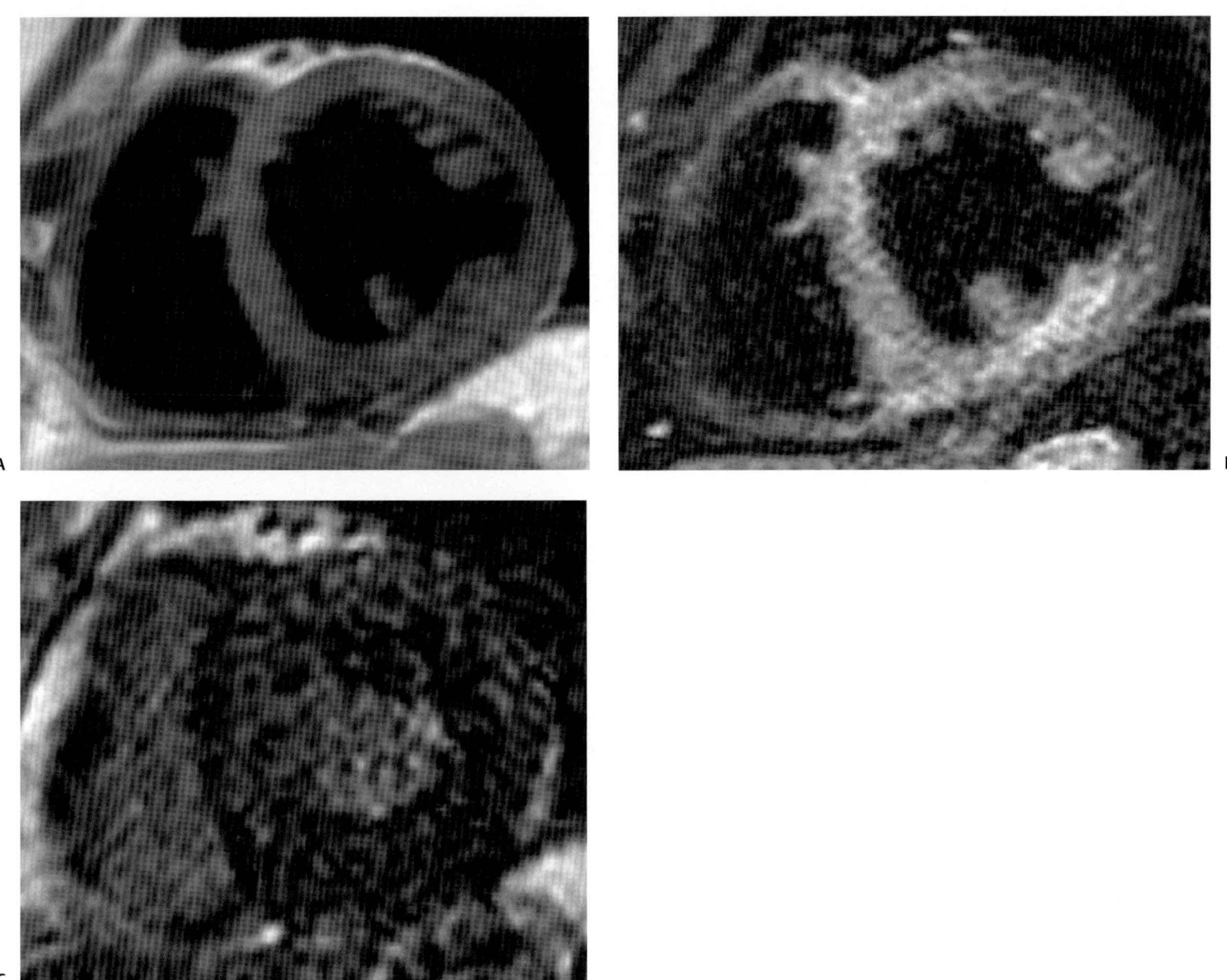

Clinical Presentation

A 37-year-old woman presents with arrhythmia and a recent syncopal event.

■ Imaging Findings

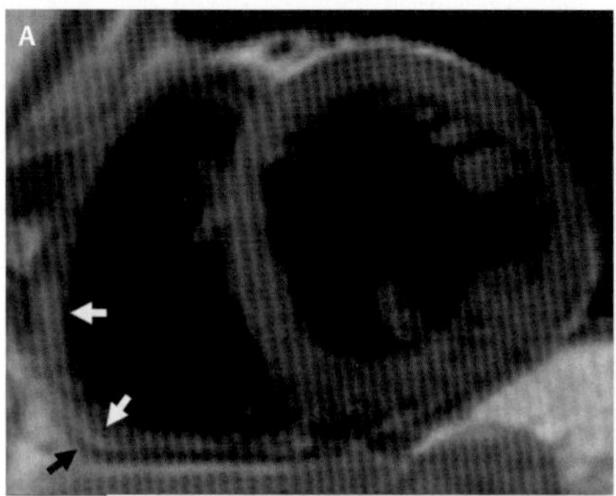

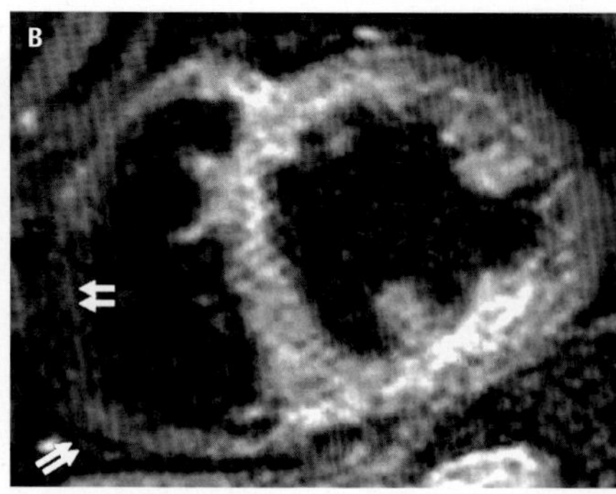

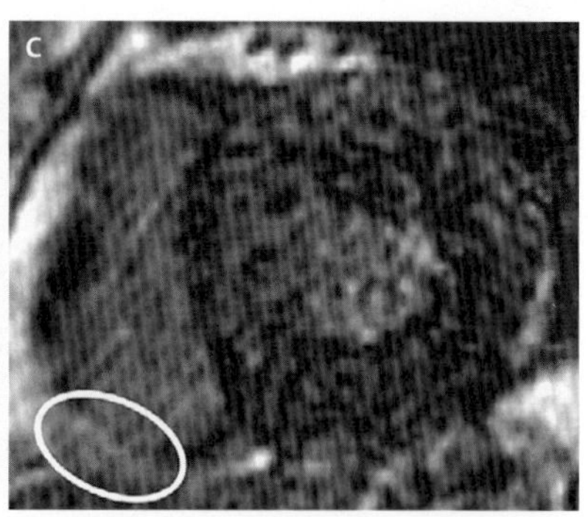

(A) In the short-axis view, with a T2-weighted spin echo sequence, there is abnormal hyperintense signal in the myocardium in the free wall, extending to the inferior wall (*white arrows*). The fatty tissue is surrounded by the myocardium; the epicardial myocardium has normal intermediate signal (*black arrow*). **(B)** After a fat saturation pulse is applied (double inversion recovery), the hyperintensity in the myocardium now has low signal (*double white arrows*), indicating the presence of fat. **(C)** Ten minutes after gadolinium is administered intravenously, inversion recovery images reveal delayed hyperenhancement of the abnormal right ventricular (RV) myocardium at the junction of the free wall and the inferior RV wall (*white oval*).

■ Differential Diagnosis

- ***Arrhythmogenic right ventricular cardiomyopathy (ARVC):*** ARVC is also known as arrhythmogenic right ventricular dysplasia (ARVD). This disease is uncommon but important because it may result in sudden death in young, otherwise healthy individuals.
- *RV myocarditis:* Myocarditis is an inflammatory or infectious process that almost always affects the left ventricle (LV).
- *Malignant lymphoma infiltration:* Diffuse large B-cell lymphoma (DLBCL) is the most common type of cardiac lymphoma; it invades the myocardium and infiltrates or forms nodular masses in the pericardium. The right side of the heart is the most common site of cardiac lymphoma.

■ Essential Facts

- Abnormal heart rhythms result in clinical symptoms such as palpitations and syncope, and even sudden death.
- Fatty and fibrous replacement is seen in the RV and less often the LV myocardium.
- The term *cardiomyopathy* is used because the disease has a genetic basis; familial inheritance is autosomal-dominant, with involvement of chromosomes 1, 2, 14, and 17.

■ Other Imaging Findings

- Normal myocardium is of uniform thickness and intermediate gray color on spin echo images.
- Fat is hyperintense on spin echo and proton density images and is hypointense when a fat saturation pulse is applied.
- Myocardial thinning, dyskinesia, and even aneurysm formation are additional findings.
- Fibrous tissue enhances with gadolinium.
- Magnetic resonance imaging (MRI) is a key imaging modality in the diagnosis of ARVC.
- Fat suppression sequences increase the specificity and conspicuity of myocardial fatty infiltration.

✔ Pearls & ✘ Pitfalls

✔ ARVD/ARVC diagnosis is based on a patient having major and/or minor criteria: two major, one major and two minor, or four minor criteria.

✔ Major criteria:
- MRI: severe dilatation and reduction of the RV ejection fraction or localized RV aneurysms and dyskinesis
- Endocardial biopsy: fibrofatty infiltration of the RV myocardium
- Electrocardiogram (ECG) abnormalities: epsilon waves or prolonged QRS complex
- Necropsy or surgery: familial disease

✔ Minor criteria:
- MRI: mildly dilated RV or reduced ejection fraction, mild segmental RV dilatation or regional hypokinesia
- ECG abnormalities: inverted T waves and late potentials
- Arrhythmia: ventricular tachycardia, frequent ventricular extrasystole
- Family history: premature sudden death due to suspected ARVD, positive family history

✘ MRI is not diagnostic of ARVC, but it can support the diagnosis.

Case 35

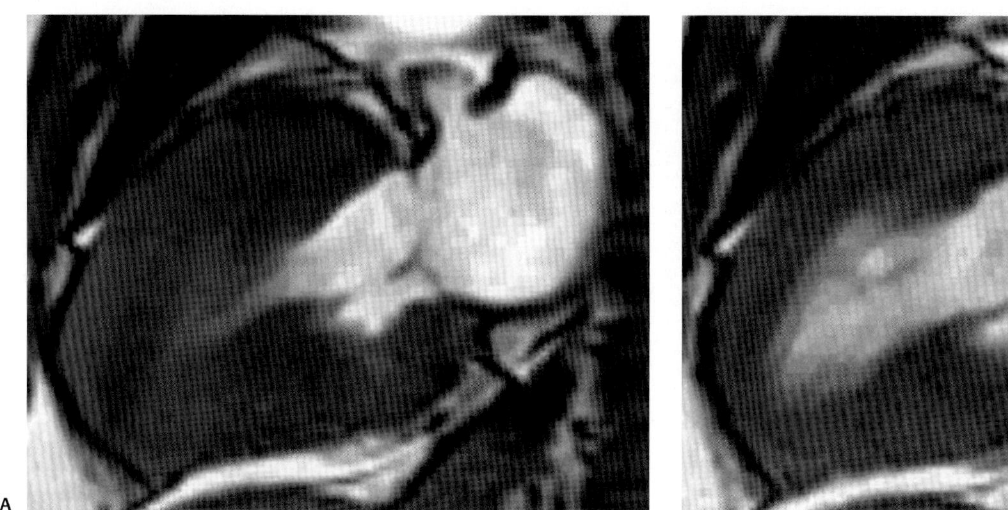

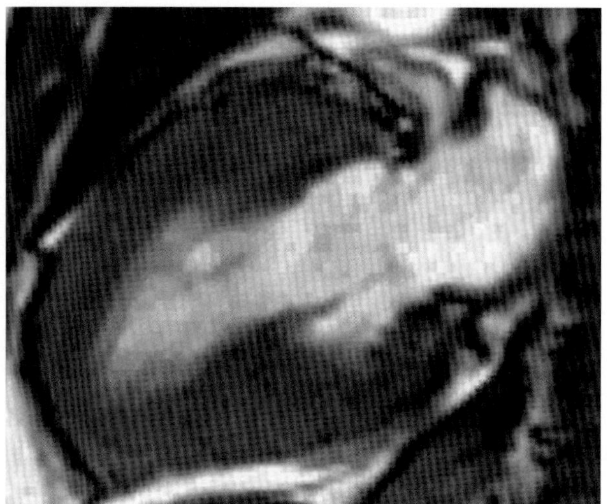

A B

Clinical Presentation

A 30-year-old man presents with familial heart disease, syncope, and palpitations. The patient has a decreased glomerular filtration rate (GFR).

Imaging Findings

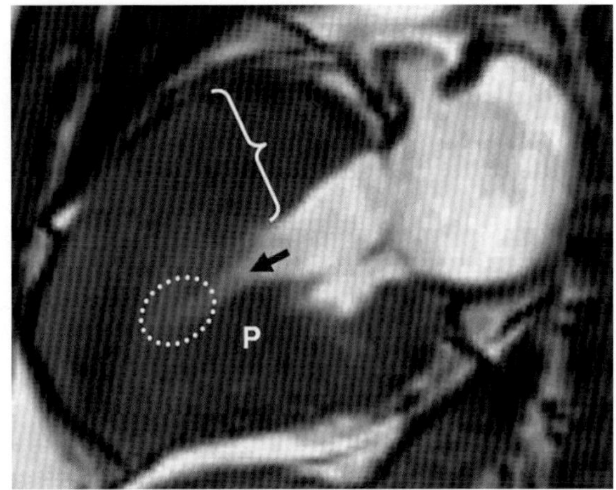

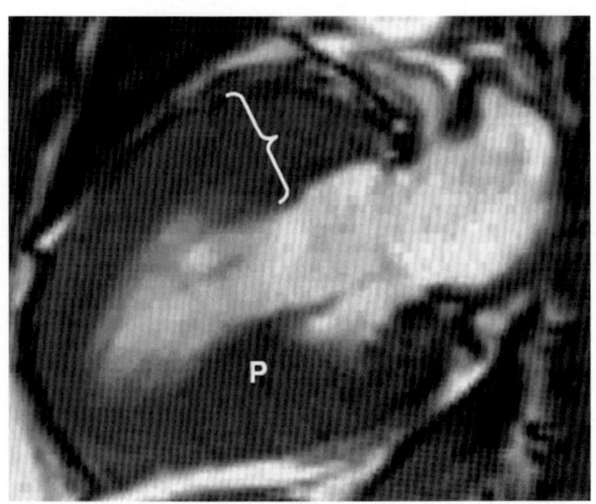

(A) In this systolic vertical long-axis view of the left ventricle (LV), the anterior (*white bracket*) and inferior walls, including the inferior papillary muscle (P), are markedly thickened. The signal of the myocardium is normal. During systole, the middle of the LV chamber is nearly obstructed, leaving the apical portion of the chamber isolated (*dotted white ellipse*).

(B) During diastole, thickening of the anterior wall (*white bracket*) remains, and the inferior walls, including the abnormally broad-based attachment of the inferior papillary muscle (P), are again seen. The degree of thickening is minimally less than in systole. The patient did not receive gadolinium because of decreased GFR.

Differential Diagnosis

- ***Hypertrophic obstructive cardiomyopathy (HOCM) with middle chamber obstruction:*** HOCM comprises a group of primary diseases of the myocardial cell sarcomere, which results in hypertrophy of the myocardium.
- *Myocarditis:* The myocardium may be thickened focally, usually involving the lateral and apical walls of the LV.
- *Dilated cardiomyopathy:* The LV chamber is small in this patient. Typically, in dilated cardiomyopathy, it is thinned, not thickened.

Essential Facts

- The myocardial sarcomere, the smallest functional unit of a muscle cell, is affected.
- HOCM is the most common type of inherited (congenital) cardiac disorder, with an estimated prevalence of 1 in 500.
- Autosomal-dominant with variable penetrance is the most common mode of inheritance and is seen in 50 to 60% of cases.
- More than 150 mutations of 10 genes have been characterized.
- Most cases of HOCM are expressed in adolescence or early adulthood but may be delayed until midlife or later.
- Clinically the disease manifests as systolic or diastolic dysfunction, left ventricular outflow tract (LVOT) obstruction, arrhythmia, or sudden cardiac death.
- Sudden cardiac death typically occurs in adolescents or young adults.

Other Imaging Findings

- Characteristic hypertrophy of the LV myocardium may be symmetric or asymmetric.
- One or both of the papillary muscles will be hypertrophic.
- Occasionally, the right ventricular myocardium is also affected.
- Asymmetric hypertrophic disease is most common; the majority of cases involve the anteroseptal wall.
- Seventy-five to 90% of patients have patchy, mid-myocardial enhancement that does not conform to the distribution of a coronary artery.

✔ Pearls & ✘ Pitfalls

✔ LV wall thickness, which is usually > 30 mm, should be measured at end-diastole, in the short axis.

✔ Obstruction of the apex, middle of the LV chamber, or LVOT can completely isolate the apex, which may be relatively dilated.

✘ Make certain that the wall measurements are not made in an oblique plane, which may result in exaggeration of wall thickness.

Case 36

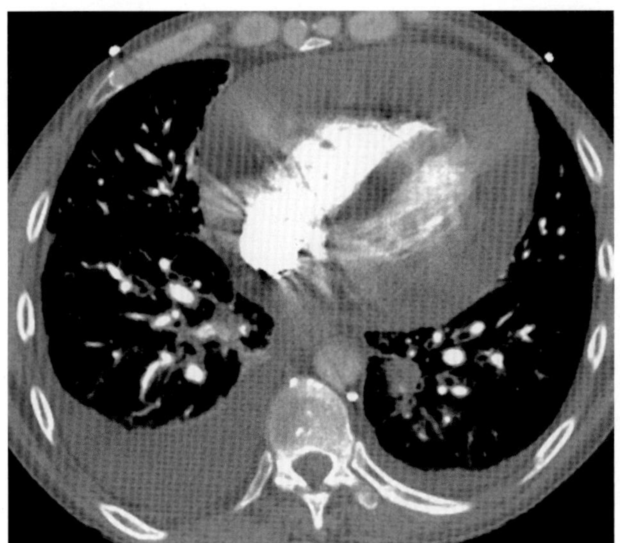

A

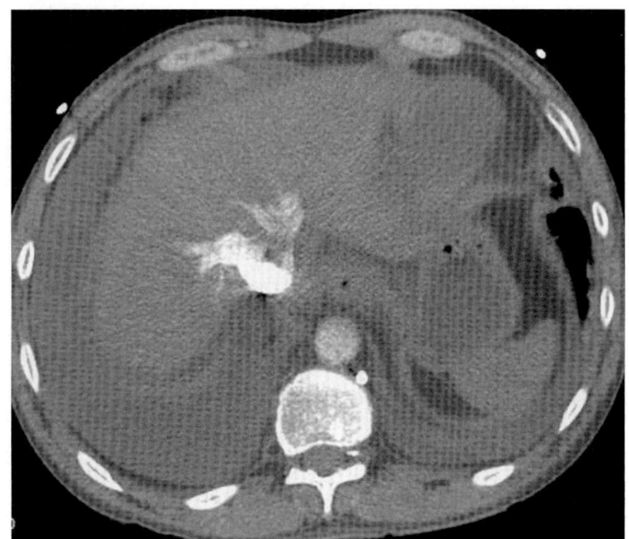

B

■ Clinical Presentation

A 50-year-old man with a history of lung cancer presents with worsening shortness of breath, distended neck veins, tachycardia, and hypotension that worsens during inspiration.

Imaging Findings

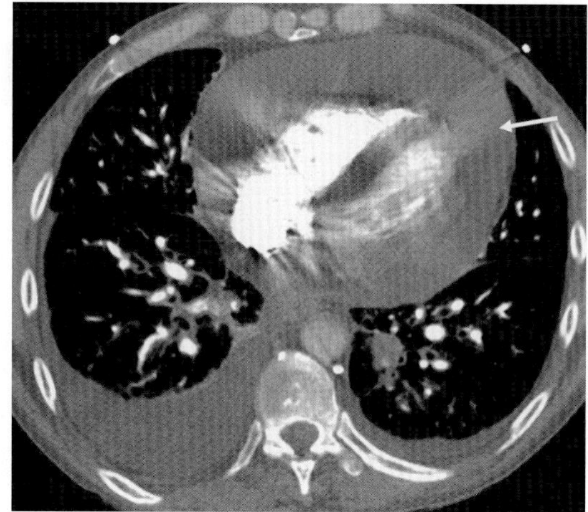

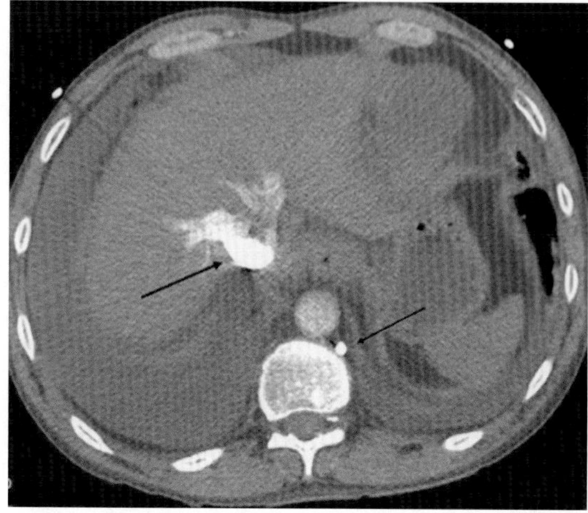

(A,B) Contrast-enhanced computed tomography (CT) of the chest: Axial images of the lower thorax and upper abdomen demonstrate a large pericardial effusion compressing the heart, with large pleural effusions and contrast reflux from the right atrium to the inferior vena cava (IVC) and hepatic veins. Also note contrast reflux into the azygos vein.

Differential Diagnosis

- ***Cardiac tamponade:*** The presence of a pericardial effusion with compression of the right ventricle (RV) and distended IVC and hepatic veins, along with the constellation of clinical findings of pulsus paradoxus, tachycardia, and distended neck veins, is consistent with tamponade physiology.
- *Constrictive effusive pericarditis:* In patients with pericardial constriction, including those with constrictive effusive pericarditis, the RV may be compressed and the systemic venous pressure increased, but abnormal pericardial thickening with some amount of pericardial effusion is present.
- *Right-sided congestive heart failure (CHF):* There are some physiologic abnormalities that are common to CHF and cardiac tamponade. In both conditions, there is impaired function of the RV and dilated IVC and hepatic veins. A significant difference is that unlike in tamponade, in which the RV is compressed, in right-sided CHF it is usually dilated.

Essential Facts

- Cardiac tamponade is defined as slow or rapid compression of the heart due to pericardial accumulation of fluid, pus, blood clots, or gas as a result of effusion, trauma, or rupture of the heart.
- Occasionally, tumor and hernia can compress the heart and present with the same physiologic consequences.
- Pulsus paradoxus is defined as a drop of > 10 mm Hg in systolic pressure during inspiration, due to an increase in right heart filling at the expense of left heart filling. It is the clinical hallmark of cardiac tamponade.
- The pericardial content reaches the limit of pericardial reserve volume, increasing the pericardial pressure (> 20 mm Hg), with compression of the cardiac chambers, which become smaller. This limits the cardiac inflow, which decreases the stroke volume, cardiac output, and ultimately blood pressure.
- Most important imaging findings include pericardial effusion (or content), dilated IVC, right atrial collapse (which may be absent in regional cardiac tamponade as in this case), and signs of increased systemic venous pressure.
- Clinical diagnosis of cardiac tamponade is often missed.
- Echocardiography has a sensitivity of 38 to 60% and specificity of 50 to 100% for this diagnosis.

Other Imaging Findings

- In the presence of pericardial effusion, flattening of the anterior surface of the heart and compression of the RV are important computed tomography (CT) findings in favor of restricted filling of the RV and cardiac tamponade.

✔ Pearls & ✘ Pitfalls

✔ The rate of accumulation of the pericardial effusion is more significant for the development of cardiac tamponade than the size or composition of the pericardial effusion. Volumes as small as 100 mL if rapidly accumulated can produce tamponade physiology; large volumes of fluid (2000 mL) can be better tolerated if accumulation is slow.

✘ Several findings that have been reported on CT associated with cardiac tamponade, including enlargement of the superior vena cava, dilation of the IVC, periportal lymphedema, reflux of contrast into the hepatic veins and azygos vein, and dilatation of the hepatic and renal veins, are not specific and can be seen in other conditions.

Case 37

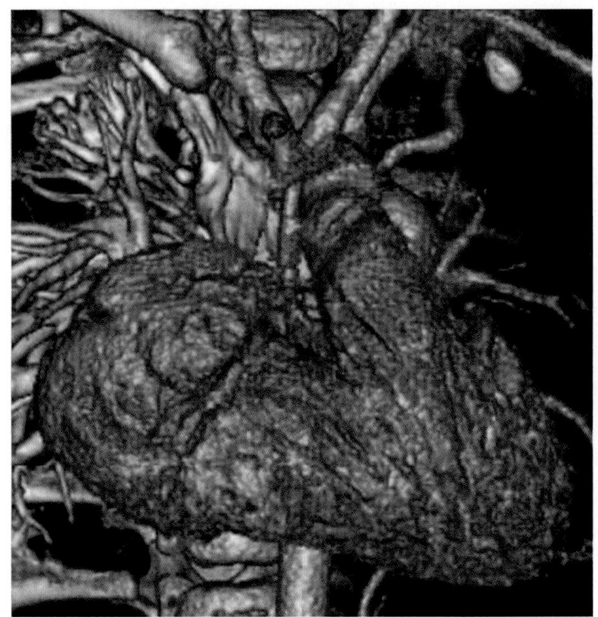
A

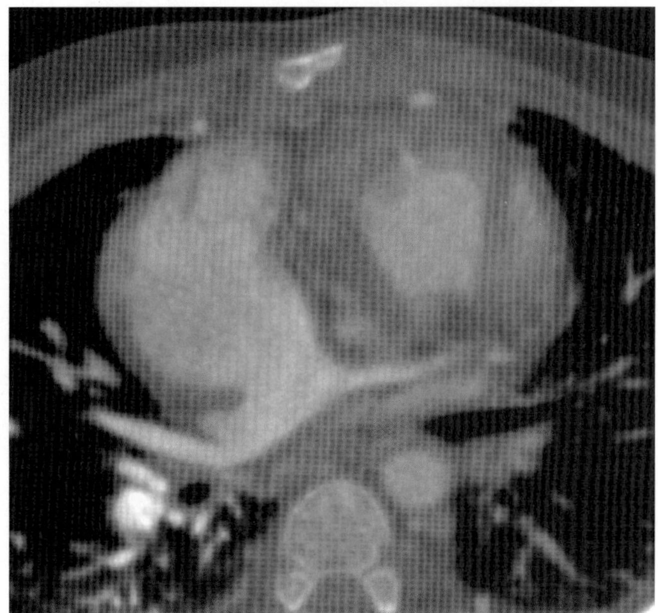
B

Clinical Presentation

A cyanotic 2-day-old male infant is severely distressed (in extremis) and has an abnormal echocardiogram.

Imaging Findings

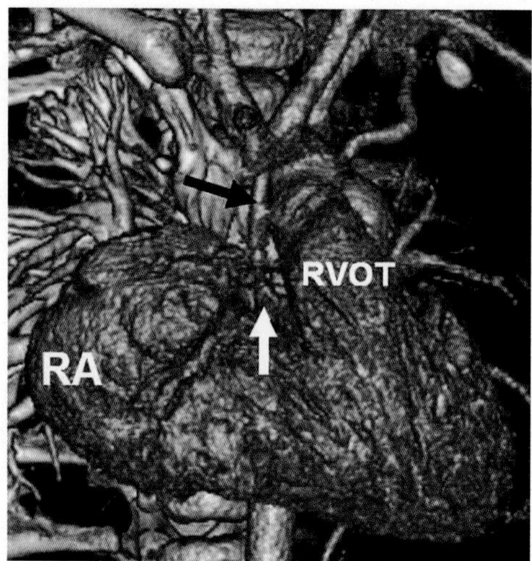

A

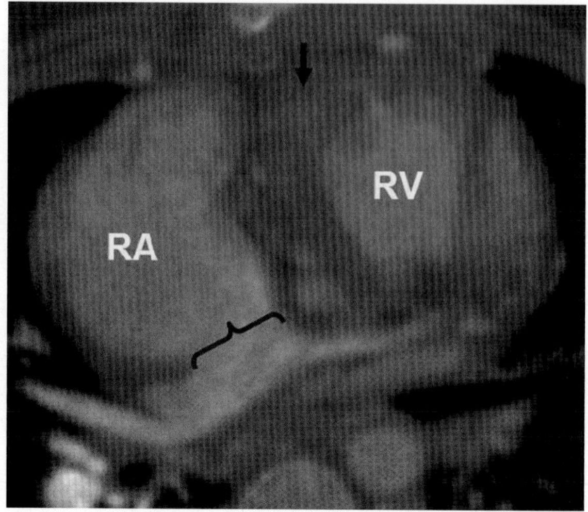

B

(A) A three-dimensional surface-rendered image of the heart shows the very tiny-caliber aortic valve (*white arrow*) and the ascending aorta (*black arrow*). The right ventricular outflow tract (RVOT) is of normal caliber, much larger than that of the ascending aorta. The right atrium (RA) is mildly enlarged, with a rounded border that can be a distinctive finding on chest radiographs. **(B)** An axial computed tomography image of the heart shows a large atrial septal defect (ASD: *bracket*). The pulmonary veins drain into the left atrium; the rounded border of the enlarged right atrium (RA) is again noted. The right ventricle (RV) is the only visualized ventricular chamber; it has a thickened, hypertrophied wall (*black arrow*).

Differential Diagnosis

All three may occur in newborns and can be associated with cyanosis.

- ***Hypoplastic left heart syndrome (HLHS):*** All of the left-sided cardiac structures (mitral valve, left ventricle [LV], aortic valve, and ascending aorta) are small. The caliber of the ascending aorta is only large enough to supply the coronary arteries.
- *Isolated hypoplasia of the aorta:* Diffuse narrowing of the aortic arch is the most common form.
- *Interrupted aortic arch:* The ascending aorta is very small but continuous; there is no interruption of the aorta.

Essential Facts

- Mitral valve stenosis limits flow of blood into the LV.
- The LV is small because of the lack of blood inflow, which normally stimulates growth of the chamber.
- The aortic valve and ascending aorta therefore do not receive blood flow; these structures are consequently very small.
- Origins of the coronary arteries are usually normal.
- In utero, retrograde flow of blood from the pulmonary arteries through the posterior descending artery (PDA) to the ascending aorta supplies the coronary arteries.
- Postnatal closure of the PDA can result in severe ischemia or myocardial infarction as blood flow to the coronary arteries is cut off. Therefore, myocardial perfusion in this congenital heart disease lesion is considered "ductal-dependent."
- An ASD must be present to allow decompression of pulmonary vein flow from the left atrium.
- When the ASD is restrictive, severe pulmonary venous hypertension is present.
- If the ASD is widely patent, the pulmonary vascular pattern is usually normal.

Other Imaging Findings

- The cardiac silhouette can be small or enlarged based on the size of the RA, which is more prominent when there is a restrictive ASD.
- When LV hypoplasia is severe, the apex of the heart is not formed by the LV, and the cardiac silhouette is abnormal.

✔ Pearls & ✘ Pitfalls

✔ Patients are dependent upon patency of the ductus arteriosus.
✔ Even mild pulmonary venous hypertension should be reported promptly to the cardiologist and neonatologist.
✔ In patients with aortic valve or aortic stenosis, with normal or only mildly reduced LV volume, a two-ventricle repair can be attempted.
✔ Fetal circulation allows normal in utero development.
✘ Postoperative imaging is most often directed to determining shunt patency. Kinking of the Blalock–Taussig shunt graft is a not uncommon complication.

Case 38

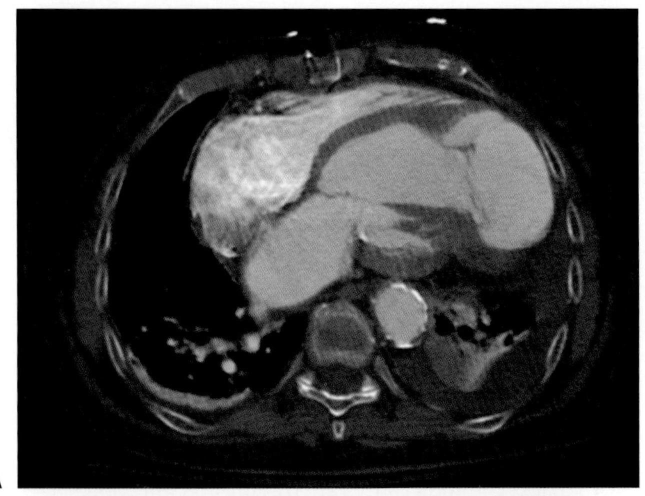
A

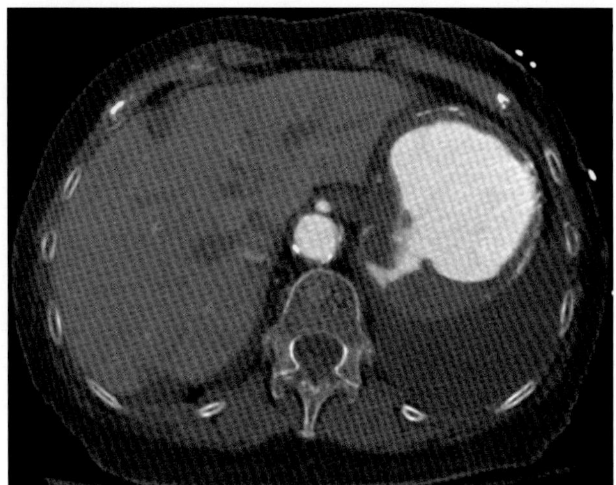
B

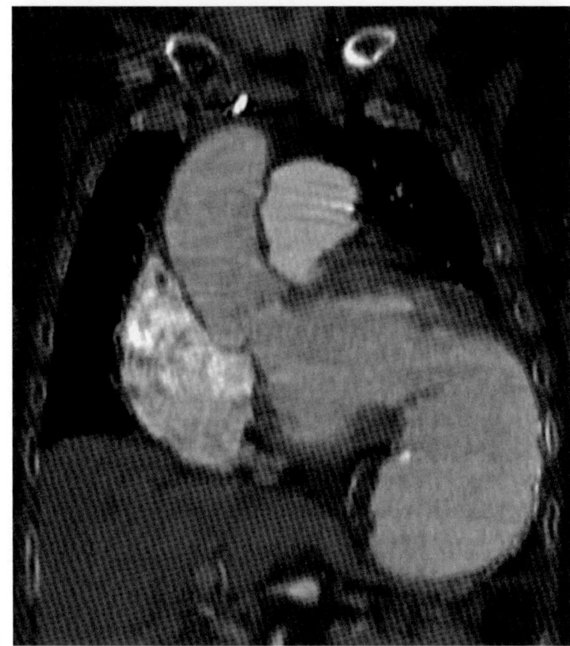
C

Clinical Presentation

Chest discomfort and dyspnea on exertion in an 86-year-old woman with a history of acute myocardial infarction

Imaging Findings

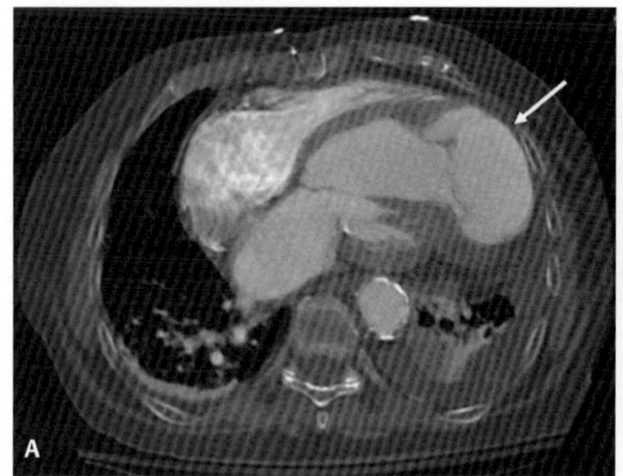

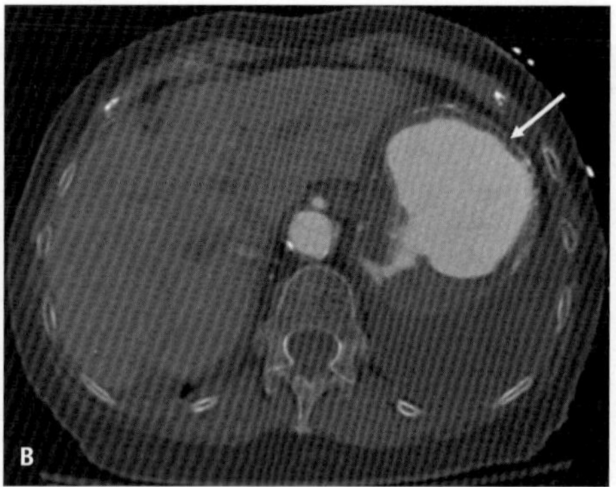

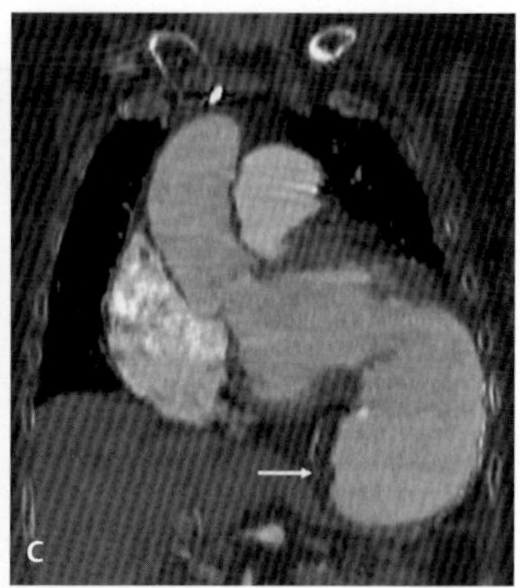

(A,B) Axial and **(C)** coronal re-formation computed tomography images reveal a large and partially calcified saccular structure at the left ventricular (LV) apex (*arrow*). This fills with contrast and communicates with the lumen of the LV through a relatively narrow mouth.

Differential Diagnosis

- ***False aneurysm of the left ventricle (FALV):*** LV pseudoaneurysms (or false aneurysms) form when cardiac rupture is contained by adherent pericardium or scar tissue. Pseudoaneurysms typically produce a bulge in the aortic contour, are discontinuous with the ventricular wall, and fill through an orifice or neck that is smaller than the aneurysmal sac.
- *True aneurysm of the LV:* A true LV aneurysm is contained by endocardium or myocardium. It represents a segment of the LV wall that protrudes beyond the expected outline of the ventricular wall. True aneuryms more often develop on the anterior wall of the LV, and they do not have a narrow neck between the dilated portion and the rest of the ventricle.
- *Dilated cardiomyopathy:* A dilated LV can also be seen in the presence of dilated cardiomyopathy. In such cases, there is global enlargement of the heart and relatively homogeneous myocardial thickness.

Essential Facts

- FALV is an uncommon complication of acute myocardial infarction, seen in 0.1% of cases.
- FALVs have a high tendency to rupture (45%).
- The most common location of FALVs is on the posterior and diaphragmatic wall of the LV.
- FALVs are commonly related to right coronary artery obstruction and inferior wall myocardial infarction.
- The cavity of the false aneurysm is frequently bigger than the ventricle.
- Wall stress that depends on LV pressure and radius and loss of myocardial integrity from prior myocardial infarction are the most important determinants of cardiac rupture.
- After myocardial infarction, complication from a surgical procedure, in particular mitral valve replacement, is the second most common cause.
- Other, less common causes are trauma and infection.
- Posterior pseudoaneurysms are twice as common as anterior pseudoaneurysms.
- Patients without surgery have a high mortality rate (10–50%) in the weeks after diagnosis.
- Among those surviving without surgery, the cumulative incidence of ischemic stroke is high (~10% per year) and results from the stagnant blood flow that leads to thrombosis.

Other Imaging Findings

- Transthoracic echocardiography is the most-studied imaging modality with respect to the differentiation between a true and a false aneurysm of the LV. The mean ratio of the ventricular wall orifice to the cavity diameter is < 0.5 for false aneurysms and close to 1.0 for true aneurysms.

✔ Pearls & ✘ Pitfalls

✔ Postoperative mortality rates after surgical repair of FALV are also high and range from 13 to 29%.

✘ LV diverticula are rare congenital anomalies consisting of localized protrusion of myocardium and endocardium and cardiac chamber lumen arising from the free wall of the LV. They may be similar in appearance to small FALVs.

Case 39

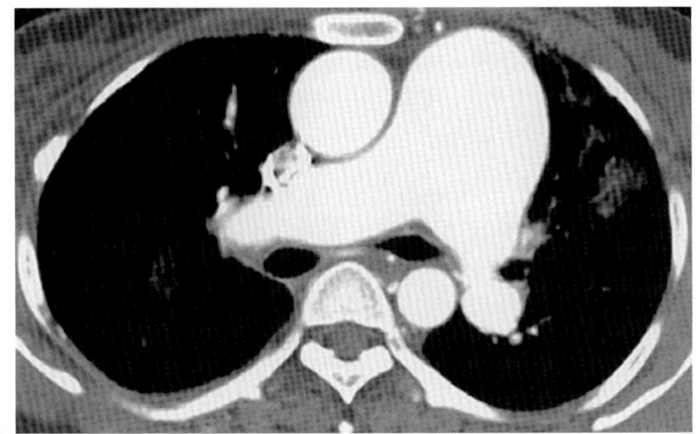

A

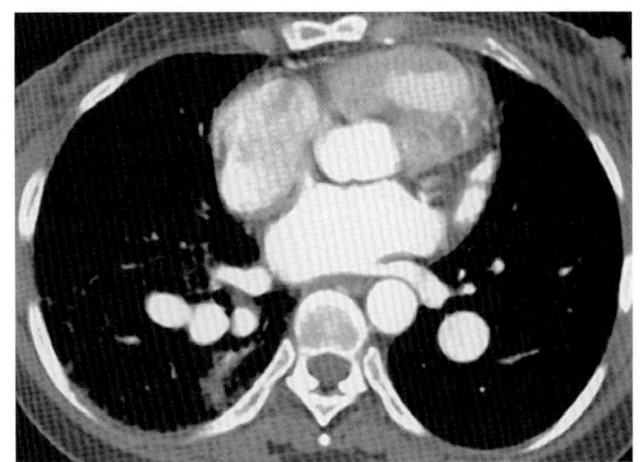

B

Clinical Presentation

Progressive exertional dyspnea and lower extremity edema in a 39-year-old woman

Imaging Findings

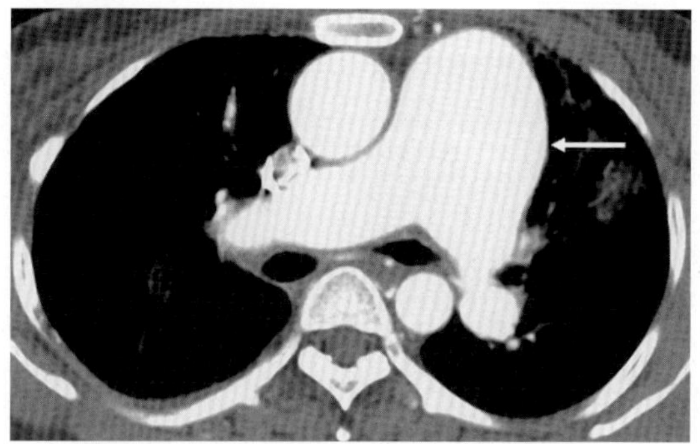

A

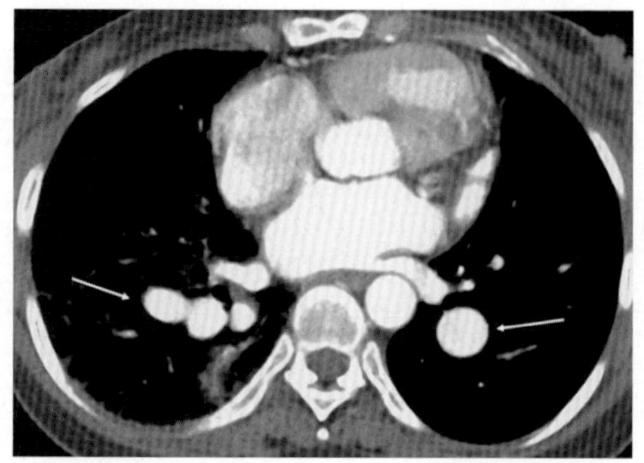

B

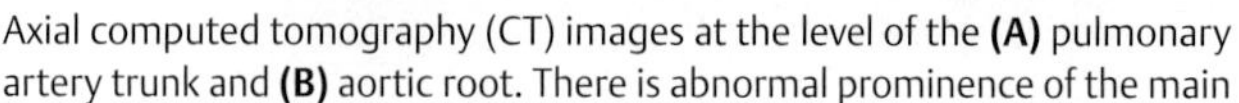

Axial computed tomography (CT) images at the level of the **(A)** pulmonary artery trunk and **(B)** aortic root. There is abnormal prominence of the main trunk, specifically the central and peripheral pulmonary arteries, consistent with pulmonary arterial hypertension (PAH).

Differential Diagnosis

- ***Pulmonary arterial hypertension:*** Abnormal prominence of the pulmonary arteries is consistent with precapillary (arterial) pulmonary hypertension.
- *Pulmonary artery aneurysm:* An aneurysm is usually defined as a focal dilatation of an artery involving all three layers of the vessel wall, exceeding 1.5 times the normal caliber of the vessel. Different conditions have been associated with aneurysm of the pulmonary arteries, including pulmonary valvular stenosis, PAH, vasculitis, infection, Marfan syndrome, and trauma.

Essential Facts

- PAH is defined as the presence of mean pulmonary arterial pressure > 25 mm Hg and pulmonary capillary wedge pressure (or left ventricular end-diastolic pressure) < 15 mm Hg.
- PAH is a progressive condition that finally leads to right ventricular failure. A common clinical presentation includes exertional dyspnea that is usually progressive over a long period of time, chest pain, syncope, and signs of right heart failure (lower extremity edema, hepatomegaly, and ascites).
- The mean age at diagnosis is 40 years (range, 36–50 years).
- Characteristic pathologic abnormalities in the small-caliber pulmonary arteries progress from intimal, medial, and adventitial proliferation to plexogenic changes characterized by endothelial proliferation, myofibroblast accumulation, and necrotizing arteritis.
- Characteristic findings in PAH on chest radiographs, CT, or magnetic resonance imaging (MRI) include abnormal dilatation of the central pulmonary arteries with tapering of the vessels as they run along the periphery.
- On conventional radiography, PAH is diagnosed when the transverse diameter of the right interlobar pulmonary artery is > 15 mm in women or > 16 mm in men.
- On CT and MRI, the upper limit of normal of the main pulmonary artery is 29 mm. Dimensions above this value are highly suggestive of PAH (sensitivity, 87%; specificity, 89%; positive predictive value, 97%).
- Calcifications of the pulmonary arterial wall are uncommon, and when present they are usually associated with chronic, severe PAH.

Other Imaging Findings

- On CT, a segmental artery-to-bronchus ratio > 1:1 in three of four lobes has 100% specificity for the diagnosis of PAH.

✔ Pearls & ✘ Pitfalls

✔ The different forms of PAH can be categorized in five groups:
- Group 1: idiopathic, familial PAH associated with such conditions as collagen vascular disease, systemic-to-pulmonic shunts, and pulmonary veno-occlusive disease
- Group 2: PAH associated with left heart disease
- Group 3: PAH associated with lung disease and/or hypoxemia
- Group 4: PAH due to chronic thrombotic or embolic disease
- Group 5: PAH due to miscellaneous conditions (tumor, fibrosing mediastinitis, etc.)

✘ Pulmonary artery systolic pressure can be estimated noninvasively by Doppler ultrasound, but the standard error of the estimate is large (5–8 mm Hg).

Case 40

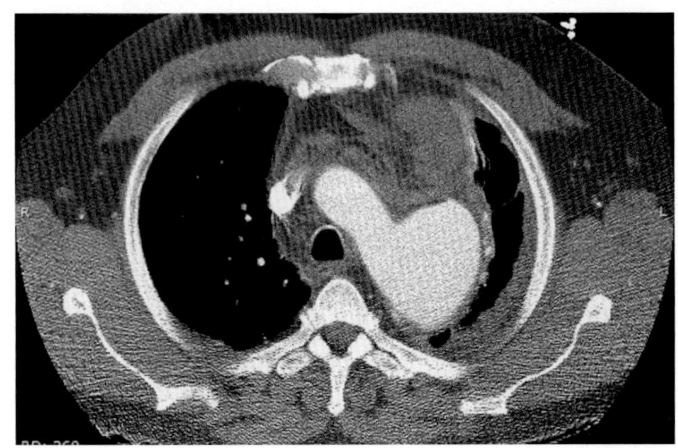

A

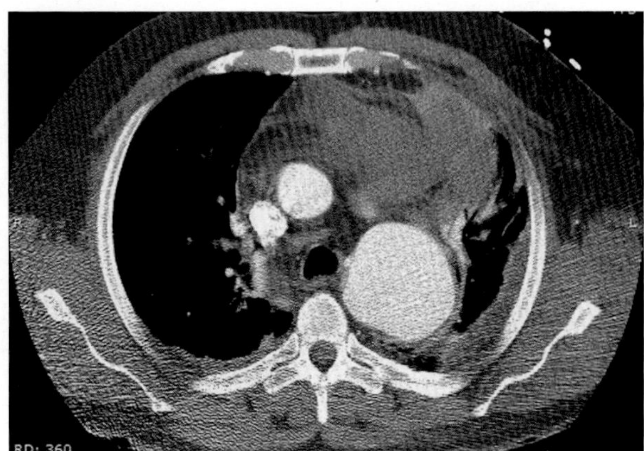

B

Clinical Presentation

A 47-year-old man presents with acute chest pain and syncope.

Imaging Findings

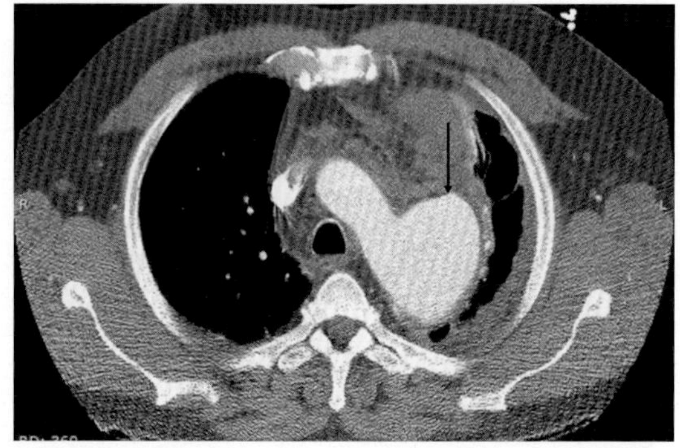
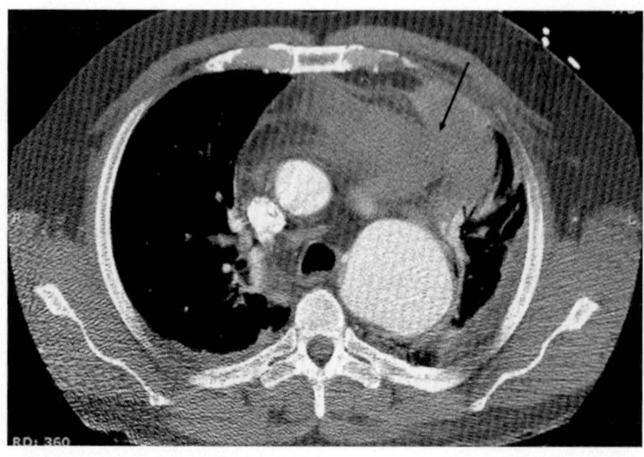
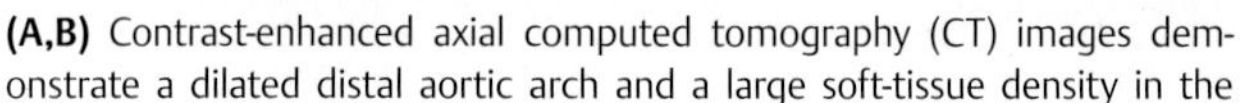

(A,B) Contrast-enhanced axial computed tomography (CT) images demonstrate a dilated distal aortic arch and a large soft-tissue density in the mediastinum adjacent to the dilated aorta with stranding of the mediastinal fat, consistent with a hematoma and associated left-sided pleural effusion.

Differential Diagnosis

- ***Ruptured thoracic aortic aneurysm:*** Contrast-enhanced multidetector CT shows an aneurysm of the distal aortic arch with extensive bleeding, hematoma formation in the mediastinum, and pleural effusion.
- *Unruptured aortic aneurysm with an associated mediastinal tumor:* The association of a mediastinal soft-tissue density and an aortic aneurysm raises the question of a tumor. The irregular density and stranding of the mediastinal mass with associated pleural effusion in this case are typical of hematoma, not of an associated tumor.

Essential Facts

- Thoracic aortic aneurysms have a high incidence of rupture (47%).
- The rupture of aortic aneurysms has a very high rate of mortality (77–95%).
- The risk for rupture increases with the size of the aneurysm.
- The average size of ruptured thoracic aneurysms is 6 cm.
- Thoracic aortic aneurysms' growth rate (0.42 cm/yr) is higher than the growth rate of abdominal aortic aneurysms (0.25 cm/yr). Aneurysms of the aortic arch have the fastest expansion rate.
- Surgical intervention is considered when the aneurysm size exceeds 5.5 cm for the ascending aorta and 6.5 cm for the descending aorta.
- Aneurysms of the ascending aorta or aortic arch may rupture into the mediastinum or pericardium, whereas aneurysms of the descending aorta may rupture into the left pleural space.
- Aortic aneurysms associated with pain are more likely to rupture. Expansion of an aortic aneurysm causes pain.

Other Imaging Findings

- Imaging findings of rupture of a thoracic aortic aneurysm include high-attenuation fluid in the mediastinum, pleural space, or pericardium and mediastinal fat stranding.

✔ Pearls & ✘ Pitfalls

✔ Laplace's law ($T = P \cdot r$) states that the wall tension (T) in an aortic aneurysm is equal to the transmural pressure (P) multiplied by the radius (r). If the radius increases for a constant pressure, wall tension increases proportionally. This creates a vicious cycle of increased tension, further dilation, and more tension.

✘ A small, contained aortic leak may be difficult to diagnose. Close application of the aneurysm to the spine and lateral draping of the aneurysm around a vertebral body suggest a weak and deficient aortic wall.

Case 41

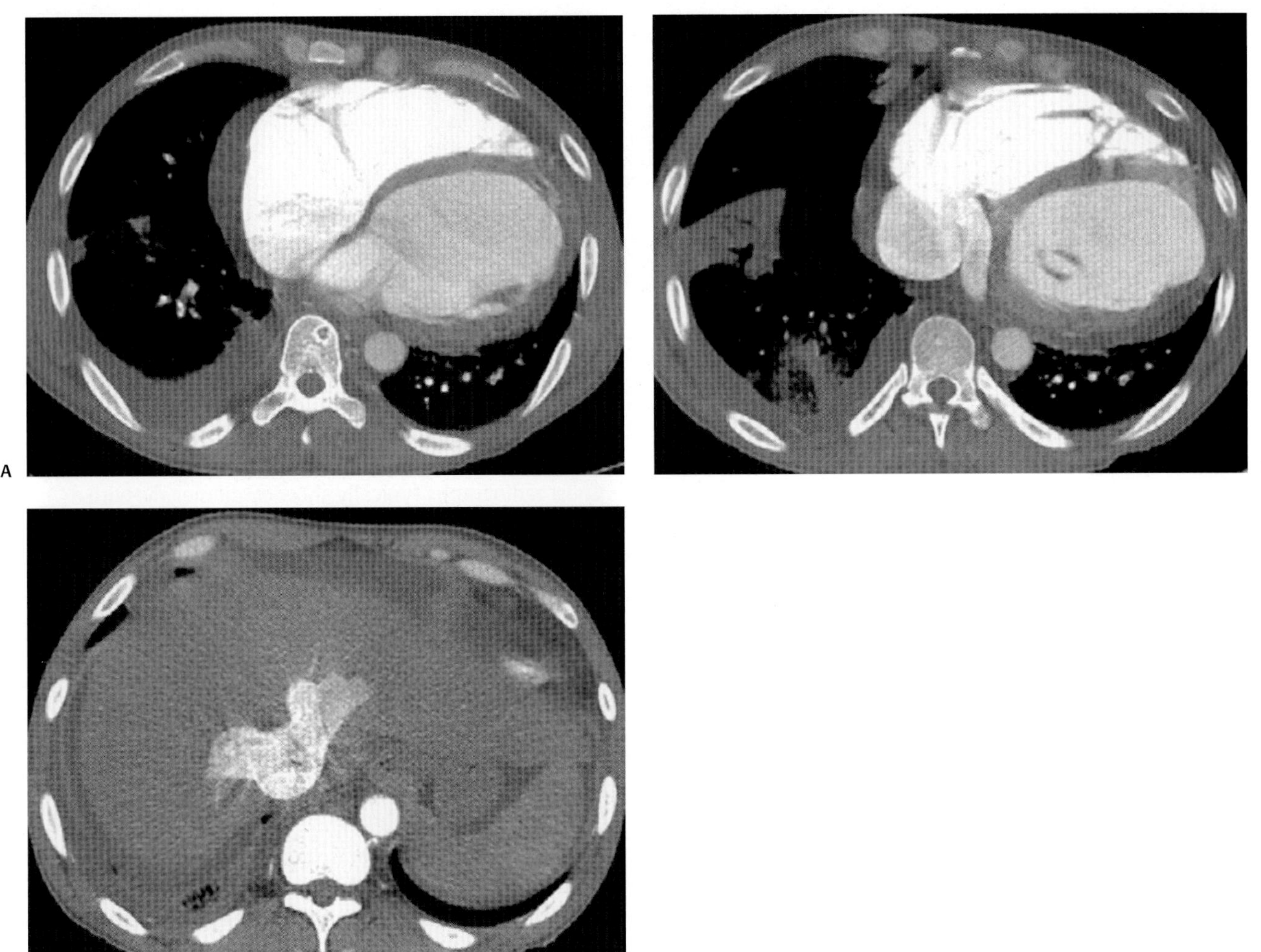

Clinical Presentation

A 45-year-old man with a past medical history of acquired immunodeficiency syndrome (AIDS) presents with dyspnea on exertion and orthopnea.

Imaging Findings

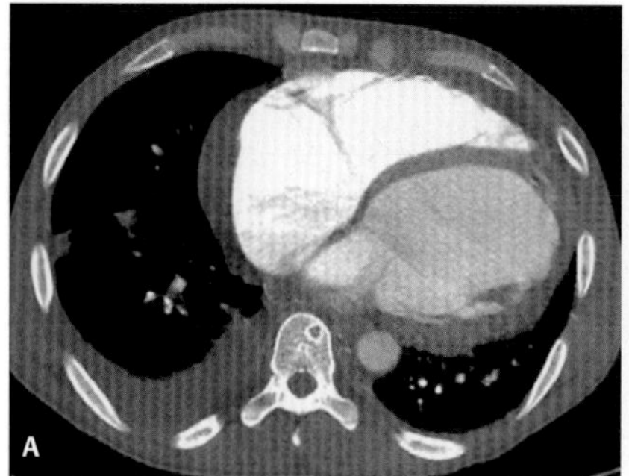

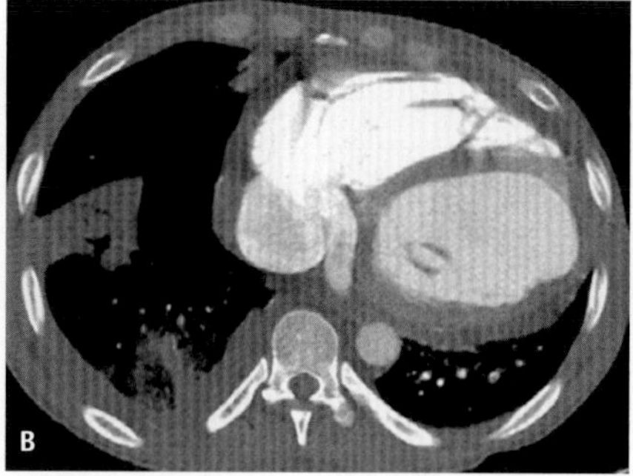

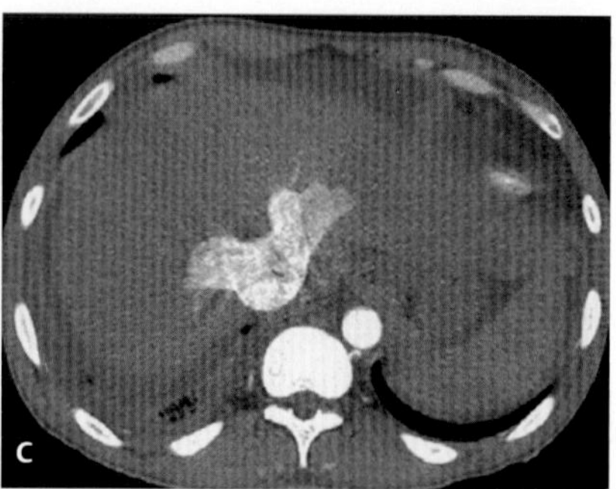

(A–C) Contrast-enhanced computed tomography (CT) images show an abnormally dilated heart with biventricular enlargement, dilated inferior vena cava and coronary sinus, and reflux of contrast from the right atrium into the hepatic veins. A moderate amount of right-sided pleural fluid is also noted.

Differential Diagnosis

- ***Dilated cardiomyopathy (DCM):*** DCM is characterized by ventricular and sometimes atrial dilatation, with impaired systolic contraction of one or both ventricles (left ventricular ejection fraction < 40%). Ventricular wall thickness is usually normal or slightly reduced, and a variable degree of congestive vascular changes may be appreciated.
- *Restrictive cardiomyopathy:* Restrictive cardiomyopathy is characterized by a normal-size heart and normal thickness of the pericardium. The myocardial wall may be normal or exhibit symmetric thickening, which may produce normal or slightly reduced ventricular volume.

Essential Facts

- DCM is common, with a prevalence of 1 in 2500. It is the third most common cause of heart failure and is responsible for more than 10,000 deaths each year in the United States.
- The traditional classification of cardiomyopathies divides them in three groups: dilated, hypertrophic, and restrictive.
- DCM also can be divided into two broad categories: primary (or familial) and secondary (e.g., ischemic, hypertensive, and viral).
- Fifty percent of cases of DCM are idiopathic. Causes of secondary DCM include infection, ischemic heart disease, infiltrative diseases, peripartum cardiomyopathy, human immunodeficiency virus (HIV) infection, and substance abuse.
- About 25% of cases of idiopathic DCM have been found to be familial, with a complex and heterogeneous pattern of inheritance, but mainly autosomal-dominant.
- Ventricular enlargement and systolic dysfunction lead to progressive heart failure, arrhythmias, thromboembolism, and sudden death.
- Most affected patients are between 20 and 60 years old.

Other Imaging Findings

- Chest radiographs typically show cardiomegaly, with a variable degree of vascular congestion. Depending on the degree of congestive heart failure, pleural effusion may also be present.
- Echocardiography is an important element in the evaluation of DCM. It helps in delineating the anatomy and function of the heart and is excellent in the evaluation of cardiac valves, which may be affected.

✔ Pearls & ✘ Pitfalls

✔ The distinction between ischemic and nonischemic DCM is important, with prognostic and patient management implications. Multidetector CT angiography is an accurate imaging modality for the differentiation between these two categories.

✘ Clinical differentiation among dilated cardiomyopathy, restrictive cardiomyopathy, and constrictive pericarditis is difficult.

Case 42

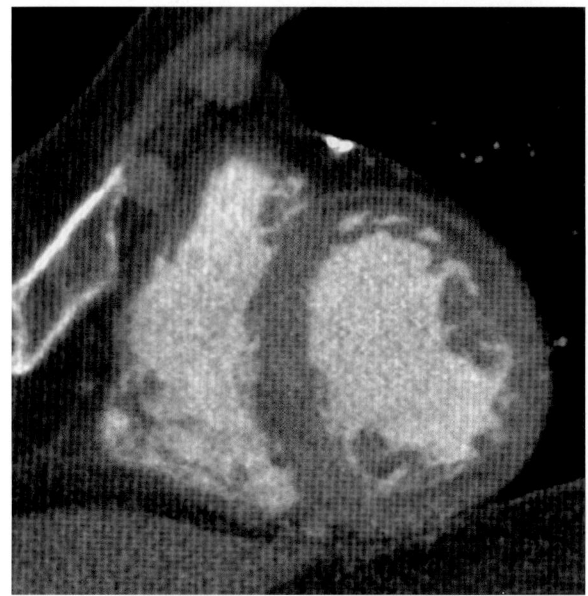

A

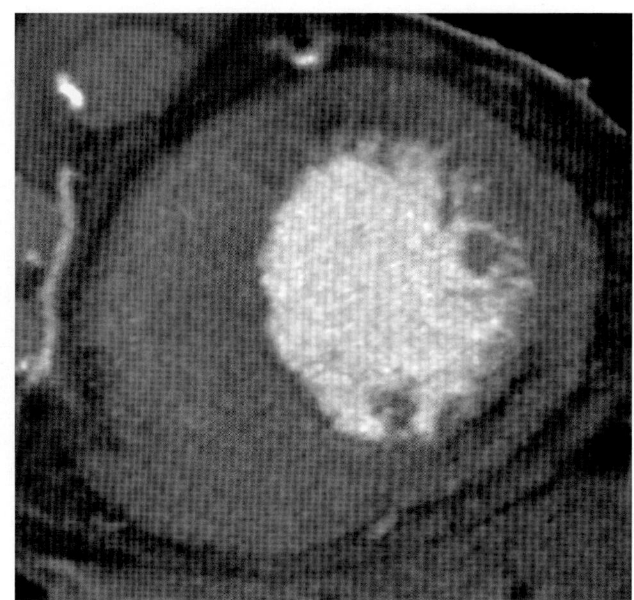

B

Clinical Presentation

Two patients are shown, each with a history of myocardial infarction.

Imaging Findings

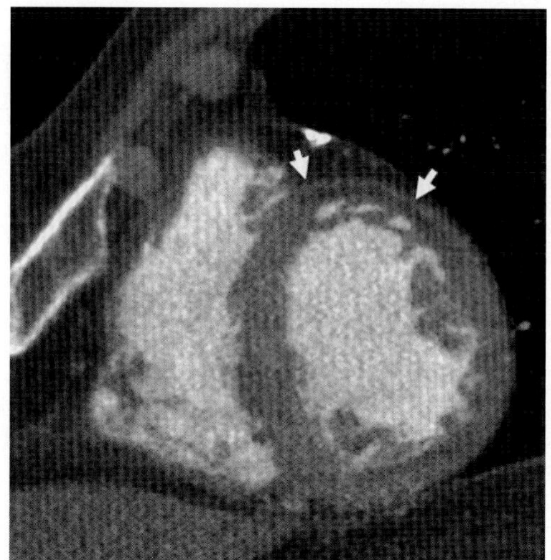
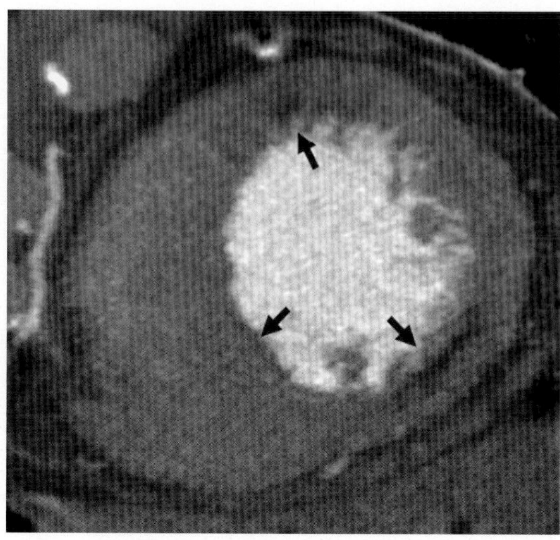

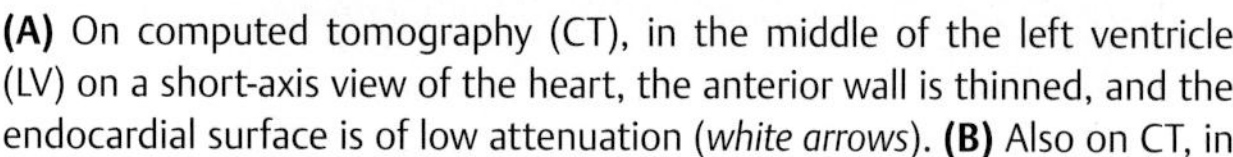
(A) On computed tomography (CT), in the middle of the left ventricle (LV) on a short-axis view of the heart, the anterior wall is thinned, and the endocardial surface is of low attenuation (*white arrows*). **(B)** Also on CT, in the second patient, the short-axis image shows several foci of low attenuation in the endocardium of the LV (*black arrows*). The myocardium is not thinned.

Differential Diagnosis

- ***Chronic infarct of the anterior wall of the LV and acute infarct versus ischemia:*** In the first patient, the anterior wall of the myocardium is thinned and is low attenuation, findings of remote infarction. In the second patient, the myocardial attenuation abnormality is limited to the endocardial surface, and the LV myocardium is normal thickness. These findings could represent a perfusion defect that could be due to ischemia or infarction. Because there is no wall thinning, the findings are likely acute.
- *Hypertrophic cardiomyopathy:* The myocardium is not thickened. The LV chamber is usually small in hypertrophic cardiomyopathy.
- *Ischemic cardiomyopathy:* Dilatation of the LV chamber can be seen in patients with ischemic cardiomyopathy, but myocardial signal/attenuation should remain normal on nonenhanced images.

Essential Facts

- The anterior and anterolateral myocardium of the LV is supplied by the left anterior descending (LAD) artery, by a diagonal branch of the LV, or in some people by an intermediate branch (ramus anteromedius) from the left main coronary artery.
- The lateral and inferolateral LV myocardium is supplied by the left circumflex (LCX) coronary artery.
- The inferior and inferoseptal LV myocardium is supplied by the right coronary artery (RCA).
- Normal myocardium has a homogeneous attenuation and uniform thickness on CT.
- Perfusion defects may affect the endocardial surface or extend into the middle myocardium.

Other Imaging Findings

- The first patient has also undergone coronary artery bypass with his left internal mammary artery grafted to the LAD artery. Metal surgical clips are the cause of very high attenuation just cephalad to the anterior wall scar.
- In the second patient, multifocal abnormalities indicate the likelihood of multivessel coronary artery disease.
- In the more commonly seen right-sided coronary artery dominance, all three coronary arteries would be diseased.
- If this patient has left-sided dominance of the coronary artery tree, the findings could be due to two-vessel disease.

✔ Pearls & ✘ Pitfalls

✔ Examine the coronary arteries to diagnose "cutoff" or occlusion of a vessel.

✔ Look for collateralization of coronary artery branches from other epicardial coronary arteries or from transmyocardial collaterals.

✔ The LV myocardium should be examined in short-axis, vertical, and horizontal long-axis cardiac imaging planes to detect wall thinning, myocardial attenuation abnormalities, and wall motion abnormalities.

✘ The standard axial plane will not allow one to examine coronary artery vascular territories accurately.

Case 43

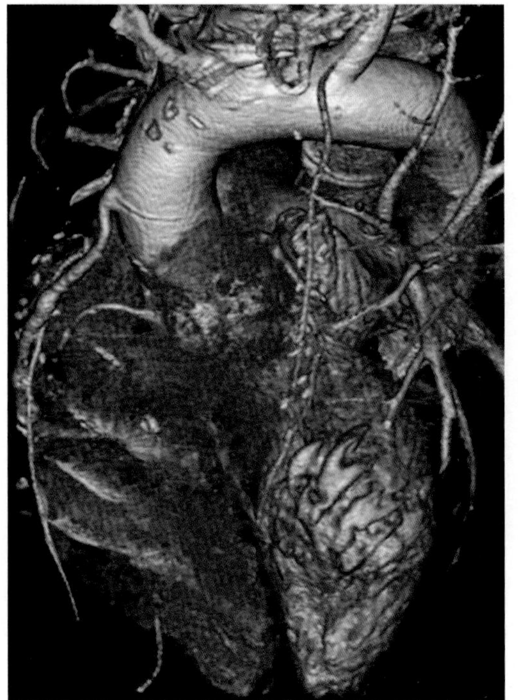

A

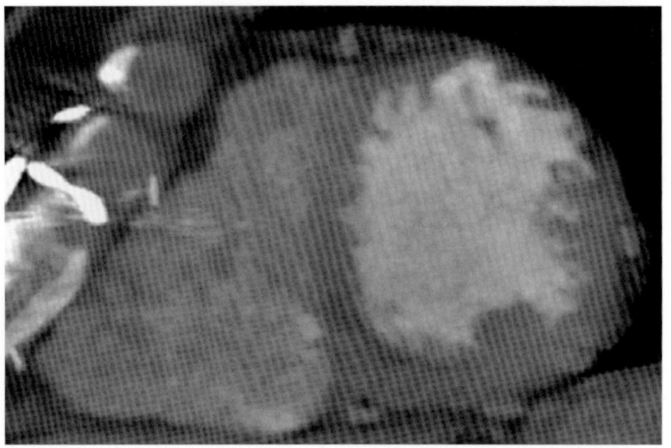

B

Clinical Presentation

A 93-year-old man with a history of myocardial infarction and left internal mammary artery (LIMA) coronary artery bypass graft (CABG)

Imaging Findings

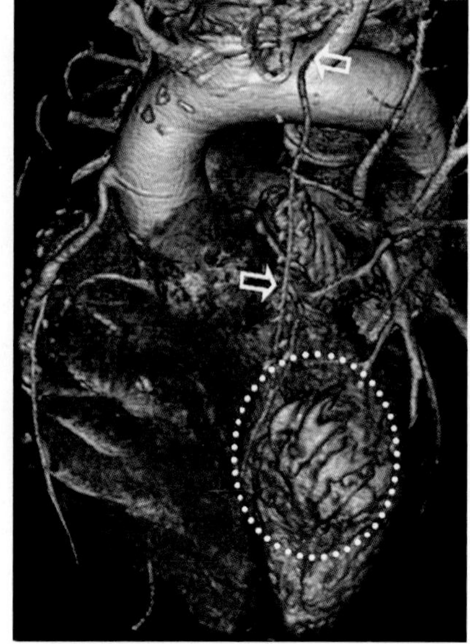

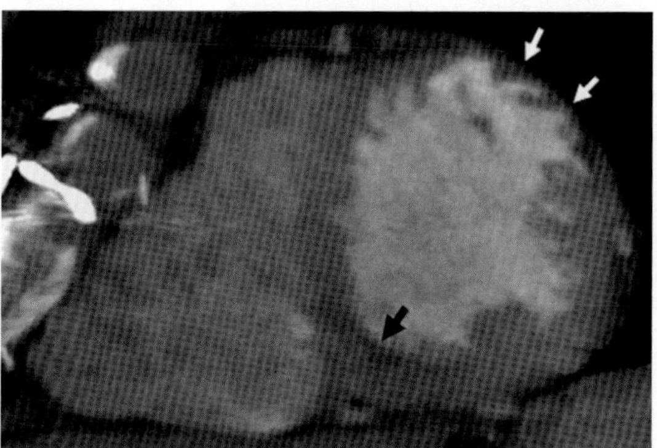

(A) Three-dimensional surface-rendered image of the heart shows focal abnormality of the endocardial surface of the anterolateral wall of the left ventricle (LV: *dotted white ellipse*). An LIMA bypass graft courses from its origin on the left subclavian artery toward the left anterior descending (LAD) artery (*open arrows*). Numerous surgical clips lie on either side of the LIMA.

(B) In a short-axis view, focal anterolateral wall thinning is marked (*white arrows*) at the site of an old infarction. Low attenuation of the endocardial surface of the inferolateral wall (*black arrow*) also represents an infarct, although there is no wall thinning.

Differential Diagnosis

- ***Chronic anterolateral LV wall infarction and LIMA CABG:*** The focal smoothing of the endocardial surface of the LV chamber and wall thinning are secondary to prior infarction. The CABG from the LIMA to the LAD artery is patent.
- *Hypertrophic cardiomyopathy:* The myocardium is not thickened; it is thinned. The LV chamber size is normal.
- *Ischemic cardiomyopathy:* There is likely no ischemia in other portions of the LV, given the normal chamber size.

Essential Facts

- Electrocardiography (ECG)-gated multidetector computed tomography (CT) has very high sensitivity and specificity for detecting coronary artery stenosis.
- ECG-gated multidetector CT is also a highly effective, noninvasive method for detecting patency or occlusion of arterial and venous CABGs.
- The anterolateral wall of the LV is supplied by the LAD artery, by a diagonal branch of the LV, or in some people by an intermediate branch (ramus intermedius) from the left main coronary artery.
- Normal myocardium has a homogeneous attenuation and uniform thickness on CT.

Other Imaging Findings

- Calcified and noncalcified atherosclerotic disease can be easily distinguished on multidetector CT.
- Areas of infarcted myocardium show thinning and typically low attenuation, which may represent fat or fibrous tissue replacing or infiltrating the myocardium.
- Wall motion abnormalities may be clearly shown when ECG-gated multidetector CT is performed retrospectively.

✔ Pearls & ✘ Pitfalls

✔ Examine the coronary arteries to diagnose "cutoff" or occlusion of a vessel.

✔ Look for collateralization of coronary artery branches from other epicardial coronary arteries or from transmyocardial collaterals.

✔ The LV myocardium should be examined in short-axis, vertical, and horizontal long-axis cardiac imaging planes to detect wall thinning, myocardial attenuation abnormalities, and wall motion abnormalities.

✘ The standard axial plane will not allow one to examine the coronary artery vascular territories accurately.

Case 44

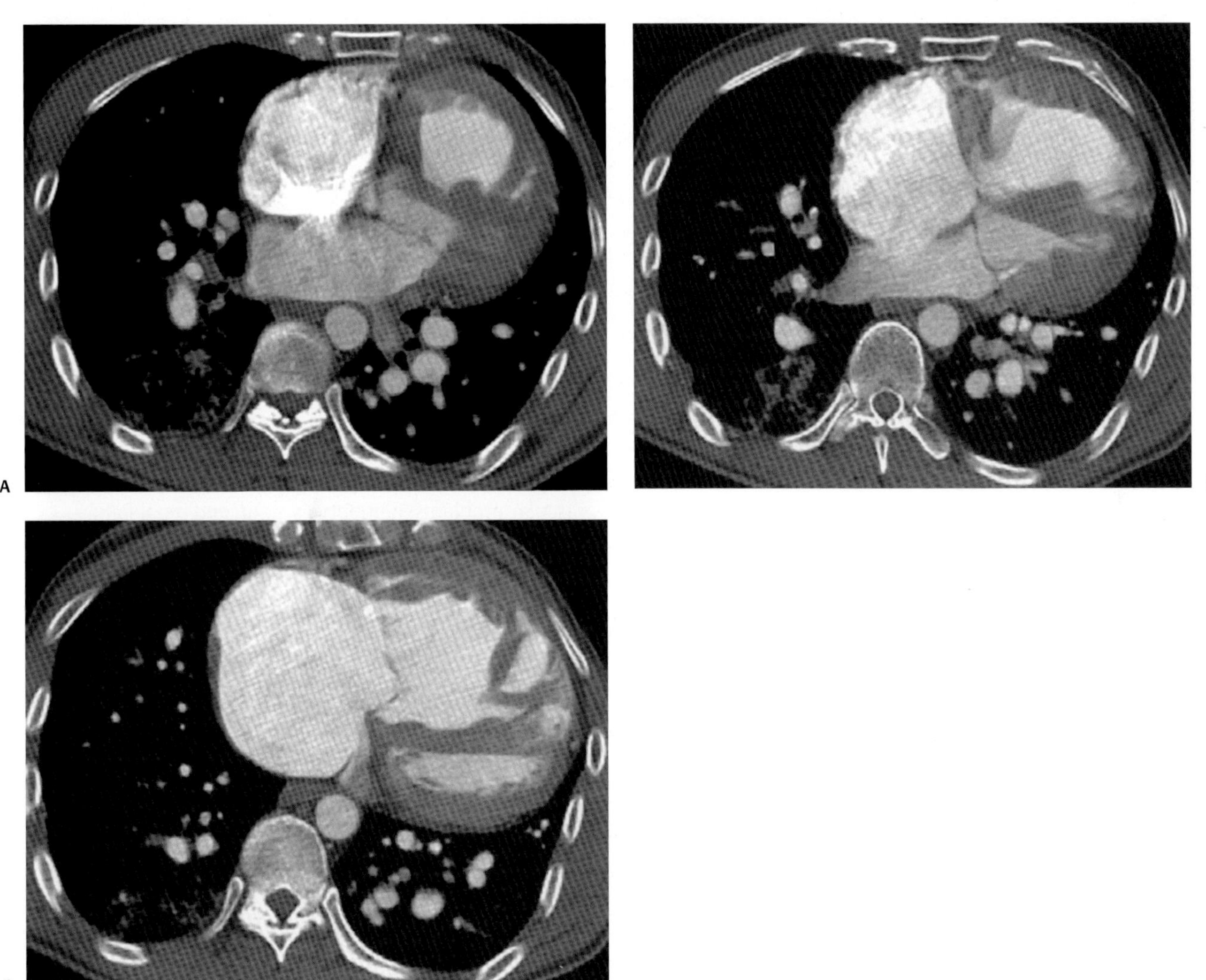

Clinical Presentation

Shortness of breath and cyanosis in a 32-year-old man

Imaging Findings

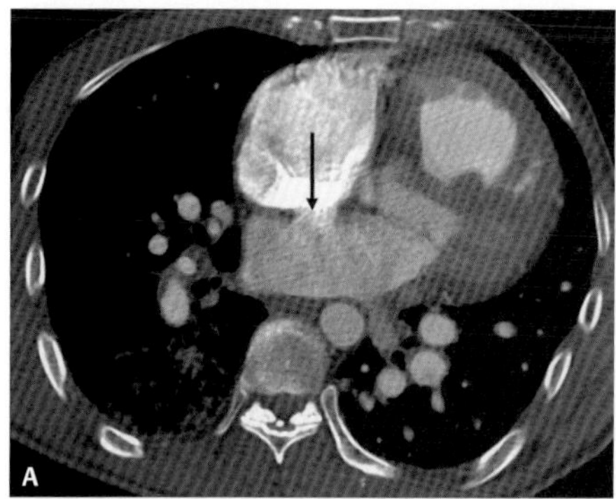
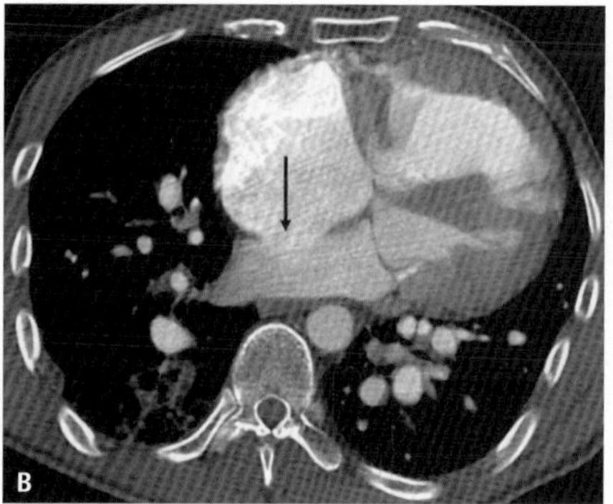
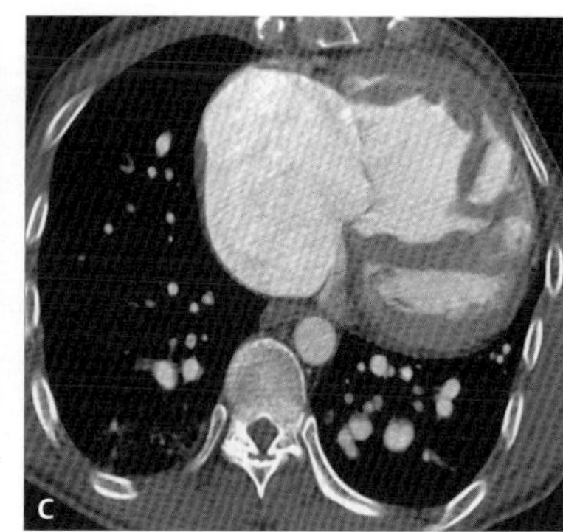

(A–C) Contrast-enhanced computed tomography images show a large defect of the central portion of the interatrial septum, right atrial and ventricular enlargement with significant hypertrophy of the right ventricle, and prominent pulmonary vasculature consistent with increased pulmonary flow.

Differential Diagnosis

- ***Eisenmenger syndrome secondary to a large atrial septal defect (ASD):*** The presence of a large left-to-right shunt that causes severe pulmonary vascular disease and pulmonary hypertension with resulting reversal of the direction of the shunting constitutes Eisenmenger syndrome.
- *Idiopathic pulmonary hypertension:* The changes in the pulmonary vasculature observed in idiopathic pulmonary hypertension, as well as the hypertrophic changes on the right ventricle, can be similar to those found in intracardiac shunts. The integrity of the interatrial and interventricular septa, as well as the absence of abnormal communication between the great vessels, helps in making the diagnosis.

Essential Facts

- Depending on the size and location of the intracardiac shunt, ~8% of patients with congenital heart disease and 11% of those with left-to-right (systemic-to-pulmonary) intracardiac shunt develop Eisenmenger syndrome.
- Congenital heart disease problems more commonly associated with Eisenmenger syndrome include ventricular septal defect, ASD, atrioventricular defect, patent ductus arteriosus, and dextro-transposition of the great arteries.
- The chronic left-to-right shunting exposes the pulmonary vasculature to increased blood flow and increased pressure.
- The pulmonary vasculature develops medial hypertrophy of the arteries, intimal proliferation and fibrosis, and occlusion of the capillaries.
- Later, in the irreversible stage, plexiform lesions of the arterial wall and necrotizing arteritis develop.
- This creates an increased pulmonary vascular resistance secondary to obliteration of much of the pulmonary vascular bed, and when it exceeds the systemic resistance, the systemic-to-pulmonary shunt is reversed to a pulmonary-to-systemic shunt. Cyanosis is then clinically manifest.
- Complications include thromboembolic events, cerebrovascular problems, hemoptysis, gout, and renal failure.
- The long-term prognosis is better than in other forms of pulmonary hypertension: 80% of affected patients are alive at 10 years after diagnosis, regardless of the location of the defect.

Other Imaging Findings

- Additional imaging features of Eisenmenger syndrome are abnormally enlarged pulmonary arteries consistent with arterial (precapillary) pulmonary hypertension, severe hypertrophy of the right ventricle, and enlarged right atrium.

✔ Pearls & ✘ Pitfalls

✔ Patients with long-standing left-to-right shunting who develop Eisenmenger syndrome are highly symptomatic, with multiorgan system compromise manifested by cyanosis, bleeding, thrombotic diathesis, ischemia, increased risk for bacterial endocarditis, cerebral abscess, and heart failure.

✘ There is confusion in the literature between Eisenmenger syndrome and Eisenmenger complex. The association of ventricular septal defect with dextro-transposition of the aorta without any pulmonary stenosis or hypoplasia, as was originally described by Dr. Victor Eisenmenger, constitutes the Eisenmenger complex. The broader concept of a larger intracardiac left-to-right shunt, with secondary pulmonary hypertension, has come to be known as Eisenmenger syndrome.

Case 45

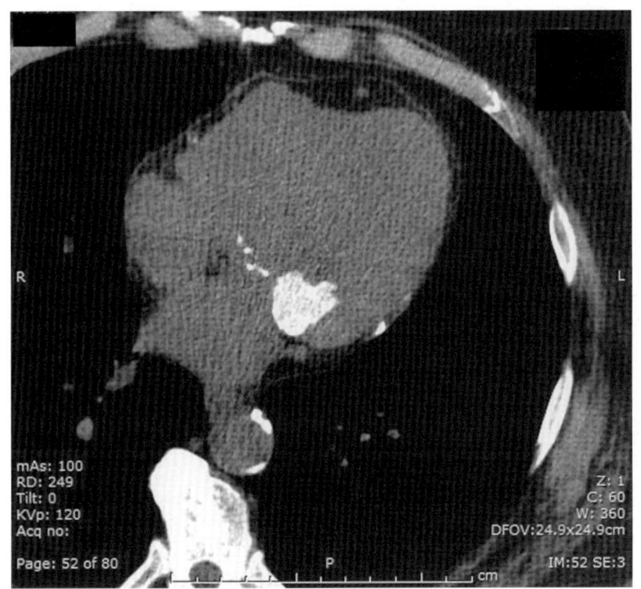

A

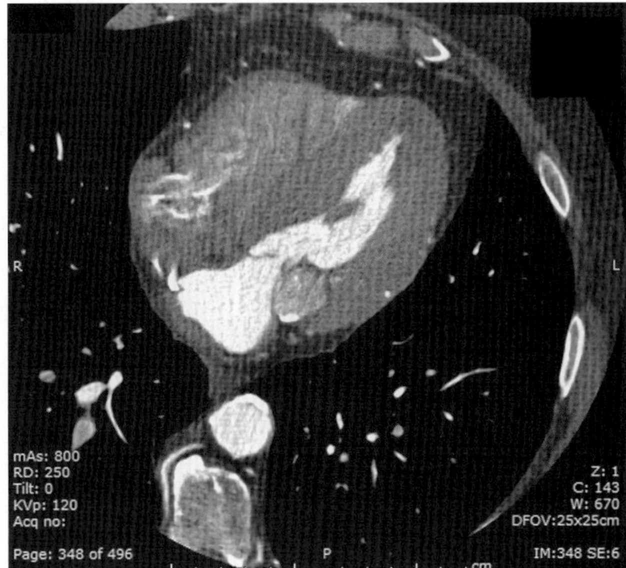

B

Clinical Presentation

A 75-year-old man presents with an “abnormal cardiac mass” on an echocardiogram.

Imaging Findings

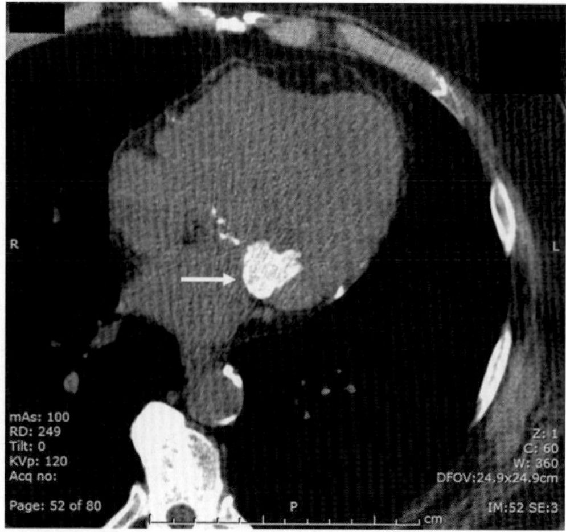

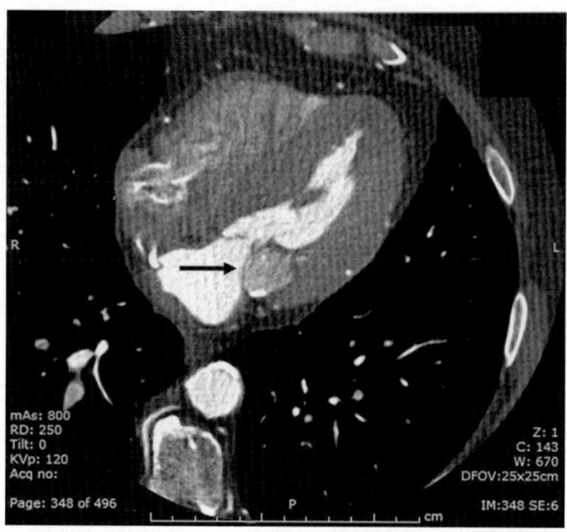

Cardiac-gated computed tomography (CT) angiography: **(A)** non-contrast- and **(B)** contrast-enhanced axial images. An irregular nonenhancing masslike calcification is visualized on the posterolateral aspect of the mitral valve annulus, producing a mild degree of distortion and mass effect on the mitral valve.

Differential Diagnosis

- ***Caseous calcification of the mitral annulus:*** Caseous calcification of the mitral annulus is characterized by large, round, tumorlike, broad-based calcification, usually on the posterior mitral annulus.
- *Mitral annulus granuloma/abscess:* Chronic infectious or inflammatory processes in the heart can also present with a diffuse or irregular pattern of calcification.
- *Myxoma:* Cardiac myxomas can present with variable degrees of calcification. They are usually more pedunculated and attached to the interatrial septum, close to the fossa ovalis.

Essential Facts

- Caseous calcification of the mitral annulus is rare.
- The reported prevalence is ~0.07% in patients undergoing echocardiography and 2.7% in a necropsy series.
- The mean age of affected patients is 65 years.
- Women are affected three times more often than men.
- In the majority of cases, this is an incidental finding with no clinical significance, but association with mitral stenosis and regurgitation has been reported.
- On echocardiography, it appears as a round or oval, tumorlike calcification of the posterior mitral annulus, with a central area of echolucency resembling liquefaction.
- Calcification may be denser in the periphery.
- Histologic analysis of this calcific content reveals an acellular basophilic substance free of germs and neoplastic or inflammatory elements that resembles toothpaste.
- This most likely represents a variant of degenerative mitral annular calcification, which is typically seen in elderly individuals.

Other Imaging Findings

- The lesion is usually broad-based, seems homogeneous on noncontrast CT, and is nonenhancing after contrast injection.

✔ Pearls & ✘ Pitfalls

✔ In patients being considered for surgical repair of the mitral valve, the diagnosis of caseous calcification of the mitral annulus is an important finding, as the bland, toothpaste-like density of this area may predispose to a higher rate of postoperative complications.

✘ Detection of cardiac calcifications on magnetic resonance imaging is unreliable, given the limitation inherent to this technology for the detection of calcium. When the lesion is large enough, a low-signal-intensity mass may be evident in cases of caseous calcification of the mitral annulus.

Case 46

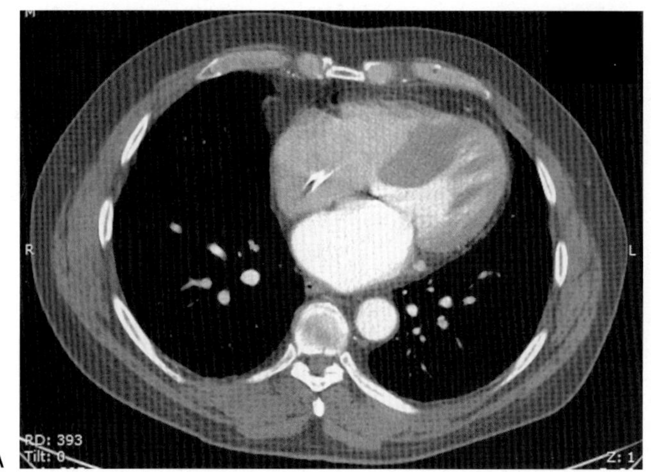

A

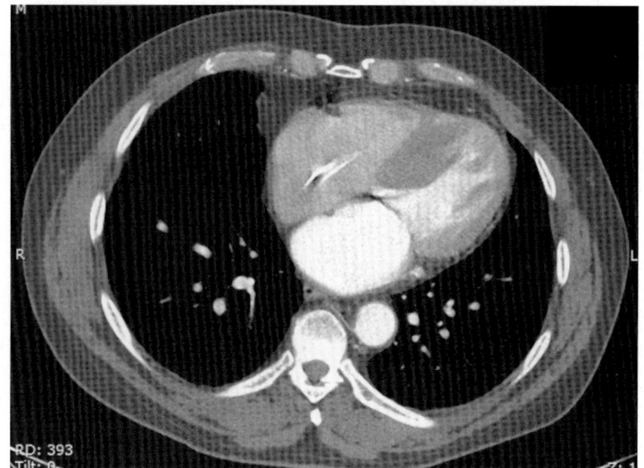

B

Clinical Presentation

A 26-year-old man presents with dyspnea and palpitations.

Imaging Findings

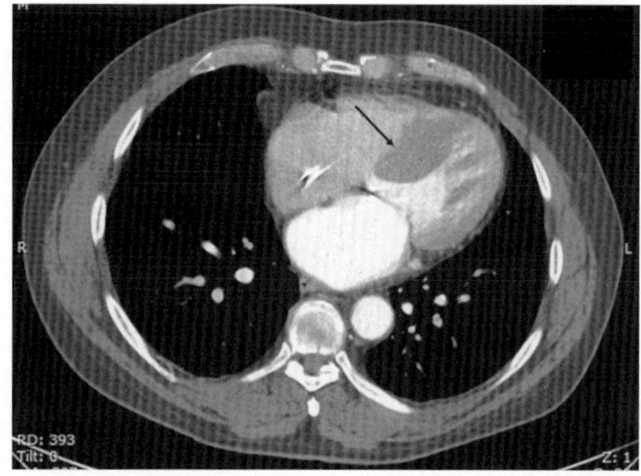

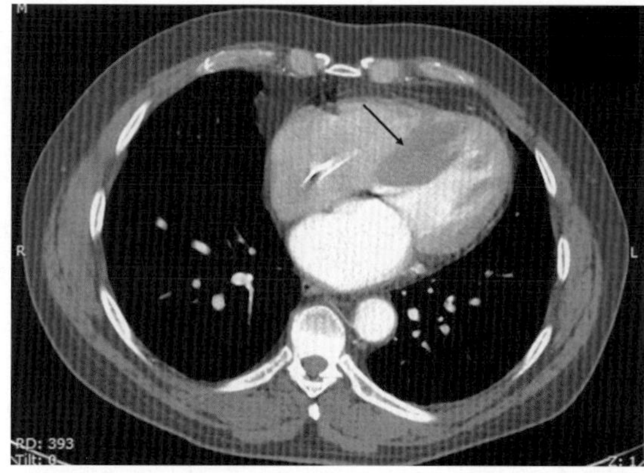

(A,B) Contrast-enhanced axial computed tomography (CT) images at two different levels reveal an abnormally thickened interventricular septum compared with the lateral wall of the left ventricle (LV), slightly reducing the lumen of the LV chamber.

Differential Diagnosis

- ***Hypertrophic cardiomyopathy (HCM):*** This is a genetic disorder exhibiting mendelian autosomal-dominant inheritance with variable penetrance (50%), or it develops as a sporadic condition, characterized by inappropriate LV hypertrophy, often with LV outflow tract obstruction and a disorganized cellular myocardium. The abnormal thickening of the subaortic septum produces a pressure gradient that creates diastolic dysfunction, impairs ventricular filling, and increases filling pressure.
- *Concentric hypertrophy of the LV:* Chronic arterial hypertension is associated with LV hypertrophy, which typically involves the myocardium in a diffuse fashion, different from the more focal distribution found in HCM.
- *Interventricular septum tumor:* Occasionally, primary or secondary tumors can sit in the interventricular septum, producing a focal thickening. Metastatic tumors more often present this way. Clinical history and abnormal patent of enhancement during CT or magnetic resonance imaging can help to differentiate between these conditions.

Essential Facts

- HCM is the most common cause of sudden death in young people, including competitive athletes.
- Histologic examination of these hearts reveals myocardial cellular disorganization and myocardial fiber disarray.
- HCM can be divided into obstructive and nonobstructive types, depending on the degree of obstruction of the LV outflow tract.
- The obstructive form is associated with a Bernoulli effect, which induces anterior mitral valve movement toward the septum during systole.
- Most patients have abnormal diastolic function.
- The molecular basis for this condition is a defect in any one of 10 genes encoding the sarcomeric protein of the myocardial cells.
- The overall prevalence in the general population is low (0.1–0.2%). Abnormal morphologic changes are more commonly seen in 25% of first-degree relatives of patients with the disorder.
- Clinical manifestations include sudden death, syncope, arrhythmia, dyspnea, orthopnea, angina, palpitations, and heart failure. The annual mortality rate is 1%.
- Men are affected more often than women.
- HCM most commonly presents in the 3rd decade of life.

Other Imaging Findings

- In HCM, a small LV cavity secondary to the marked hypertrophy of the myocardium may also be present.

✔ Pearls & ✘ Pitfalls

✔ During echocardiography, the key finding in the obstructive form of HCM is the anterior motion of the anterior mitral valve leaflet during systole and the asymmetric septal hypertrophy, with a ratio of septal wall thickness to posterior wall thickness of > 1.4:1.0.

✘ Apical HCM is a distinct type of HCM with a predilection for the apical region of the LV. It has a better prognosis, is commonly associated with hypertension, and is rarely associated with sudden cardiac death.

Case 47

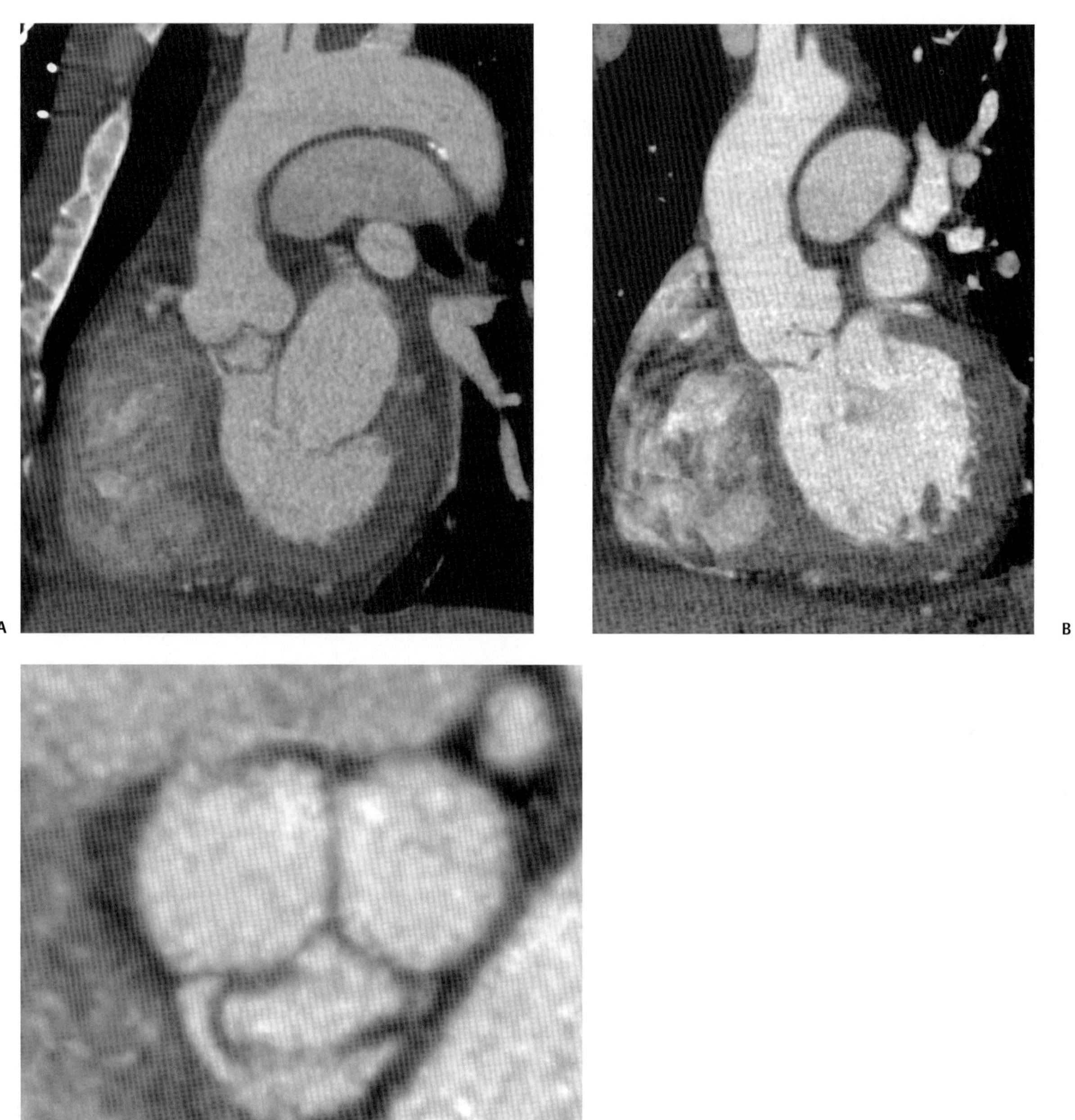

Clinical Presentation

A 45-year-old man presents with chest pain and new onset of a murmur. Echocardiography shows severe aortic insufficiency.

Imaging Findings

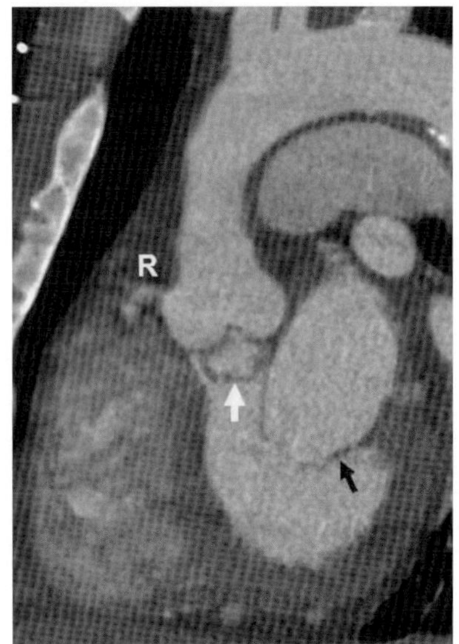

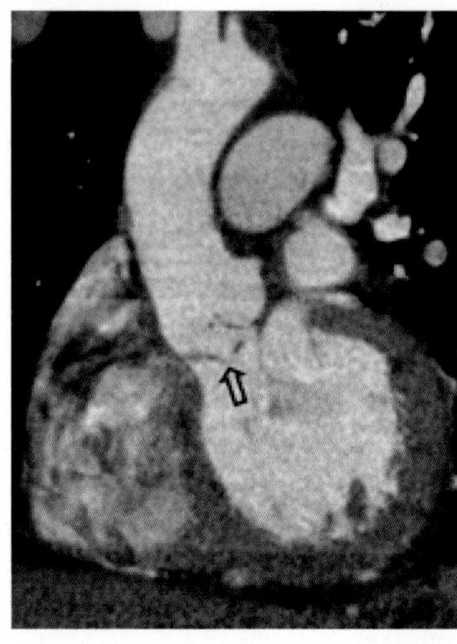

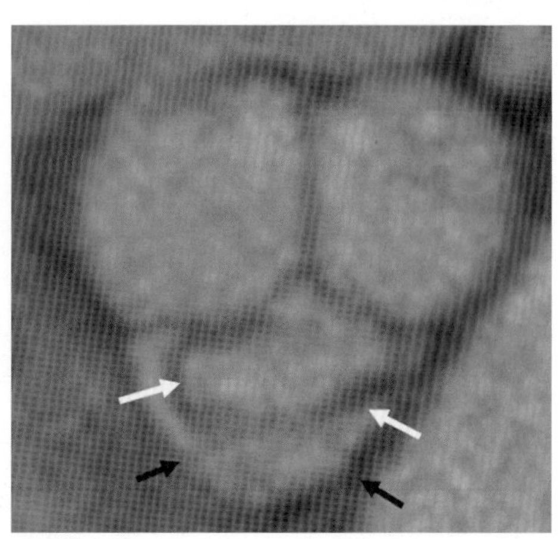

A B C

(A) A sagittal oblique view of the aortic valve and ascending aorta shows a linear low-attenuation structure (*white arrow*), which is the noncoronary cusp of the valve, at the level of the aortic valve, extending into the left ventricular (LV) outflow tract. The posterior leaflet of the mitral valve (*black arrow*) and origin of the right coronary artery (*R*) are shown. **(B)** A coronal oblique view of the aortic valve and ascending aorta is rotated 90 degrees from **(A)**. The linear low attenuation structure (*open black arrow*) in the LVOT is the noncoronary cusp of the aortic valve. **(C)** An axial oblique, en face view of the aortic valve shows a curvilinear density of the noncoronary cusp of the aortic valve (*white arrows*), which has been avulsed from the wall of the sinus of Valsalva (*black arrows*).

Differential Diagnosis

- ***Avulsion of a cusp of the aortic valve:*** Dissection of the thoracic aorta may begin with or secondarily involve the aortic valve. When dissection is limited to the aortic valve, the valve is incompetent, resulting in a murmur.
- *Vegetation of the aortic valve:* Vegetation of cardiac valves is most commonly seen in patients with infective endocarditis and congenital deformities of a valve.
- *Neoplasm of the aortic valve:* Papillary fibroelastomas of the aortic valve are benign neoplasms that arise from cardiac valves. When on the arterial side of the aortic valve, they can obstruct the valve, becoming a source of emboli or causing insufficiency.

Essential Facts

- Trauma is the most common cause of avulsion of a cusp of the aortic valve.
- Valval insufficiency rapidly or progressively leads to congestive heart failure or death unless surgically corrected.
- Valvuloplasty and valve replacement are surgical options.
- Avulsion of the noncoronary cusp of the aortic valve has been reported in patients with pseudoxanthoma elasticum, an inherited connective tissue disease.

Other Imaging Findings

- The tear of the intimal surface of the aorta may be the site of dissection.
- Examine the ascending aorta and origins of the coronary arteries for extension of dissection.
- The avulsed leaflet is mobile; in this case, the leaflet prolapses into the LV outflow tract during diastole.
- Severe aortic insufficiency is also present.

✔ Pearls & ✘ Pitfalls

✔ Vegetation and tumors of the aortic valve are more likely to be masslike, not linear, as is this avulsed leaflet.

✘ A non–electrocardiography (ECG)-gated computed tomography (CT) scan will fail to show the findings because of motion of the aortic valve.

✘ In patients with acute chest pain, consider magnetic resonance imaging or ECG-gated multidetector CT.

Case 48

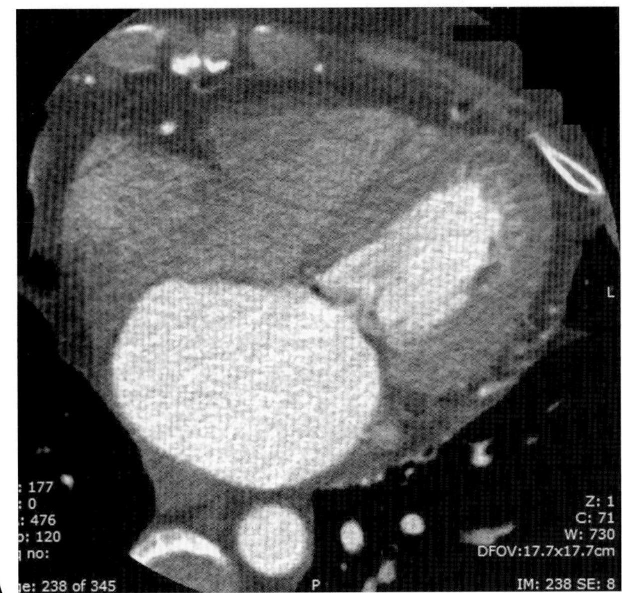

A

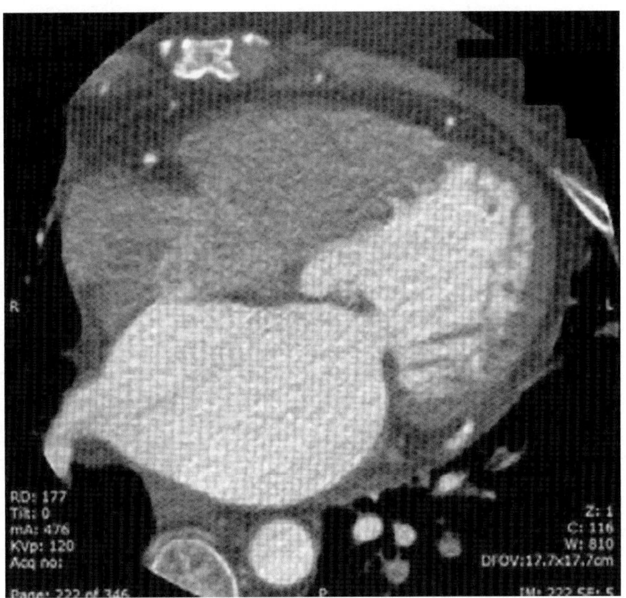

B

Clinical Presentation

A 50-year-old woman presents with dyspnea on exertion.

Imaging Findings

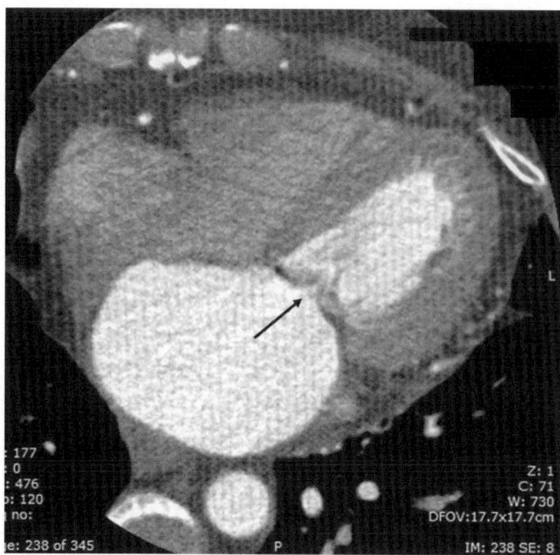

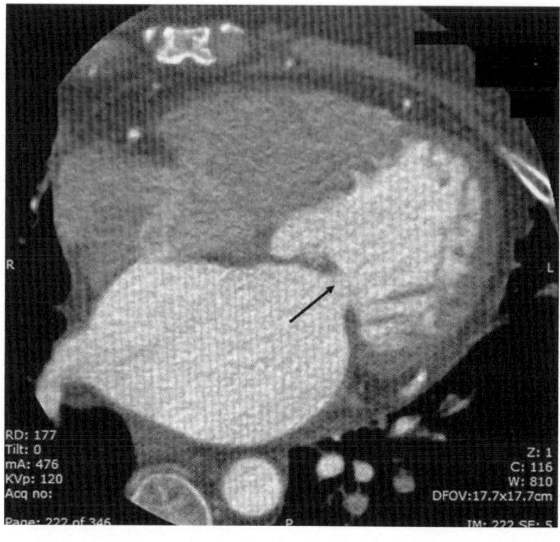

Contrast-enhanced electrocardiography (ECG)-gated cardiac computed tomography (CT) images at **(A)** 40% (systole) and **(B)** 75% (diastole). There is abnormal thickening of the mitral valve, as well as reduced opening of the leaflets during diastolic filling and a dilated left atrium, findings consistent with mitral valve stenosis.

Differential Diagnosis

- ***Mitral valve stenosis:*** On ECG-gated cardiac CT, mitral valve stenosis is identified when a usually thickened mitral valve shows limited opening during ventricular diastole. This is associated with an enlarged left atrium.
- *Mitral valve insufficiency:* Mitral valve insufficiency is characterized by abnormal opening of the mitral valve during ventricular systole.

Essential Facts

- Mitral valve stenosis is an obstruction to the left ventricular (LV) inflow at the level of the mitral valve, which prevents normal filling of the LV.
- The most common cause of mitral valve stenosis is rheumatic carditis (60–90% of cases), with a delay of up to 3 decades between the initial episode of rheumatic fever and the development of stenosis.
- Women are affected by mitral valve stenosis twice as often as men.
- Congenital deformity of the mitral valve is a less common cause and typically is seen in children.
- Occasionally, an atrial myxoma, a thrombus, or severe degenerative annular calcification produces mitral valve stenosis.
- The normal area of the mitral valve is 4 to 5 cm^2. Symptoms usually develop when the area of the affected valve is < 2.5 cm^2.
- Mitral valve stenosis produces elevation of the left atrial pressure, which is transmitted to the pulmonary veins and capillaries. This can translate into pulmonary edema.
- Pulmonary arteriolar resistance increases, and pulmonary arterial hypertension can develop.
- Presentation is usually in the 5th or 6th decade.
- Other complications are atrial fibrillation, embolic events, and hemoptysis.
- The diagnostic imaging tools of choice for mitral valve stenosis are two-dimensional and color Doppler echocardiography. These allow visualization of the morphology and mobility of the mitral valve apparatus; measurement of the valvular area, chamber size, and function; and assessment of the hemodynamic severity of the obstruction.
- Assessment of the mitral valve area in patients with mitral valve stenosis by multidetector ECG-gated cardiac CT has excellent correlation with planimetric measurements obtained by Doppler echocardiography.

Other Imaging Findings

- Mitral valve leaflet calcification visualized on cardiac multidetector CT indicates mitral valve sclerosis or stenosis. A significant correlation between the degree of mitral valve calcification on multidetector CT and the severity of stenosis has been reported.

✔ Pearls & ✘ Pitfalls

✔ Arrhythmias, in particular atrial fibrillation and atrial flutter, are common in patients with mitral valve stenosis. Older patients are more prone to this complication, which is also associated with a poorer prognosis.

✘ Mitral valve leaflet and mitral annulus calcification may coexist, but generally they are different processes, with different pathophysiology and clinical significance. Mitral valve leaflet calcification is closely associated with rheumatic heart disease. Mitral annulus calcification is more commonly a degenerative process that tends to affect elderly women.

Case 49

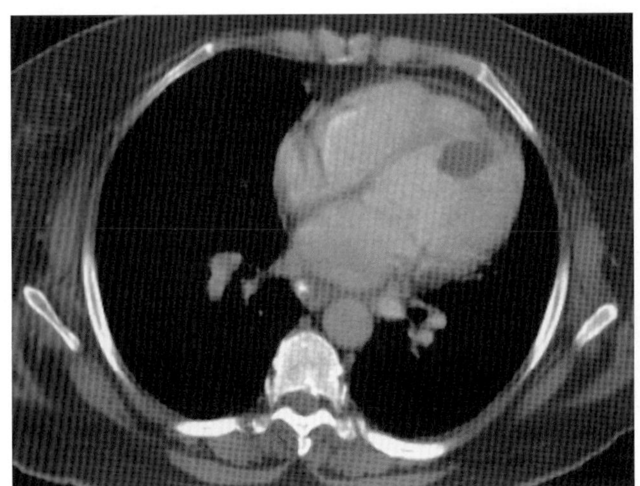

A

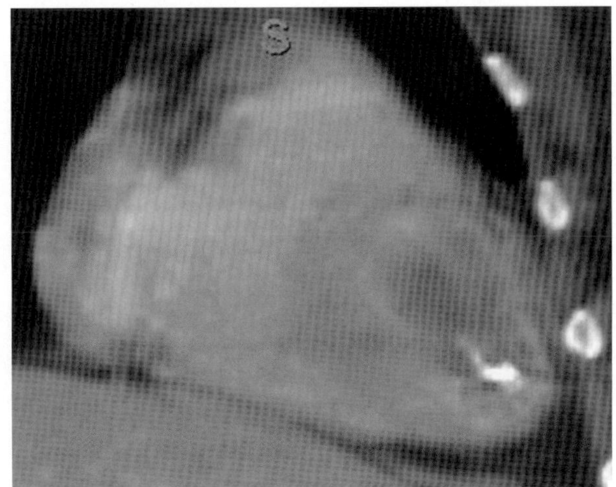

B

Clinical Presentation

A previously healthy 61-year-old woman presents with nausea and generalized upper abdominal pain in the emergency department.

Imaging Findings

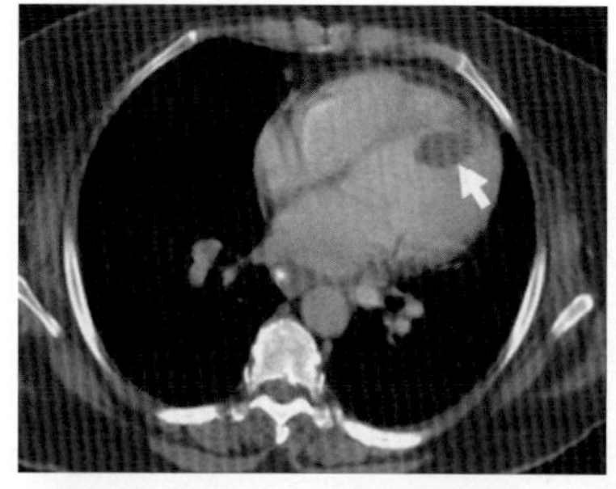
A

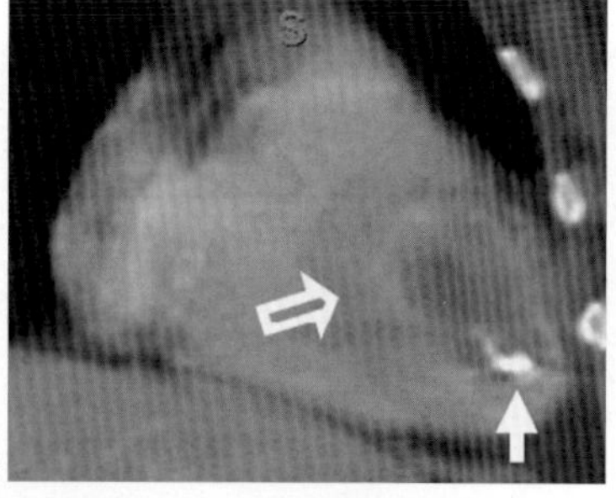
B

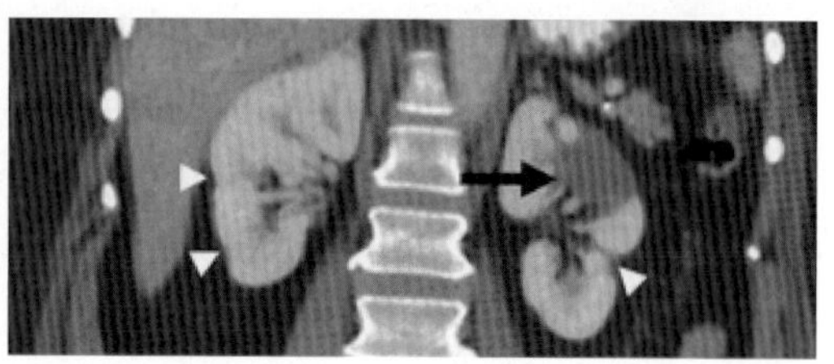
C

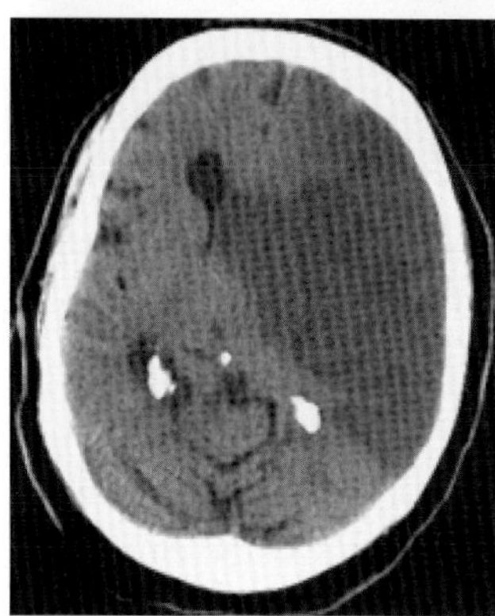
D

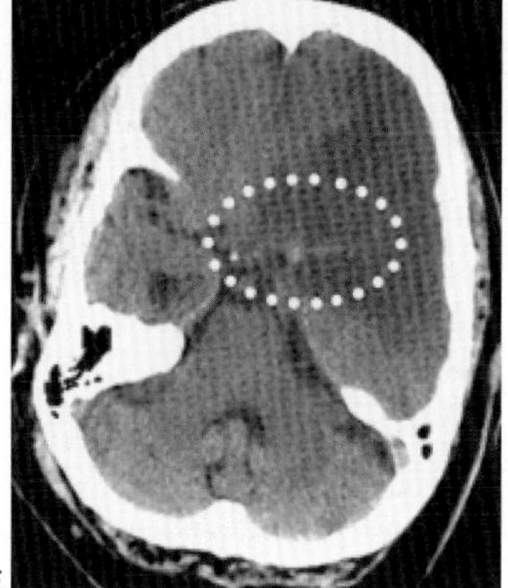
E

(A) A low-attenuation mass in the left ventricular (LV) chamber (*white arrow*) is a thrombus. The LV is dilated in this patient, who is believed to have had a myocardial infarction (MI) some time ago. **(B)** A coronal reconstructed image shows areas of different attenuation in the thrombus, which contains calcium, an indication that the thrombus has been present for a long time (*white arrow*), and concentric rings of low attenuation (*open white arrow*), which represent layers of thrombus that have formed more recently. **(C)** A wedge-shaped infarct of the left kidney (*black arrow*) is due to embolization of part of the LV thrombus and is the cause of the patient's abdominal pain. The irregularities of the renal contour (*white arrowheads*) are likely due to prior renal infarcts. **(D,E)** Subsequently, the patient developed right-sided paralysis. Brain computed tomography (CT) shows infarction of the left middle cerebral artery (MCA) territory and hyperdense thrombus in the MCA (*dotted ellipse*).

Differential Diagnosis

- ***Thrombus of the LV apex with subsequent emboli to the kidneys and brain:*** The LV chamber is dilated and contains a filling defect that is a thrombus of varying age. A thrombus in any cardiac chamber can result in embolic disease.
- *Cardiac neoplasm:* The mass in the LV is atypical of most neoplasms, as it does not have a broad attachment to the ventricular myocardium.
- *Renal carcinoma metastasis to the LV:* The CT appearance of the left renal abnormality is wedge-shaped and therefore more typical of infarction than neoplasm. Renal carcinoma can involve the heart, but more typically it extends to the heart from the renal vein and inferior vena cava into the right atrium.

Essential Facts

- Thrombi form as a result of poor ventricular function, usually from an arrhythmia or following MI.
- Anticoagulation is recommended for 3 months following MI to prevent the development of LV thrombus.
- MI to the anterior wall represents the highest risk for developing a LV thrombus.
- Thrombi can also form in patients with dilated cardiomyopathy because wall motion abnormalities result in poor movement and slow blood flow.
- Fifty percent of patients with LV aneurysm can form LV thrombi.
- LV thrombi put patients at risk for embolic disease, as likely developed in this patient's left kidney.
- The patient was therefore in danger of developing a stroke.

Other Imaging Findings

- When a thrombus is discovered in one of the cardiac chambers, embolic disease can develop in other organs.

✔ Pearls & ✘ Pitfalls

✔ Pain, altered renal function, and stroke can be signs of embolic disease in patients with a history of prior MI.
✔ Suspected embolic disease to any vascular bed should prompt a search for the source.
✘ Unknown MI, atrial fibrillation, and patent foramen ovale are possible cardiac causes of embolic phenomena.

Case 50

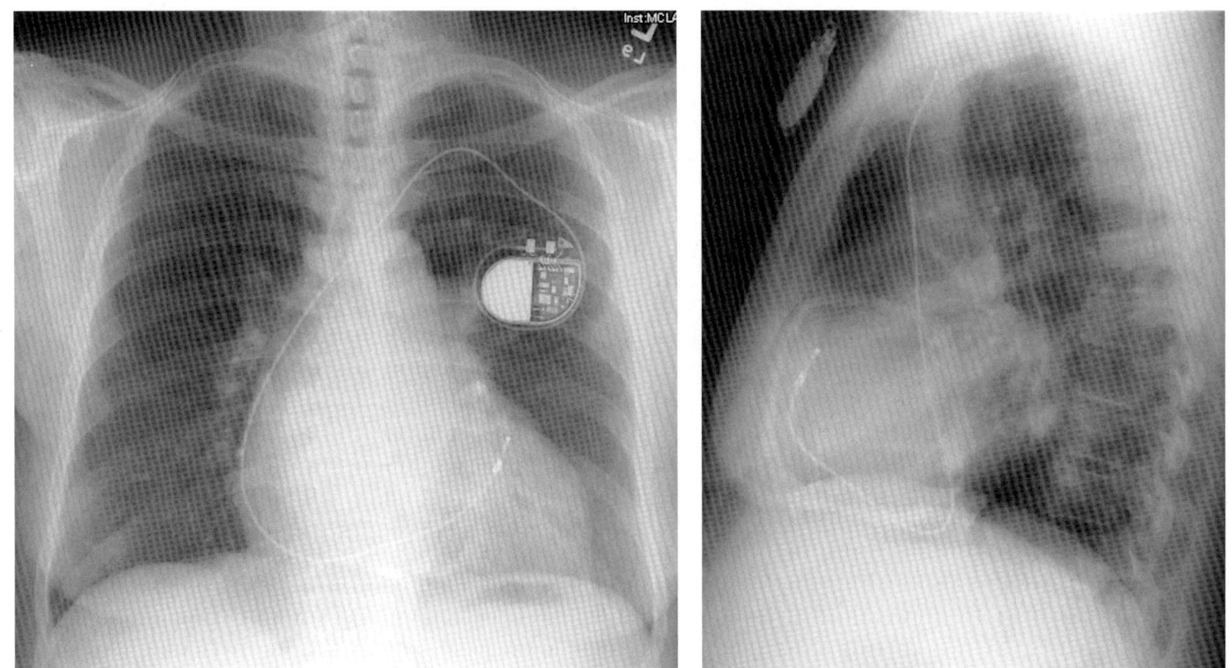

A B

Clinical Presentation

A 56-year-old woman presents with a history of chronic heart failure.

Imaging Findings

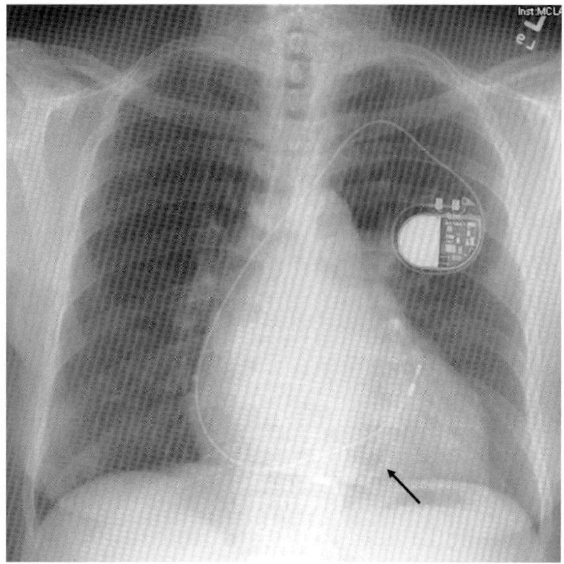
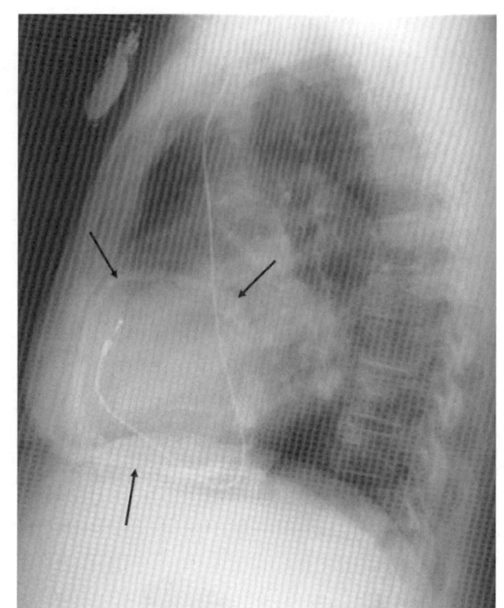

Conventional chest radiographs, **(A)** posterolateral and **(B)** lateral views. An abnormal rim of irregular calcification, better appreciated on the lateral view, is seen delineating the outer cardiac contour. The patient has a pacemaker from a left subclavian approach.

Differential Diagnosis

- ***Constrictive pericarditis:*** Fibrous or calcified thickening of the pericardium that prevents normal diastolic ventricular filling is a characteristic imaging finding of restrictive pericarditis.
- *Pericarditis without constriction:* Pericardial thickening from diverse acute and chronic inflammatory causes may occur in the absence of constrictive physiology.
- *Myocardial calcification:* Chronic inflammatory and metabolic disorders may produce myocardial calcification. Computed tomography helps to differentiate between pericardial and myocardial distribution of calcified plaques.

Essential Facts

- The most common causes are previous surgery and radiation therapy.
- Other possible causes are infectious pericarditis (e.g., tuberculosis), collagen vascular disease, and uremia.
- The physiologic effect may be constrictive physiology.
- The affected pericardium usually exceeds 4 mm in thickness, up to 10 or 12 mm.
- Irregular calcification may occur anywhere over the surface of the heart, but the largest accumulations are usually present at the atrioventricular groove.
- When constriction is present, imaging findings include ventricular deformity, with tubular small ventricles and dilated atria.
- Surgery may be needed in cases of constrictive pericarditis. Complete normalization of cardiac hemodynamics is reported in 60% of patients.

Other Imaging Findings

- In cases of calcified pericarditis with constriction, signs of impaired diastolic filling may be present, with dilatation of the inferior vena cava and hepatic veins, hepatosplenomegaly, and ascites.

✔ Pearls & ✘ Pitfalls

✔ Differentiation between constrictive pericarditis and restrictive cardiomyopathy is crucial, as the definitive treatment of restrictive cardiomyopathy is surgical (pericardiectomy or pericardial stripping).

✘ Constrictive pericarditis may be seen in patients with normal pericardial thickness (18%).

✘ Transthoracic echocardiography is limited for evaluating pericardial thickening.

Case 51

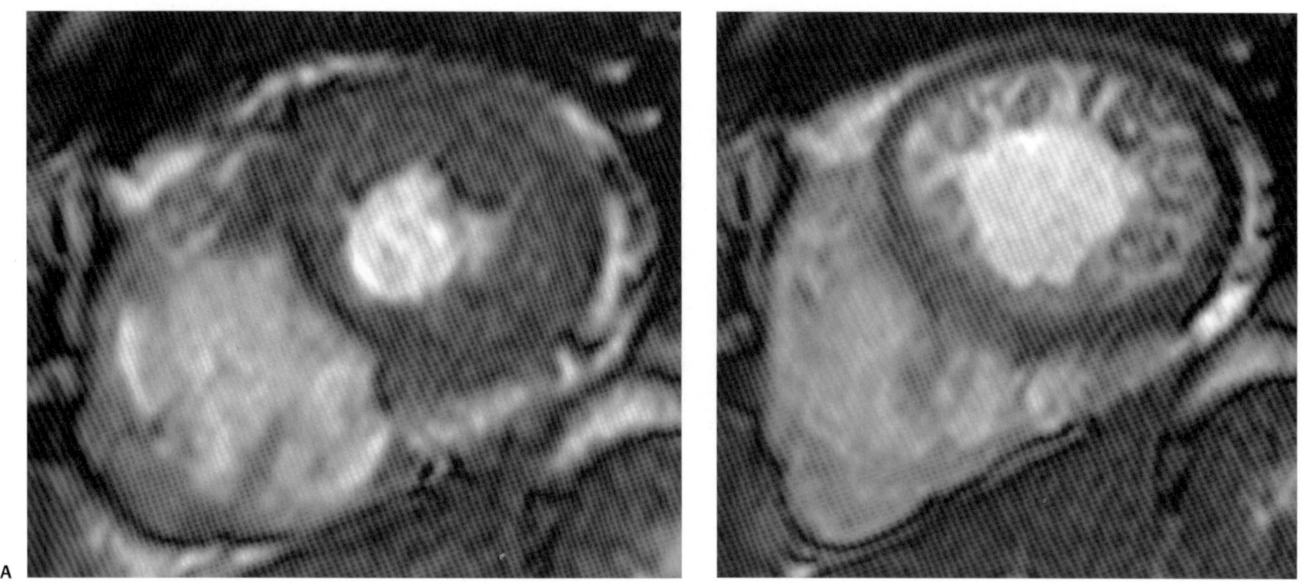

Clinical Presentation

A 31-year-old woman presents with an abnormal echocardiogram.

Imaging Findings

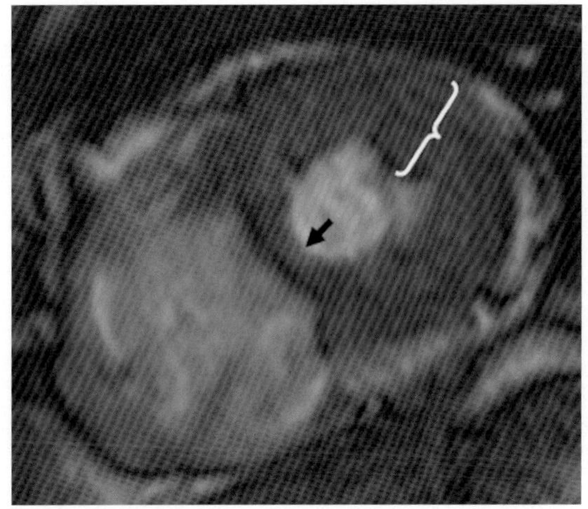

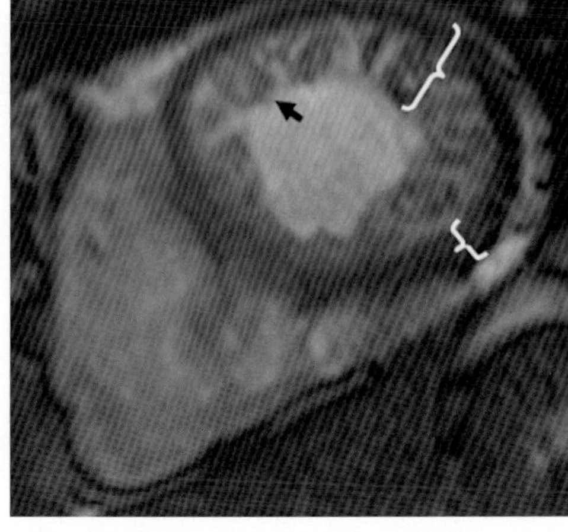

(A) In the short-axis view, at end-systole there appears to be hypertrophy of the anterior, lateral, and inferior walls of the left ventricle (LV: *white bracket*). The septal wall is much thinner (*black arrow*). **(B)** A view of the same mid LV chamber level at end diastole reveals marked abnormality throughout the LV myocardium. Although the myocardium is rather thin (*small white bracket*), numerous abnormal trabeculations (*black arrow*) are seen. The width of the thin myocardium and trabecula are equal to the wall thickness in the systolic image (*large white bracket*).

Differential Diagnosis

- ***Noncompaction of the LV myocardium:*** The LV myocardium normally undergoes a process of compaction that results in dense myocardial muscle that contracts efficiently. In this patient, the myocardium is poorly organized with exaggerated trabeculae.
- *Hypertrophic cardiomyopathy:* The myocardium is thin rather than thickened. The LV chamber is usually small in hypertrophic cardiomyopathy.
- *Ischemic cardiomyopathy:* Dilatation of the LV chamber can be seen in patients with ischemic cardiomyopathy, but myocardial thickness should remain normal.

Essential Facts

- Ventricular noncompaction is a rare disease that has most often been described in association with structural congenital cardiac disease, particularly obstructed LV or right ventricular outflow.
- Ventricular noncompaction in patients without structural congenital heart disease is rarer.
- The disease is a congenital cardiomyopathy that occurs secondary to arrested development of organized compaction of the myocardium.
- Morphologically, the LV myocardium is thinner than normal, but the trabeculation is markedly prominent. In systole, the myocardium may appear to be thickened.
- LV noncompaction can become symptomatic and be diagnosed at any time from infancy through young adulthood.
- Fibrous and elastic tissue on the endocardial surface and in the intertrabecular recesses of the LV is seen in noncompaction of the LV myocardium.
- The symptoms and signs include decreased ventricular function, ventricular arrhythmias, and endocardial thrombus formation.
- Embolic phenomena may be secondary findings.
- LV noncompaction may be familial, either X-linked or otherwise associated with the q28 region of the X chromosome. This area of the X chromosome is involved in muscular dystrophies and myopathies.
- The myocardium is described as "spongy" on gross and histologic examination.

Other Imaging Findings

- Structural congenital heart disease may be present in patients with LV noncompaction.
- All affected wall segments are hypokinetic.

✔ Pearls & ✘ Pitfalls

✔ Systolic function is decreased, which may result in increased LV end-systolic volume and decreased ejection fraction.

✔ Arrhythmia may manifest as wall motion abnormalities and exacerbate functional abnormalities.

✘ False tendons and anomalous chordae tendineae can be distinguished from the hypertrabeculation of noncompaction because they cross or span the LV chamber.

Case 52

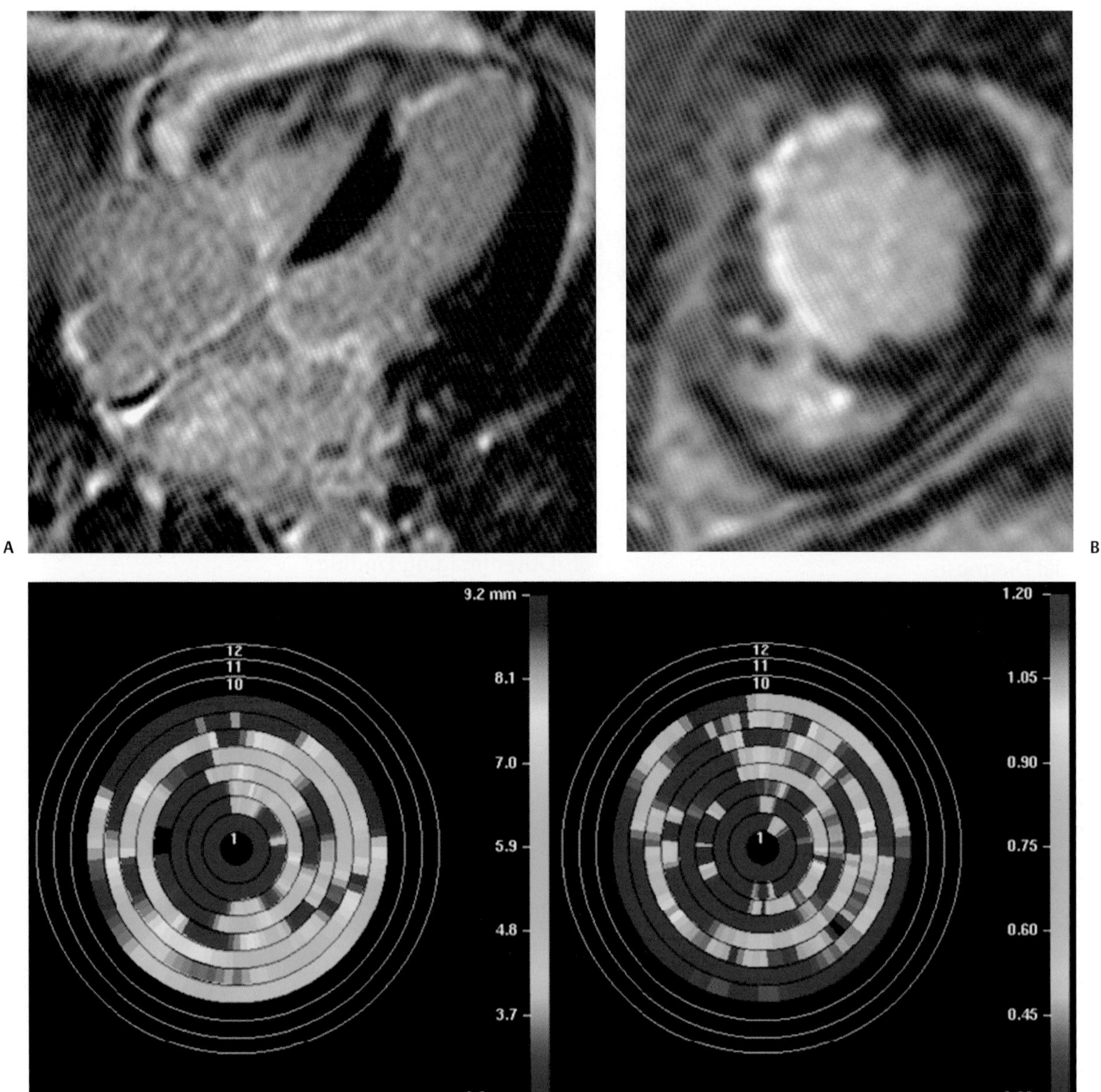

Clinical Presentation

A 93-year-old man presents with a history of myocardial infarction.

Imaging Findings

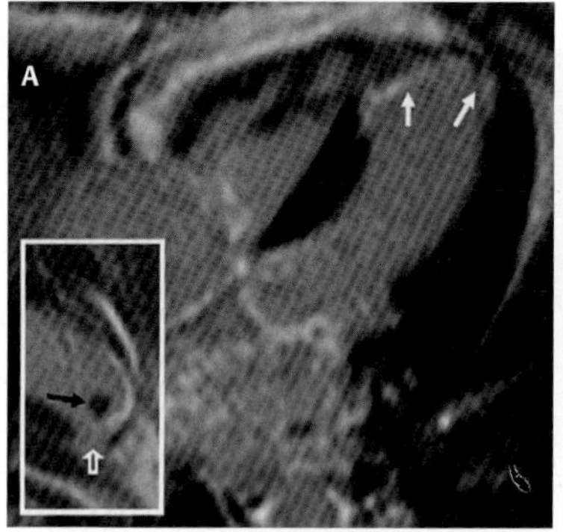

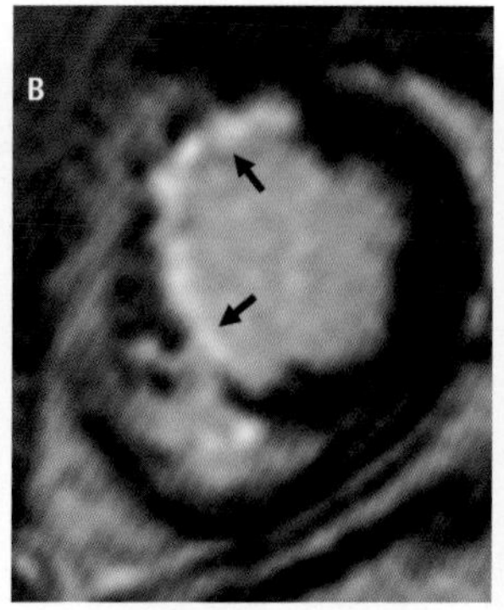

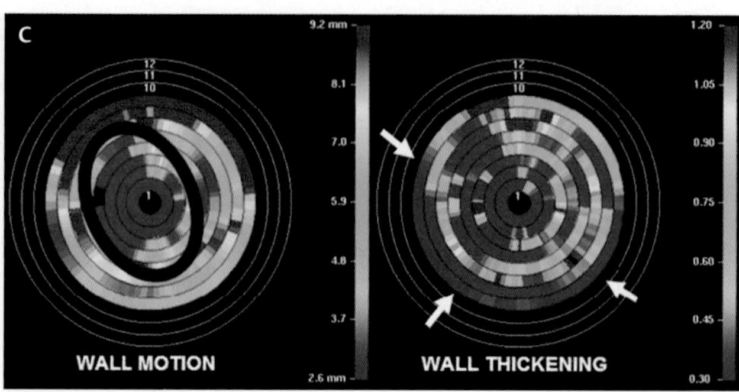

(A) In the four-chamber view, following delayed gadolinium administration, there is subendocardial enhancement at the apex (*white arrows*). In a cropped two-chamber view, a low-signal mass is in the apex of the left ventricle (LV: *black arrow*). Delayed enhancement is transmural in the inferoapical LV wall (*open white arrow*). **(B)** Near the apex, in a short-axis view, hyperintense subendocardial enhancement involves the septal and anterior walls (*black arrows*). **(C)** Color maps generated from a short-axis stack performed for functional assessment indicate the relative wall motion (*left image*) and wall thickening (*right image*) of the LV. Blue indicates hypokinesis at the LV apex (*black oval*) and poor wall thickening of much of the LV myocardium (*white arrows*). Findings correlate with the areas of infarction.

Differential Diagnosis

- ***Apical infarction, thrombus, hypokinesis, and poor wall thickening:*** Distal septal and apical wall thinning along with wall motion abnormalities and subendocardial enhancement are diagnostic of myocardial infarction (MI). An apical mass in a patient with prior MI is most likely thrombus.
- *Hypertrophic cardiomyopathy:* Although myocardial enhancement can be seen in hypertrophic cardiomyopathy, the wall is not abnormally thickened. The LV chamber is usually small in hypertrophic cardiomyopathy.
- *Myocarditis:* Myocarditis typically involves the lateral and apical walls of the LV and the pattern of enhancement which spares the subendocardial surface of the LV, involving the mid myocardium.

Essential Facts

- Most LV thrombi form within the first 2 weeks, but they can form as early as 48 hours after myocardial infarction.
- Inflammatory cells infiltrate necrotic myocardium following infarction, inducing platelet and fibrin deposition on the endocardial surface of the myocardium, thus encouraging thrombus formation.
- Inflammatory markers such as C-reactive protein may help to predict on which patients thrombi are more likely to form.
- Potential embolic complications from LV thrombi portend a poor prognosis.

Other Imaging Findings

- If the face of a clock is used for reference, 12:00 is the anterior wall, 3:00 the lateral wall, 6:00 the inferior wall, and 9:00 the septal wall.
- Dividing the myocardium into segments and using color maps can aid in the diagnosis of coronary artery disease.
- On the color maps, the LV apex is in the center, the base of the heart is the outer ring of color, and the segments in between are in the midchamber.

✔ Pearls & ✘ Pitfalls

✔ Look for areas of wall motion abnormality (akinesis, marked hypokinesis) or aneurysm as a site of thrombus formation.

✔ Calcium may be missed on magnetic resonance imaging but should be obvious on computed tomography (CT).

✘ On CT, mixing of contrast with non–contrast-enhanced blood is an unusual finding in the LV, but it may be seen in the right side of the heart.

Case 53

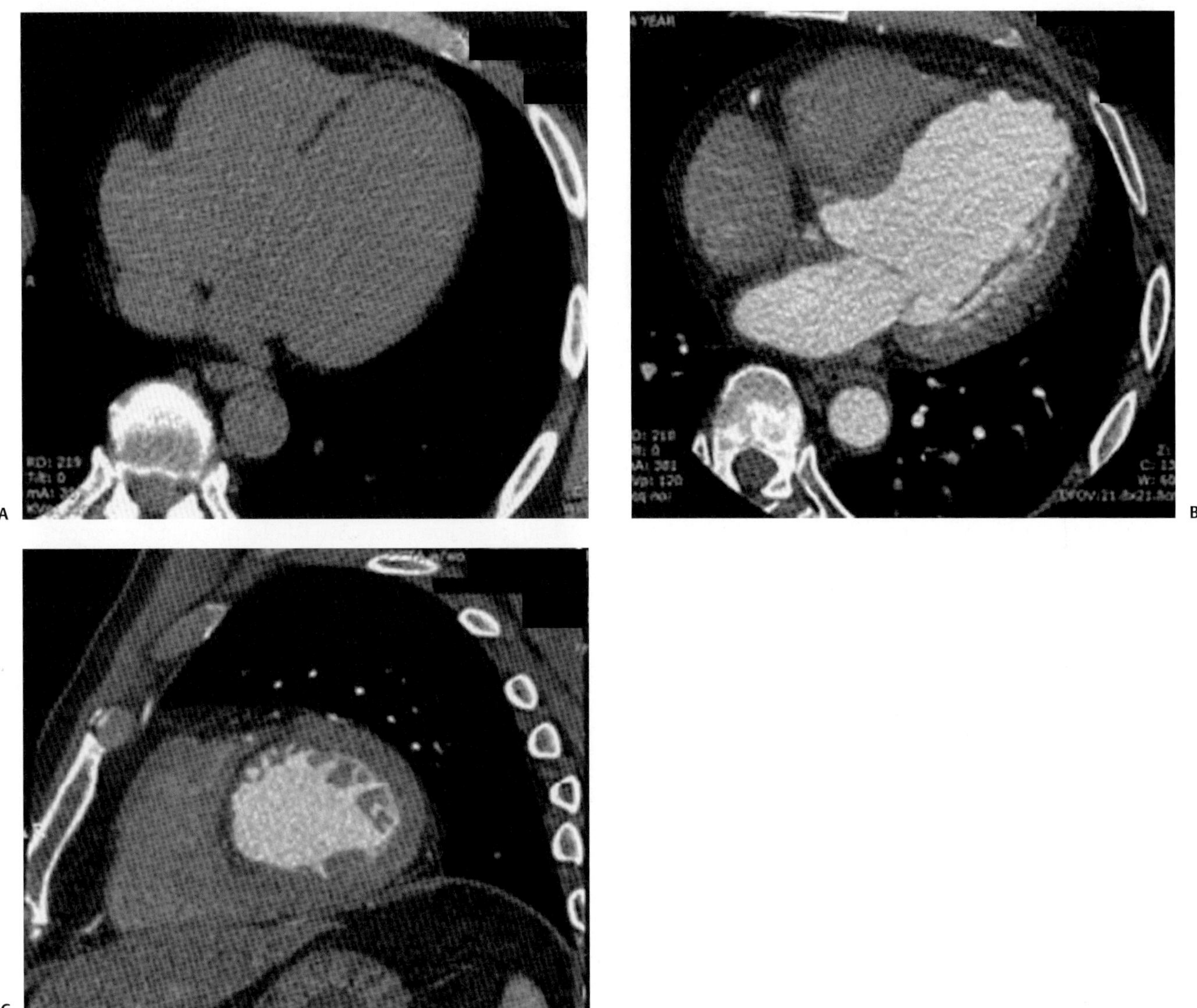

Clinical Presentation

Dyspnea on exertion and palpitations in a 54-year-old man with a history of diabetes

Imaging Findings

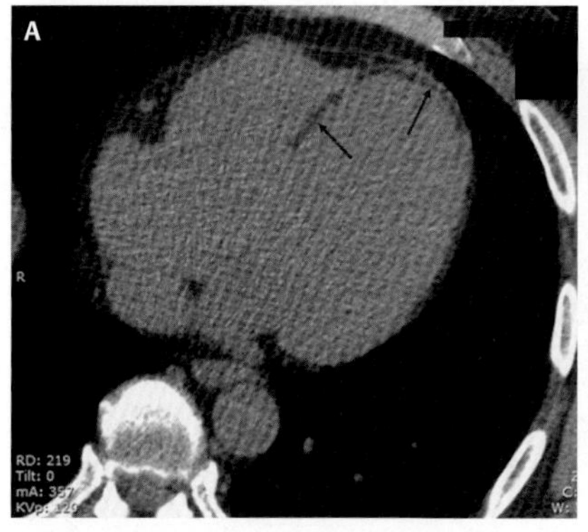

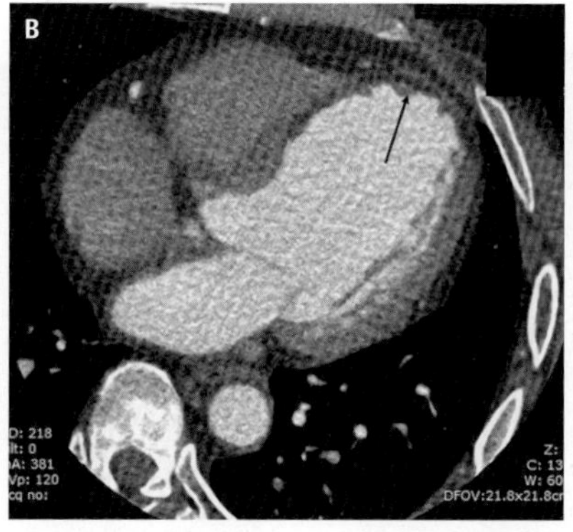

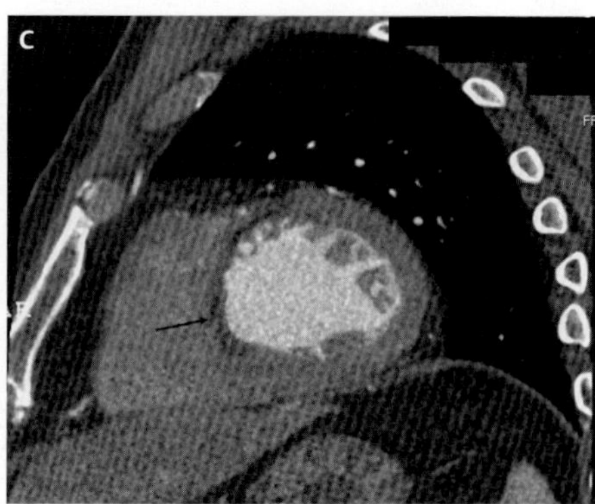

(A) Non–contrast- and **(B)** contrast-enhanced images of a cardiac-gated computed tomography (CT) angiogram show abnormal thinning, dilatation, and low-density fat infiltration of the interventricular septum and apex of the left ventricle (LV).

Differential Diagnosis

- ***Myocardial fatty replacement in old infarcted myocardium:*** Linear and curvilinear macroscopic fat deposits are visualized in an abnormally thin LV wall, which is characteristic of remote infarcted myocardium.
- *Arrythmogenic right ventricular dysplasia (ARVD):* In this condition, which typically presents in young adults, there is fibrofatty replacement of the right ventricle (RV) myocardium with secondary thinning, dilatation, poor contraction, and abnormal regional wall motion. Even though the LV can be involved (47%), the RV is the one more significantly affected.
- *Lipomatous hypertrophy of the interatrial septum:* In this condition, there is abnormal accumulation of fat in the interatrial septum. The LV myocardium and interventricular septum are not affected.

Essential Facts

- Mature adipose tissue is highly prevalent in the myocardium of healed myocardial infarcts (68–84% in pathology series). Only a minority of healed old myocardial infarcts contain no fat.
- CT shows LV myocardial fat in ~50% of patients with chronic LV infarction.
- The origin of this fat is probably fatty metaplasia of the fibrous tissue that develops in the scar of the infarcted myocardium.
- Common CT imaging features include thin linear or curvilinear fat attenuation in the subendocardial myocardium of the LV, often associated with LV wall thinning.
- Associated calcification can also be present.

Other Imaging Findings

- Noncontrast T1-weighted magnetic resonance imaging (MRI) also shows increased fat deposition in the myocardium in patient with infarcts > 6 months old.

✔ Pearls & ✘ Pitfalls

✔ The presence of linear or curvilinear fat deposition in the walls of the LV on CT (either contrast or noncontrast examination) or MRI is highly characteristic of remote and healed myocardial infarction.

✘ Post-infarction fat deposition should be differentiated from ARVD, in which fat deposition is present in the RV.

Case 54

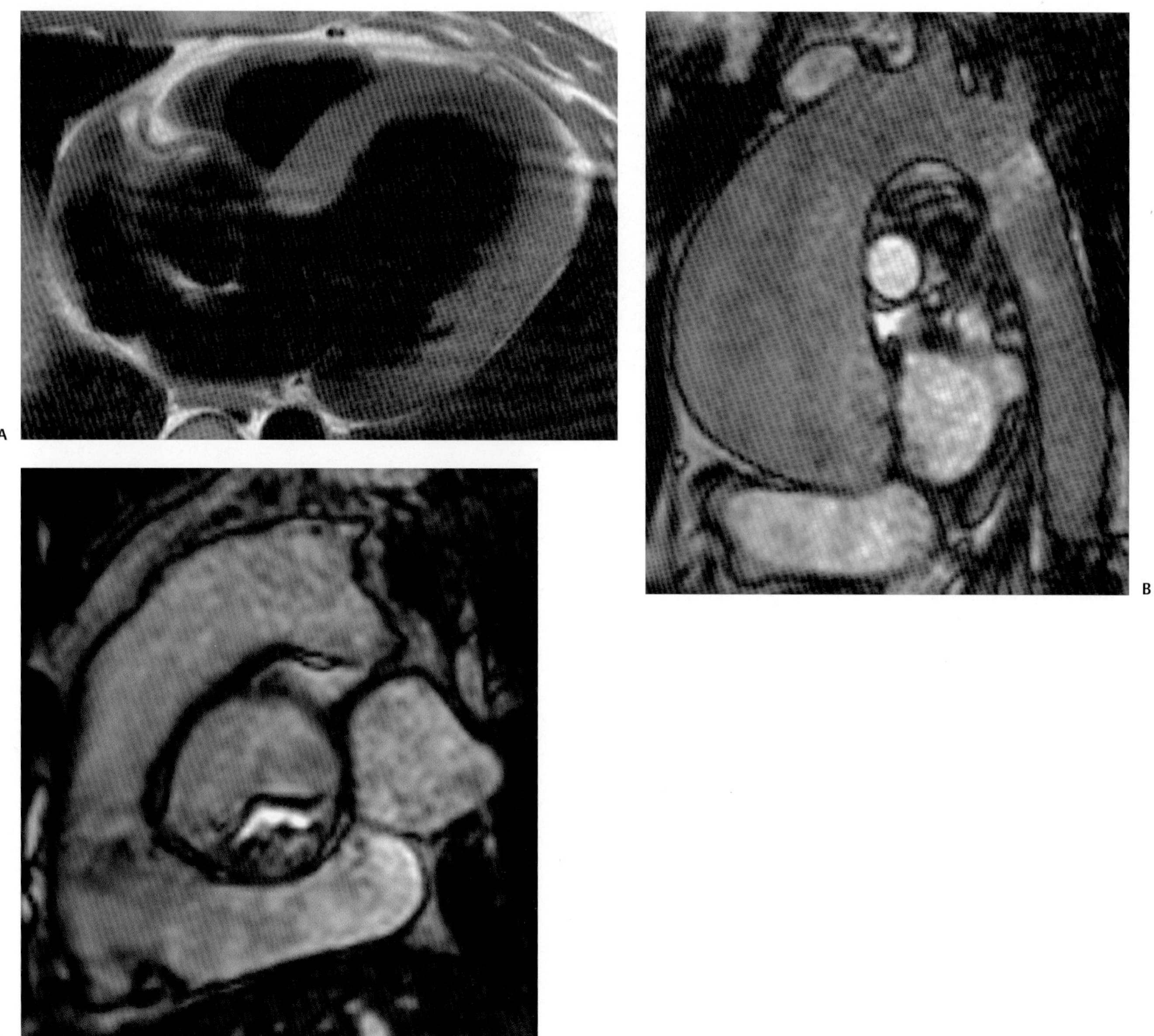

Clinical Presentation

A 65-year-old man presents with a systolic murmur and abnormal chest radiograph.

Imaging Findings

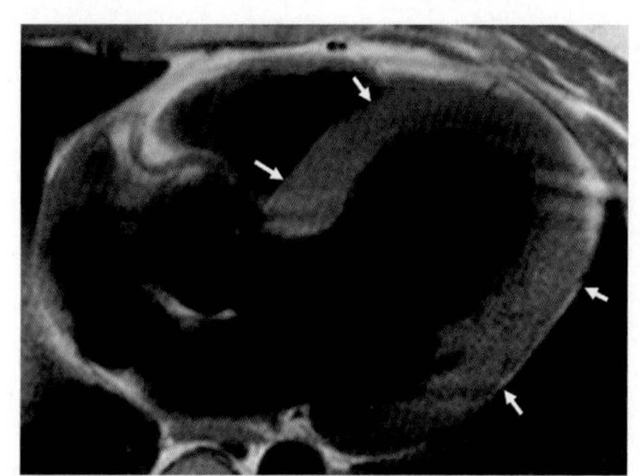

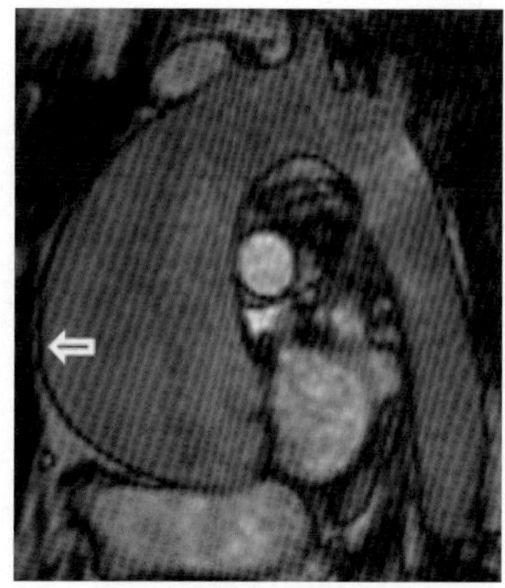

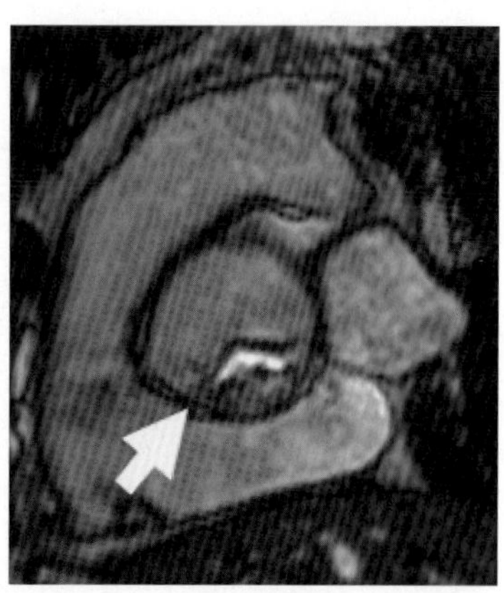

(A) An axial black blood image of the heart shows mild concentric left ventricular (LV) hypertrophy (*white arrows*). **(B)** This candy cane view of the aorta shows marked dilatation of the ascending aorta (*open arrow*) but normal caliber of the aortic arch and descending aorta. **(C)** En face view of the aortic valve during systole shows the valve leaflets do not open completely; the orifice is slitlike (*white arrow*). The edges of the valve leaflets are irregular and very low-signal because of degenerative changes, including thickening and calcification.

Differential Diagnosis

- ***Degenerative aortic valve stenosis with secondary dilatation of the ascending aorta and LV hypertrophy:*** High-velocity blood flow through the stenotic aortic valve causes dilatation of the ascending aorta. Increased work of the LV myocardium pumping blood through the stenotic valve results in hypertrophy.
- *Mild stenosis of the aortic valve:* The degree of stenosis of the aortic valve in this patient appears severe. Mild grades of aortic valve stenosis are usually asymptomatic and are unlikely to result in LV hypertrophy and dilatation of the ascending aorta.
- *Aortic aneurysm:* This patient does not have aneurysm of the ascending aorta, such as that seen in patients with atherosclerotic disease. LV myocardial hypertrophy is not associated with atherosclerotic disease.

Essential Facts

- Aortic valve stenosis may be congenital or acquired.
- Degenerative changes may be due to atherosclerotic disease or infectious endocarditis, or they may be seen in bileaflet valves that were not stenotic at birth.
- Acquired aortic valve stenosis may be due to rheumatic disease, degenerative calcific change, or infectious endocarditis.
- Symptomatic patients presenting before the 7th decade may have symptoms related to the end result of rheumatic heart disease.
- Congenital causes of aortic valve stenosis that presents in adulthood include bicuspid aortic valve, tricuspid valve with partially fused leaflets, and subvalvular or supravalvular narrowing.
- Patients with congenital aortic valvular stenosis usually present before 30 years of age.

Other Imaging Findings

- Aortic dissection may be associated with aneurysm.
- Aortic leaflet thickening may contribute to stenosis, as the thickened leaflets are less mobile.
- A muscular ridge or subvalvular membrane may be seen when the stenosis is below the valve.
- An hourglass shape of the proximal ascending aorta can be seen if the level of stenosis is supravalvular.

✔ Pearls & ✘ Pitfalls

✔ If a bileaflet aortic valve is present, examine the aortic arch and infundibulum for coarctation.

✔ Patients with the coarctation are susceptible to premature coronary artery atherosclerosis.

✘ The view of the aortic valve must be completely en face. Oblique views of the valve may lead to a false interpretation of stenosis or asymmetric development of the valve leaflets.

✘ View the leaflets in systole and diastole to assess complete opening and closing.

Case 55

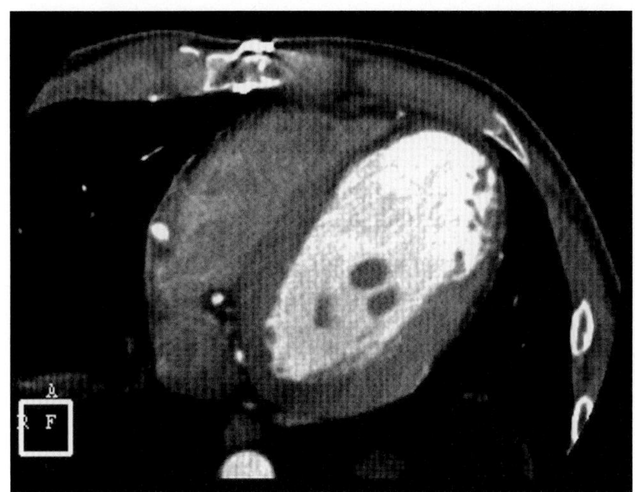

A

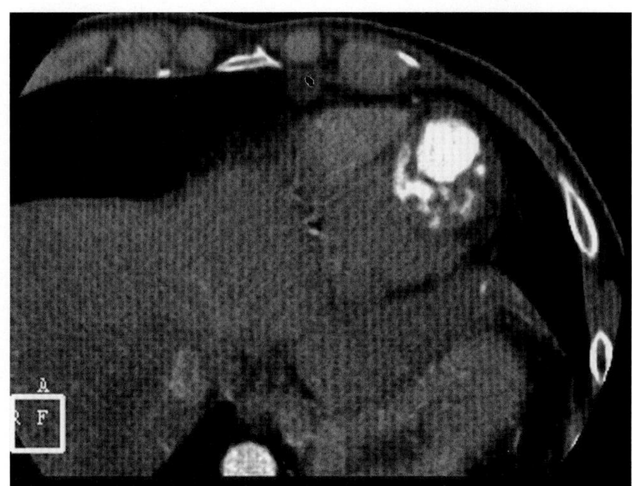

B

Clinical Presentation

Angina and dyspnea on exertion in a 55-year-old man with a coronary artery bypass graft (CABG).

Imaging Findings

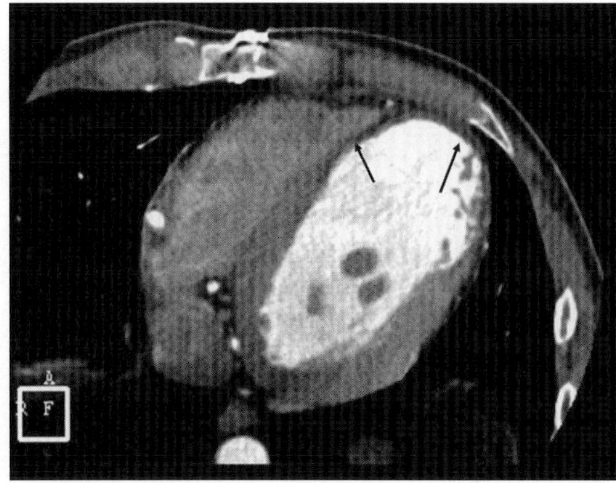

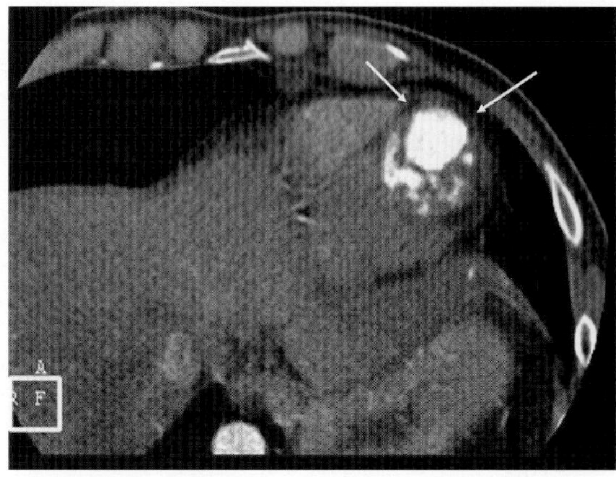

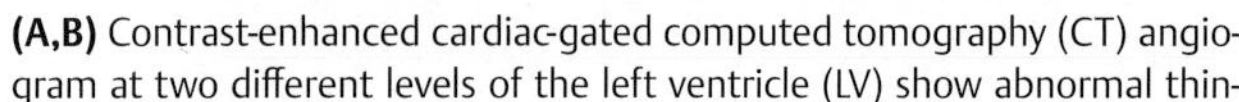

(A,B) Contrast-enhanced cardiac-gated computed tomography (CT) angiogram at two different levels of the left ventricle (LV) show abnormal thinning, dilatation, and low density with fatty replacement of the myocardium at the apex of the LV.

Differential Diagnosis

- ***True left ventricular aneurysm (LVA):*** LVA is defined as a distinct area of abnormal LV diastolic contour with systolic dyskinesia or paradoxical bulging. On CT angiogram, it usually presents as an abnormal bulge of the LV in a previously infarcted myocardium that is thin and exhibits low density.
- *LV pseudoaneurysm:* Pseudoaneurysms or false aneurysms of the LV are contained ruptures of the ventricle that typically present 1 or 2 weeks after myocardial infarction and more often occur in the vascular territory of the left circumflex artery (two thirds of cases) or secondary to cardiac surgery (one third of cases). A distinctive feature of a pseudoaneurysm is that the "mouth" of the communication with the ventricle is smaller than in a true aneurysm.
- *Dilated cardiomyopathy:* The LV can be enlarged and thinned in dilated cardiomyopathy, but involvement is usually diffuse, different from the focal thinning appreciated in a true LVA.

Essential Facts

- Between 8 and 35% of patients with an acute myocardial infarction will develop a true LVA.
- The absolute incidence of LVA is declining because of the increased use of thrombolytic agents and early revascularization techniques after an acute coronary event.
- More than 95% of LVAs result from coronary artery disease and myocardial infarction.
- Less common causes are trauma, Chagas' disease, sarcoidosis, myocarditis, and congenital or idiopathic conditions.
- LVAs can be demonstrated as early as 48 hours after infarction.
- True LVAs usually develop after transmural infarction in the vascular territory of the left anterior descending artery (88%) or, less commonly, the dominant right coronary artery.
- Associated intraluminal thrombus is common (40%).
- LVA rupture is rare, and affected patients usually have a relatively good prognosis and in general are treated medically.
- Angina, dyspnea, and arrhythmia are the most common presenting symptoms of these patients.

Other Imaging Findings

- The gold standard for the diagnosis of LVA and differentiation from false aneurysm has been left ventriculography, with demonstration of an area of dyskinesia or akinesia in the apical or apicoanterior aspect of the LV. True versus false LVAs can also be differentiated with magnetic resonance imaging.

✔ Pearls & ✘ Pitfalls

✔ Sixty percent of patients with LVAs have three-vessel coronary artery disease.

✘ True aneurysms that contain myocardial elements in their walls have a better prognosis and are treated medically; they should be differentiated from false aneurysms, which are composed of an organized hematoma contained by the pericardium, are more likely to rupture, and are treated surgically.

Case 56

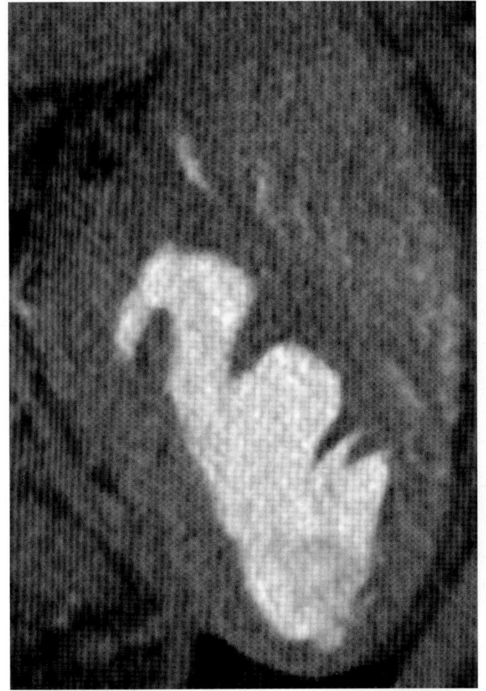

A

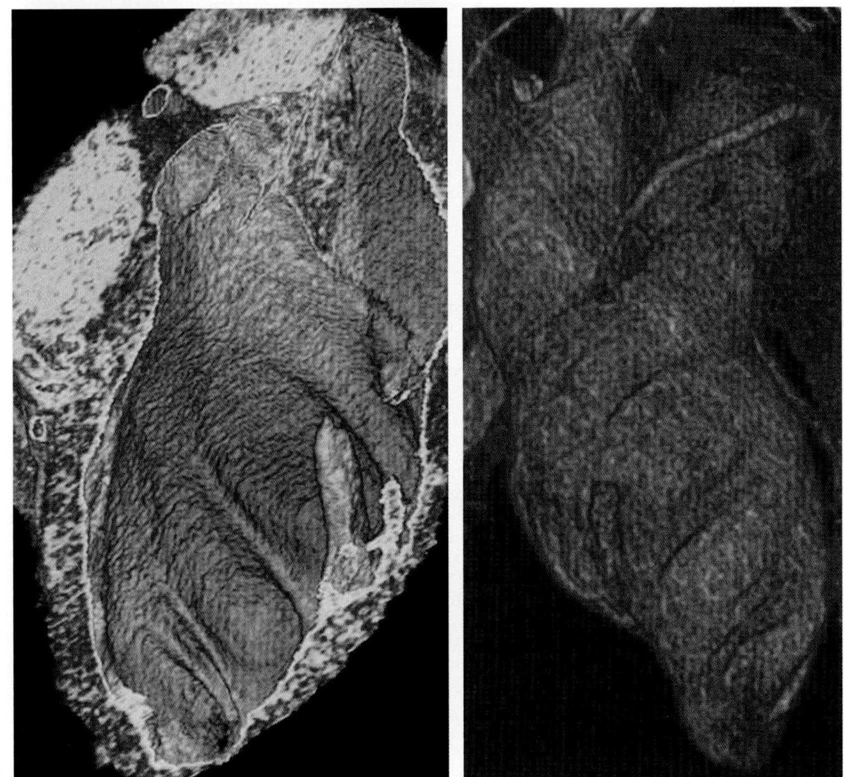

B C

Clinical Presentation

A 34-year-old man presents with mild chest pain and abnormal findings on transthoracic echocardiogram.

Imaging Findings

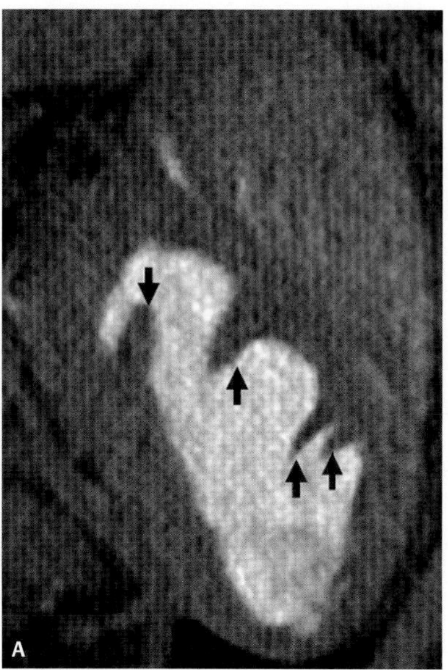

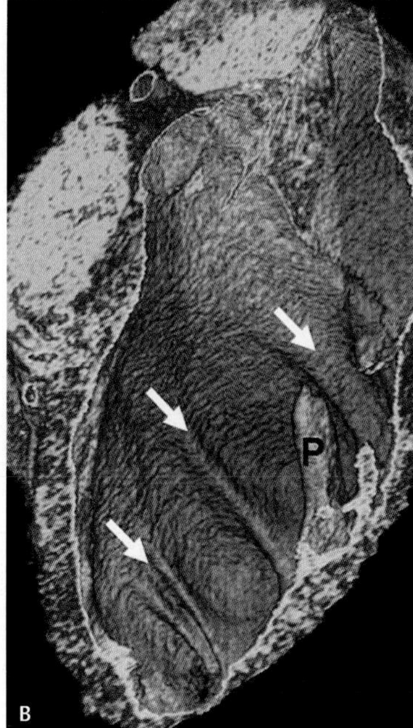

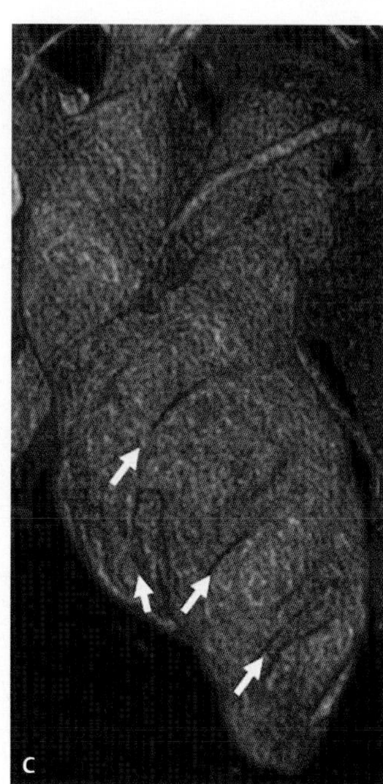

(A) Triangular myocardial structures project into the left ventricular (LV) cavity (*black arrows*) from the inferior and septal wall. **(B)** A hollowed-out view of the LV shows the myocardial projections extending into the lumen (*white arrows*) and the posterior papillary muscle (*P*). **(C)** This three-dimensional view shows the "cast" of the contrast-enhanced blood pool of the LV with filling defects from the abnormal myocardial structures (*white arrows*).

Differential Diagnosis

- ***False tendons (cords) of the myocardium:*** The LV chamber is normal thickness, but there are numerous linear cords of muscle with broad-based attachments to the myocardium that project into the LV lumen.
- *Hypertrophic cardiomyopathy:* The myocardium is not diffusely thickened. The focal thickening of the myocardium is not typical of any known cardiomyopathy.
- *LV thrombus:* The cords or tendons of the myocardium are isoattenuating to myocardium. Thrombus is often of lower attenuation and may contain calcium when chronic.

Essential Facts

- False tendons of the LV myocardium are bands of normal myocardium in an abnormal location.
- Arrhythmia, likely generated because of their abnormal orientation, is one known complication of false tendons.
- LV false tendons/false chordae tendineae ("heartstrings") are fibrous or fibromuscular bands that span across the LV from the septum to the other walls and/or papillary muscle.
- False tendons may displace papillary muscles and therefore lead to chordae or valve dysfunction.
- Although found in patients with murmurs and arrhythmias, false tendons are usually clinically silent.

Other Imaging Findings

- Wall motion abnormalities are not typical.
- The attenuation and signal intensity of false cords are identical to those of normal myocardium on all imaging modalities.

✔ Pearls & ✘ Pitfalls

✔ Unlike true chordae tendineae, false tendons do not connect to the mitral leaflets and are unrelated to the mitral valve.

✔ False chordae are believed to be anatomical variants with a developmental etiology.

✘ False tendons can be mistaken for tumors, subaortic membranes, thrombus borders, and septal hypertrophy, but their tissue characteristics should be identical to those of the remainder of the myocardium.

Case 57

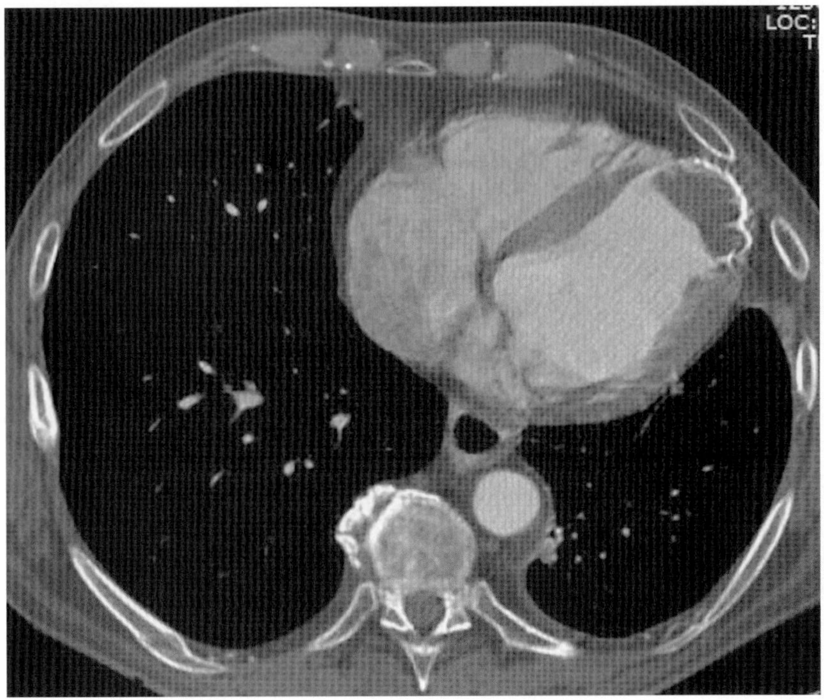

Clinical Presentation

Dyspnea and palpitations in a patient with a past medical history of myocardial infarction 7 years before

Imaging Findings

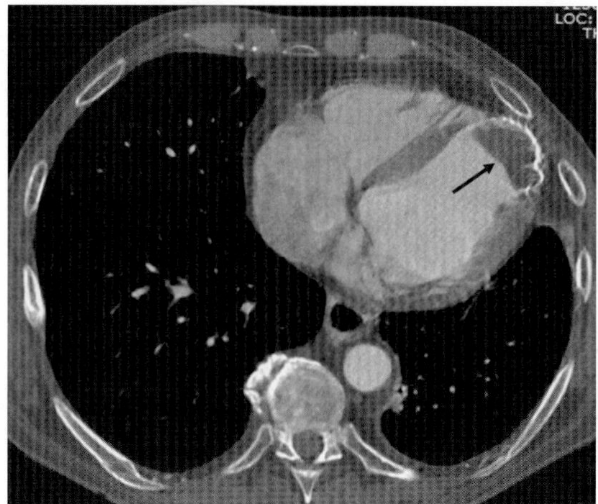

Contrast-enhanced axial computed tomography image demonstrates abnormal curvilinear calcification of the anterior and apical left ventricle (LV) with a low-density intraventricular soft-tissue mass.

Differential Diagnosis

- ***Calcified left myocardial infarction and ventricular thrombus:*** A curvilinear myocardial calcification visualized in the apex of the LV, with an associated mural thrombus, is consistent with chronic myocardial infarction and secondary thrombus formation.
- *Endomyocardial fibrosis (EMF):* EMF is a severe progressive form of restrictive cardiomyopathy that can present with linear calcification within the endocardium. When the LV is involved, a large amount of endocardial tissue produces an inflow tract and/or obliteration of the apex.
- *Pericardial calcification:* Pericardial calcifications are more commonly seen as amorphous, dense, and irregular calcium-density deposits that more commonly involve the atrioventricular and interventricular grooves in patients with prior surgery, infection, inflammation, or radiation therapy.

Essential Facts

- Calcified myocardial infarcts are more common in men than women.
- Most calcified myocardial infarcts develop in areas of severe transmural infarction with a dilated LV and commonly present with an associated ventricular aneurysm.
- Myocardial calcification requires time to develop and is seen at least 2 years after infarction occurred.
- The mechanism of calcium deposit in survivors of acute myocardial infarction is dystrophic calcification of the necrotic myocardium.
- In an autopsy series of patients with calcified myocardial infarction, the average time between infarction and death was ~13 years.
- The most common presenting clinical manifestation is heart failure. Malignant arrhythmias are the second most common clinical finding.

Other Imaging Findings

- On posteroanterior chest radiographs, post-infarction LV calcifications are seen to the left of the midline and in the region of the cardiac apex. Right ventricular calcifications are very rare.

✔ Pearls & ✘ Pitfalls

✔ LV calcification is more common in the apex and anterior wall of the LV, followed by the interventricular septum (8% of cases), in myocardial infarctions > 6 years old.

✘ Identification of myocardial or pericardial calcifications with magnetic resonance imaging is limited.

Case 58

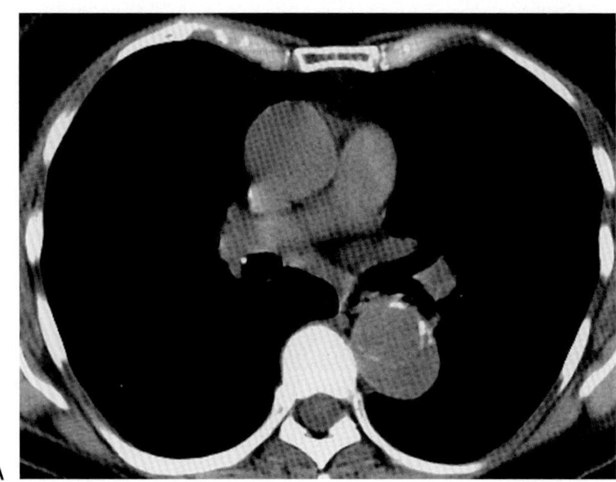
A

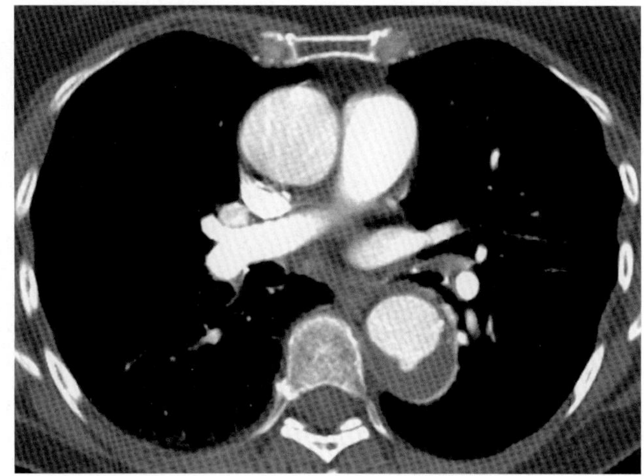
B

Clinical Presentation

A 62-year-old woman presents with chest pain

Imaging Findings

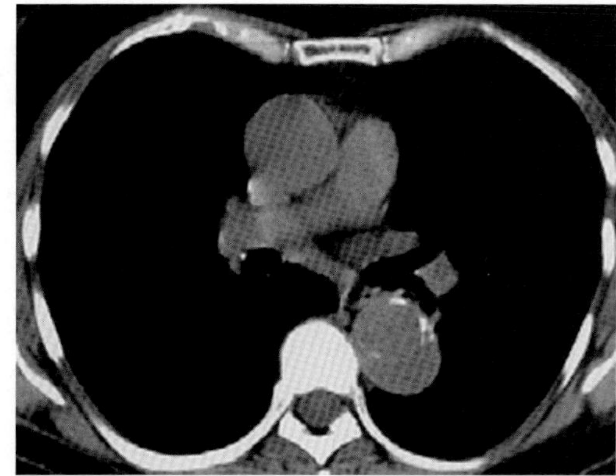

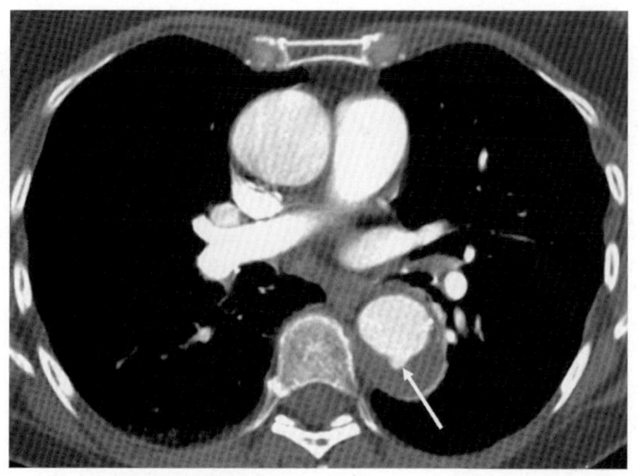

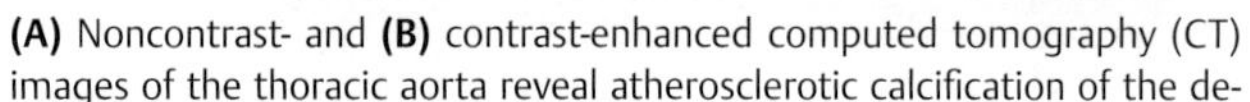

(A) Noncontrast- and **(B)** contrast-enhanced computed tomography (CT) images of the thoracic aorta reveal atherosclerotic calcification of the descending aortic wall, with an ulcerlike collection of contrast and a focal area of wall thickening.

Differential Diagnosis

- ***Penetrating atherosclerotic aortic ulcer:*** Noncontrast- and contrast-enhanced CT images show an enlarged, heavily calcified descending aorta with atherosclerotic disease. After contrast opacification of the lumen in the presence of a penetrating ulcer is confirmed, associated with an underlying intramural hematoma in the aortic wall.
- *Thrombosed aortic aneurysm:* In this case, the aorta is abnormally dilated, but the abnormal collection of contrast allows the identification of a penetrating ulcer with intramural hematoma.
- *Thrombosed aortic dissection:* A thrombosed false lumen in an aortic dissection can have a similar appearance, but the identification of a penetrating ulcer is crucial for the correct diagnosis.

Essential Facts

- An ulcerated atherosclerotic plaque disrupts the internal elastic lamina, burrowing deeply through the intima into the aortic media.
- This may precipitate a localized intramedial dissection with a variable amount of intramural hematoma within the affected aortic wall.
- Occasionally, the hematoma may progress into the adventitia, weakening the aortic wall with formation of a pseudoaneurysm, or it may rupture in the thoracic cavity.
- The process is initially asymptomatic and typically affects elderly patients with advanced atherosclerosis.
- Lesions can be single or multiple, and the most common locations are the descending thoracic aorta (89.5%) and the aortic arch.
- When the condition is symptomatic, chest or back pain is the typical presentation.

Other Imaging Findings

- On magnetic resonance imaging, the ulcer crater and associated intramural hematoma can be well visualized. On spin echo sequences, the ulcer is seen as a signal void in the thickened aortic wall. On angiographic sequences, it presents as an outpouching that connects with the aortic lumen.
- When the aortic ulcer is ruptured, the most significant imaging finding is bleeding into the thorax, mediastinum, and extrapleural space.

✔ Pearls & ✘ Pitfalls

✔ Most aortic ulcerations are asymptomatic, remain stable, and do not enlarge. About one third of them progress, generally resulting in increased aortic diameter, which may eventually end in aneurysm formation or overt aortic dissection.

✘ Atherosclerotic aortic ulcers are confined to the intima and are commonly asymptomatic. When the ulcer penetrates deeper into the aortic wall, intramural hematoma formation is present.

Case 59

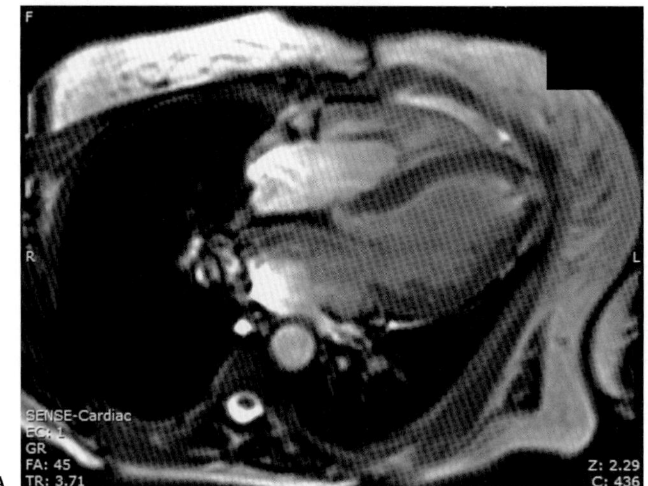

A

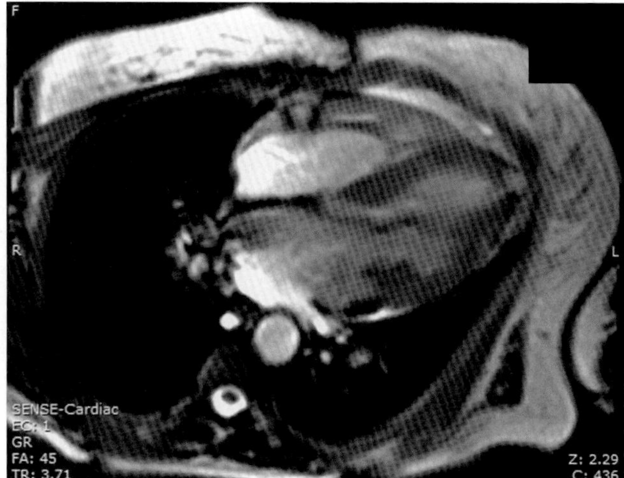

B

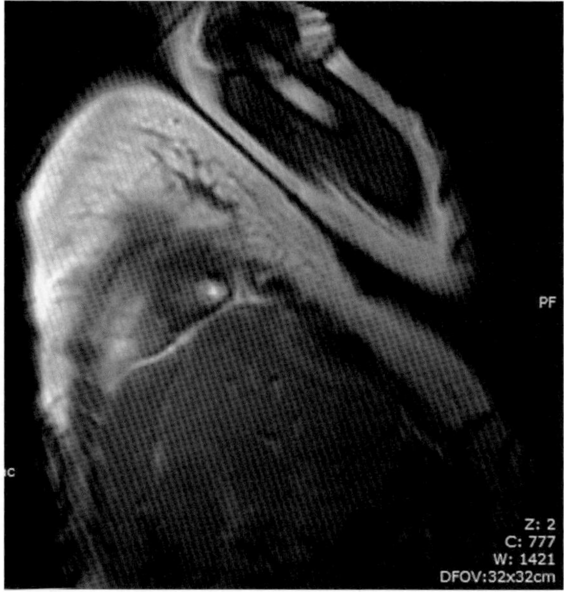

C

Clinical Presentation

Abnormal echocardiogram in a 55-year-old woman

Imaging Findings

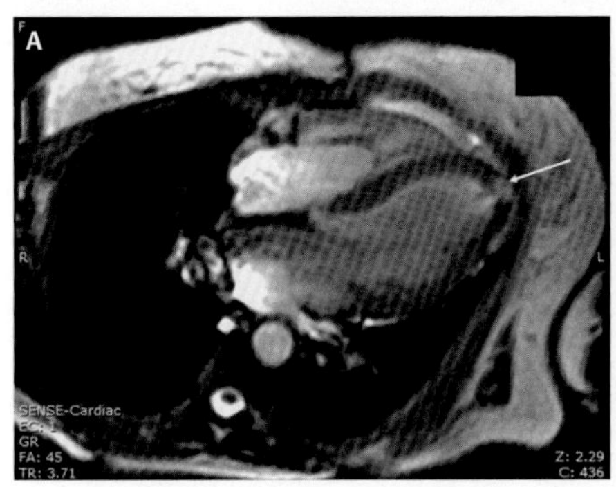

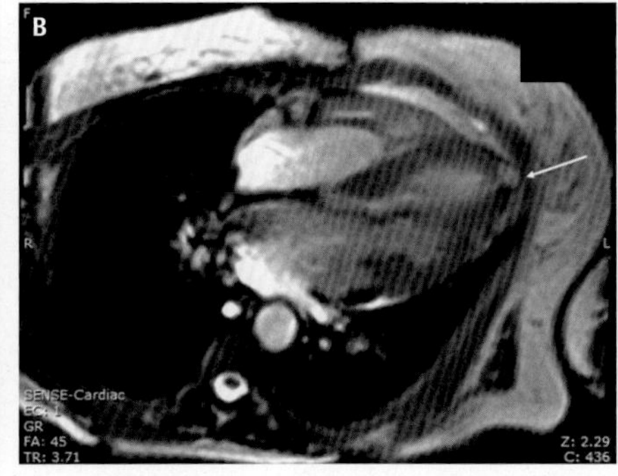

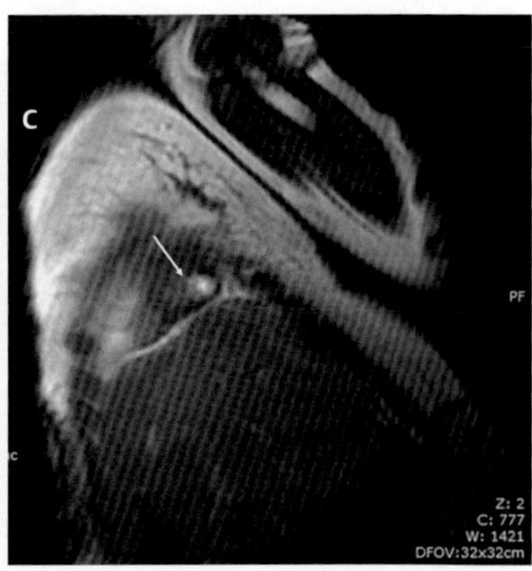

Cardiac magnetic resonance images in the **(A,B)** axial plane and **(C)** short-axis view from balanced turbo field echo sequences reveal a small saccular or diverticular formation (*arrows*) in the apex of the left ventricle (LV).

Differential Diagnosis

- ***Ventricular diverticulum:*** A congenital cardiac diverticulum most commonly occurs in the LV and usually presents as an incidental finding. It is defined as a pouch or saclike projection from the cardiac lumen. Its connection to the ventricular lumen may be wide or narrow. Histologically, the wall of the diverticulum contains all the layers of normal ventricular myocardium.
- *Ventricular pseudoaneurysm/aneurysm:* Acquired ventricular aneurysms and pseudoaneurysms result from a myocardial disease, such as myocardial infarction, myocarditis, sarcoidosis, or from trauma. Because they are not contained by normal myocardium, they exhibit abnormal contraction with bulging during diastole.
- *Isolated ventricular noncompaction:* The diagnosis of this condition requires visualization of more than three intertrabecular recesses. In this condition, there is abnormal endomyocardial morphogenesis with hypertrophy and prominent trabeculation of the LV myocardium.

Essential Facts

- There is a wide range of reported prevalence rates, from 0.04% (echocardiography) to 2.2% (computed tomography angiography).
- Ventricular diverticula are most likely congenital disorders; they have been reported to be associated with congenital anomalies, including septal defects, pulmonary stenosis, dextrocardia, and aortic valvular disease.
- Large diverticula can predispose to thrombus formation and peripheral arterial embolization.
- There are two types: muscular and fibrous. The muscular type contracts normally. Fibrous forms often are akinetic or dyskinetic.
- A wide range of diameters has been reported, from 0.5 to 9 cm, but most commonly ventricular diverticula are < 1.5 cm in diameter and feature a narrow feeding neck.

Other Imaging Findings

- Catheter angiography shows diastolic filling and systolic emptying.

✔ Pearls & ✘ Pitfalls

✔ Multidetector computed tomography has shown that congenital ventricular aneurysms are more common than previously thought. They are typically seen arising from the LV as an incidental finding.

✘ Aneurysms and pseudoaneurysms of the LV can have a similar appearance. Clinical history and functional analysis (dynamic images) are helpful to differentiate them.

Case 60

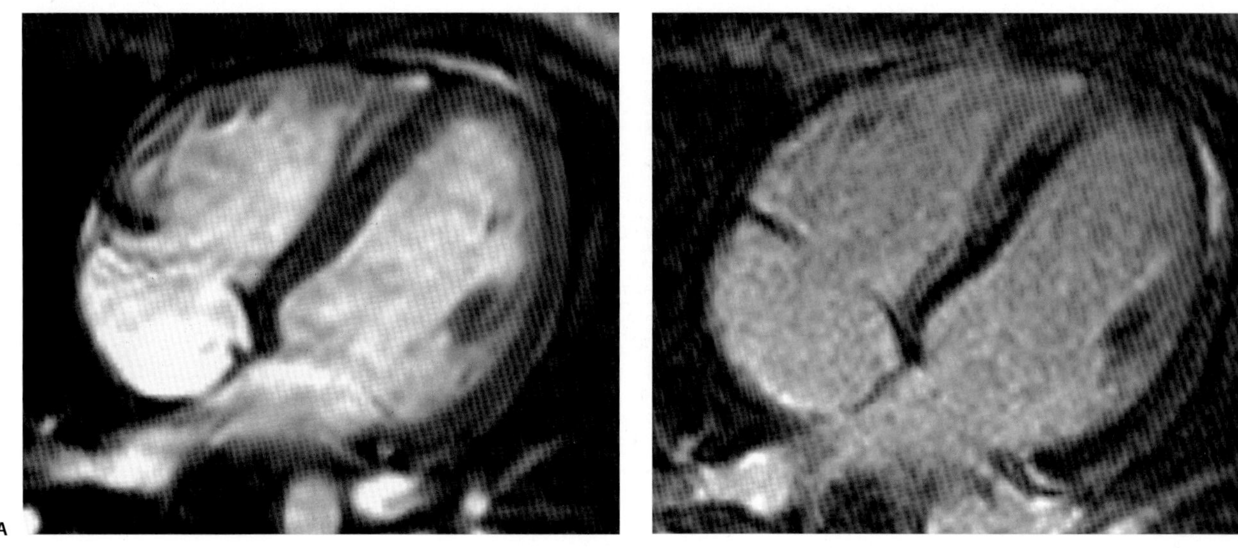

A B

Clinical Presentation

A 46-year-old woman presents with acute onset of chest pain.

Imaging Findings

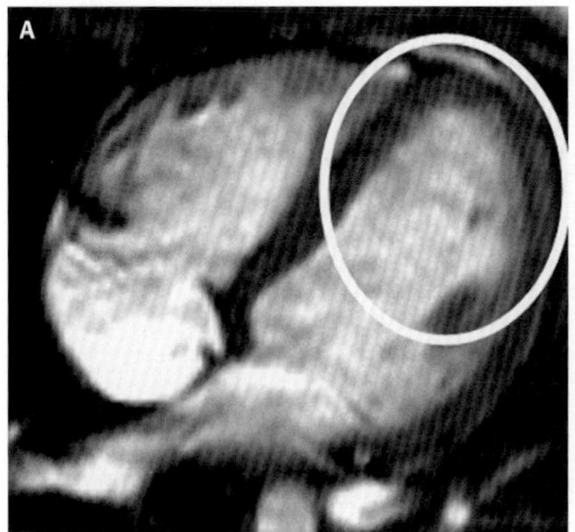

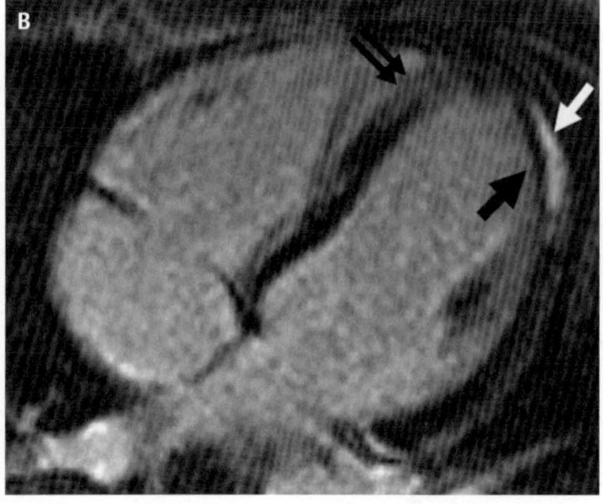

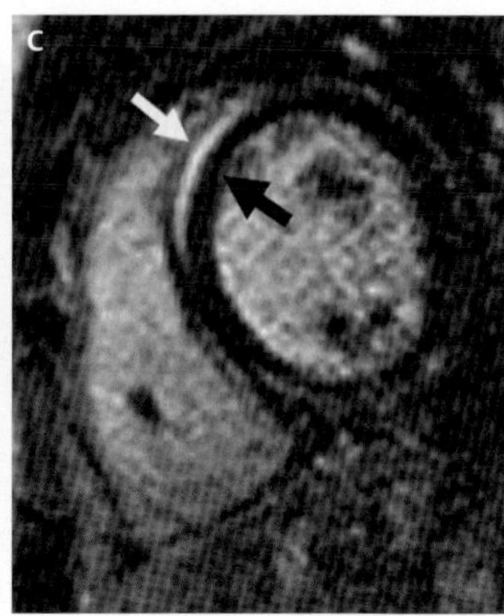

(A) In the four-chamber view, the right ventricle and left ventricle (LV) are dilated, and the distal septal and lateral walls and apex are hyperintense compared with the other segments of myocardium (*white oval*). Also note the irregular margin of the myocardium in the distal septal wall compared with the well-defined septum at the base of the heart. **(B,C)** Following intravenous administration of gadolinium, delayed images were performed in the four-chamber and short-axis views. The distal septal and lateral and anteroseptal walls are enhancing abnormally. The enhancement of the lateral and anteroseptal walls is very intense (*white arrows*) and spares the endocardial surface (*single black arrows*). The distal septal wall does not enhance as intensely, but the enhancement is transmural (*double black arrows*).

Differential Diagnosis

- ***LV myocarditis:*** The involvement of the lateral and apical walls of the LV, along with the pattern of enhancement that spares the subendocardial surface of the LV, is indicative of myocarditis.
- *Myocardial infarction:* The pattern of myocardial enhancement does not conform to a vascular territory. Lack of enhancement of the subendocardial myocardium suggests that this is an incorrect diagnosis.
- *Ischemic cardiomyopathy:* Dilatation of the LV chamber can be seen in patients with ischemic cardiomyopathy, but the myocardial signal should remain normal on nonenhanced images.

Essential Facts

- Myocarditis is an injury of the myocardium, usually an inflammatory process due to viral infection.
- Myocarditis progresses from a focal myocardial disease to generalized disease over several days, beginning with interstitial edema and lymphocyte infiltration.
- Myocarditis tends to involve the lateral and apical walls of the LV.
- The clinical and symptomatic aspects of cardiomyopathy mimic myocardial infarction.
- Myocarditis affects the myocardium in a distribution that does not follow a coronary artery vascular distribution.
- Myocardial blood flow is maintained in myocarditis.
- In late and chronic stages, myocarditis progresses to dilated cardiomyopathy.
- Patients determined to have myocarditis generally are younger and have few cardiovascular risk factors than do the typical patients with myocardial infarction.

Other Imaging Findings

- Early or first-pass contrast-enhanced magnetic resonance imaging sequences show normal myocardial perfusion in patients with myocarditis.
- Nodular hyperenhancement in the myocardium also suggests the diagnosis of myocarditis.
- The paraspinal skeletal muscles may show enhancement on postgadolinium T1 sequences.

✔ Pearls & ✘ Pitfalls

✔ Use a combination of functional precontrast imaging along with early and late postgadolinium imaging to differentiate myocarditis from myocardial infarction.

✔ Cine white blood images reveal segmental wall motion abnormalities.

✘ Focal enhancement may be subtle during the early phase of disease because of only focal myocardial involvement and minimal cellular disruption.

✘ Repeat imaging 7 to 10 days later is suggested in patients with equivocal or minimal findings. Myocarditis progresses from a focal myocardial disease to generalized disease over several days, beginning with interstitial edema and lymphocyte infiltration.

Case 61

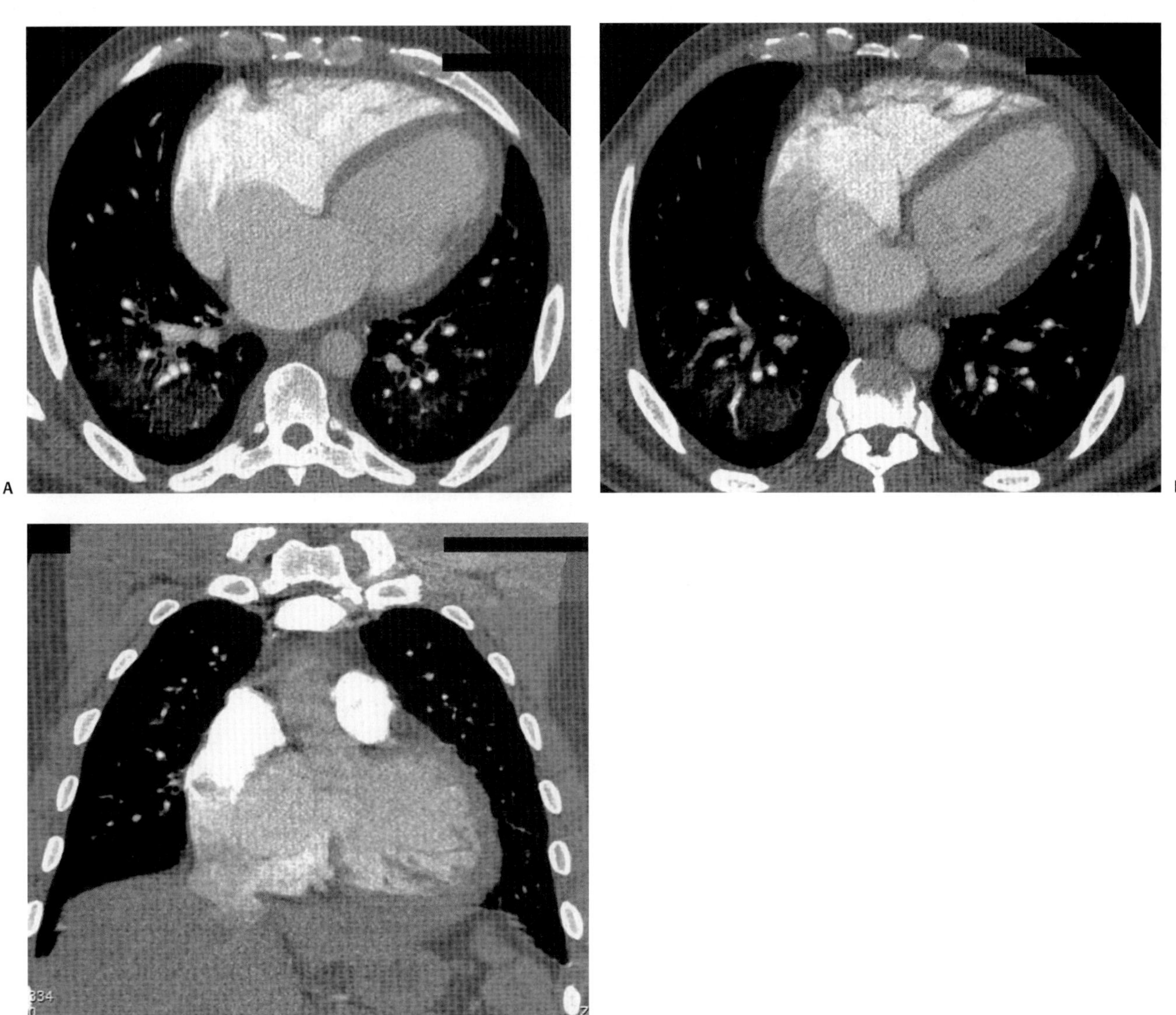

Clinical Presentation

Pulmonary embolism protocol in a 42-year-old man with chest pain (CT)

Imaging Findings

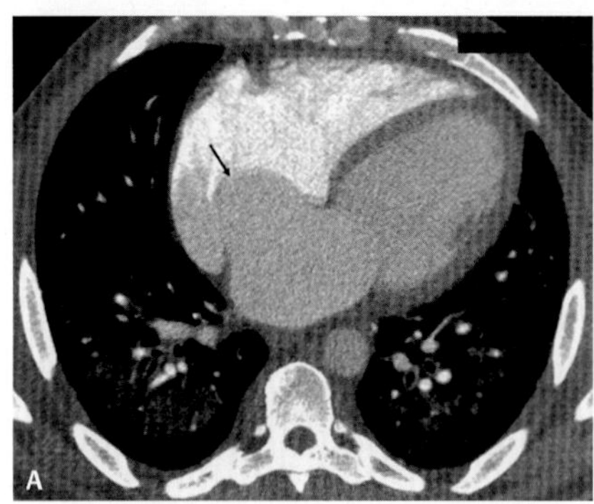

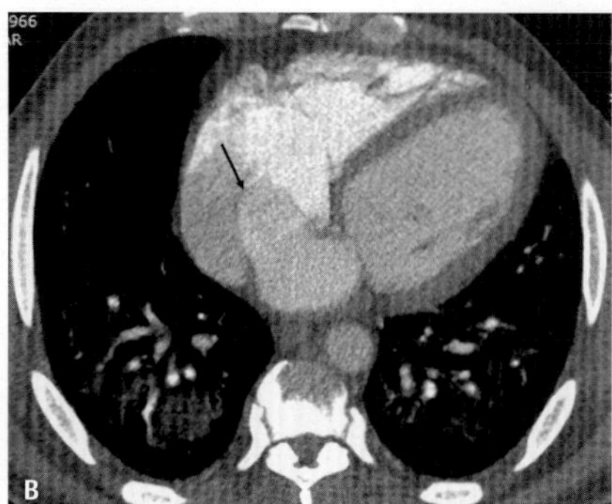

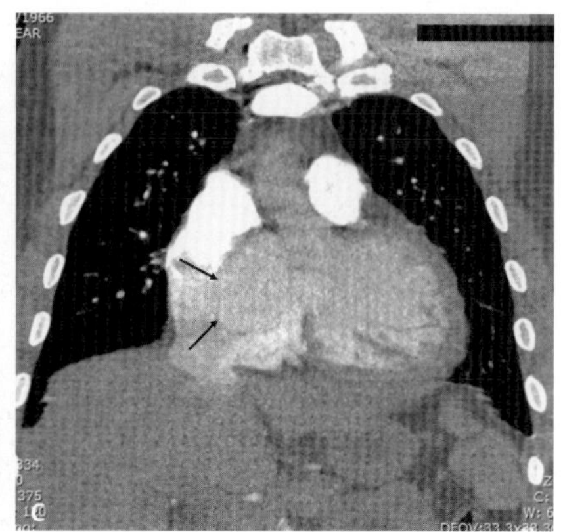

Contrast-enhanced multidetector CT **(A,B)** axial and **(C)** coronal images show an abnormal protrusion or outpouching of the interatrial septum from the expected central and midline position into the right atrium.

Differential Diagnosis

- ***Interatrial septal aneurysm (IASA):*** IASA is characterized by an abnormal protrusion of the interatrial septum toward either the right or left atrium.
- *Accessory appendage of the left atrium:* Accessory appendages of the left atrium are common (10%), more often seen as small diverticulum-like structures projecting from the right upper side of the left atrial wall.

Essential Facts

- The prevalence of IASA was between 2 and 5% in a transesophageal echoradiography (TEE) series.
- The etiology of IASA is probably congenital.
- IASA is seen as a thin linear mobile structure < 2 mm thick.
- The fossa ovalis is commonly involved.
- Most commonly, the IASA protrudes into the right atrium (90%).
- An association with interatrial shunting is common (patent foramen ovale, atrial septal defect).
- Other common associations are mitral valve prolapse (23%) and aneurysm of the sinus of Valsalva (5%).

Other Imaging Findings

- Interventricular septal aneurysm can also occur. In adults, the diagnostic criterion for interatrial or interventricular septal aneurysm is bowing of the septum > 15 mm to either side (> 5 mm in children), and the entire septum should not be involved.

✔ Pearls & ✘ Pitfalls

✔ A strong association between IASA and stroke and peripheral arterial embolism has been found (44–58%), with an increased annual stroke rate (3.8%).

✘ Identification of IASA on CT in nongated acquisition or without the saline chaser technique is very limited because of the very thin appearance of the protruding wall and similar density within the right and left atria. Similarly, transthoracic echocardiography has lower sensitivity than TEE for this diagnosis.

Case 62

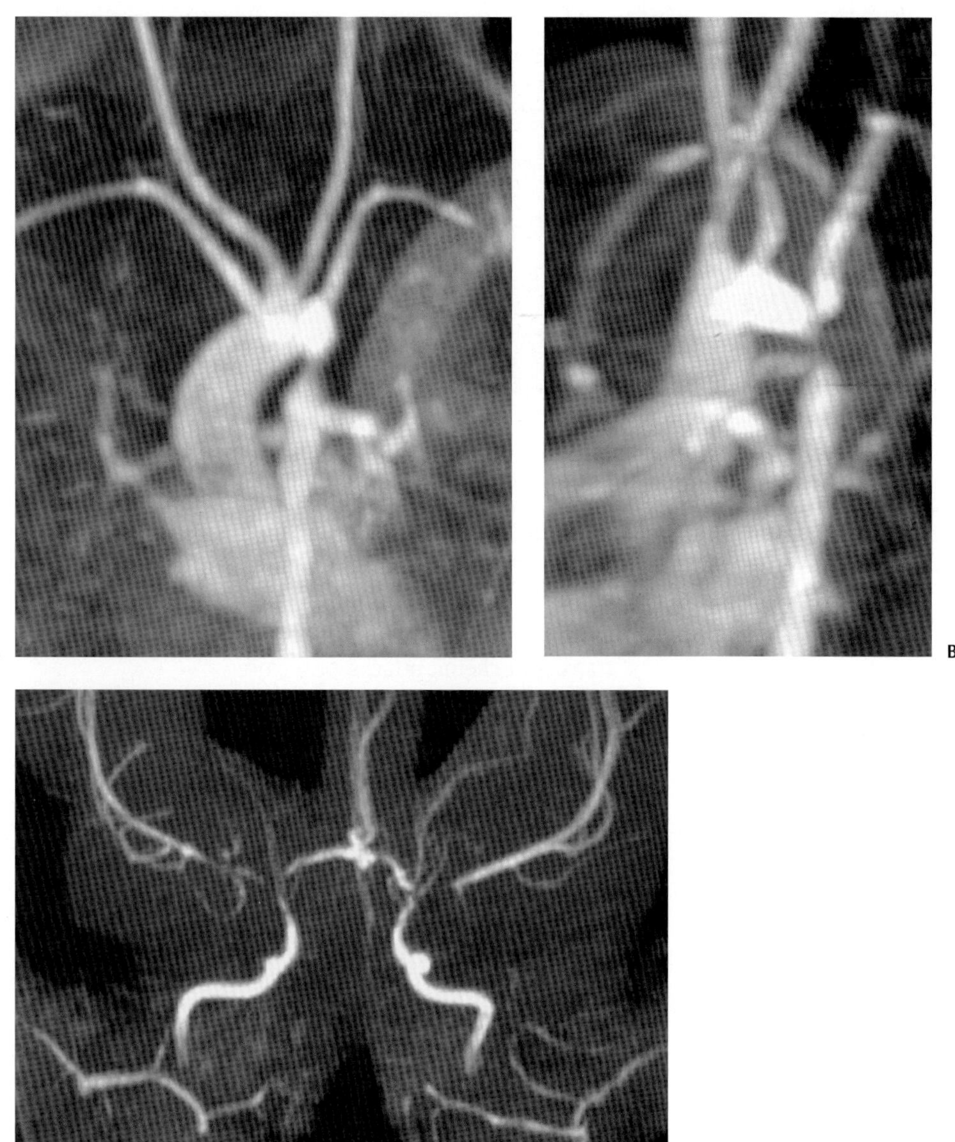

Clinical Presentation

A 4-year-old boy presents with new findings of hypertension and left-sided weakness.

Imaging Findings

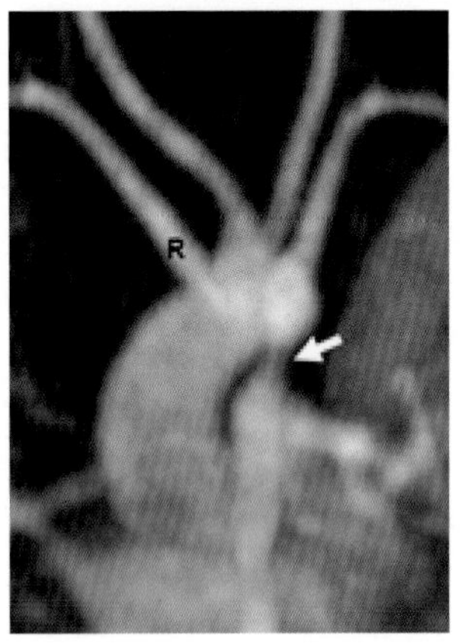

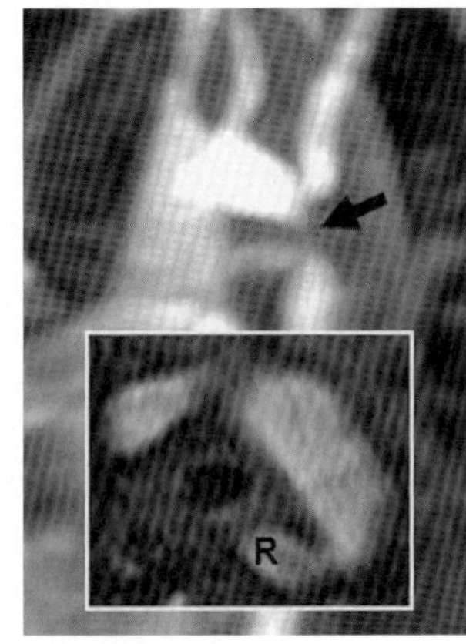

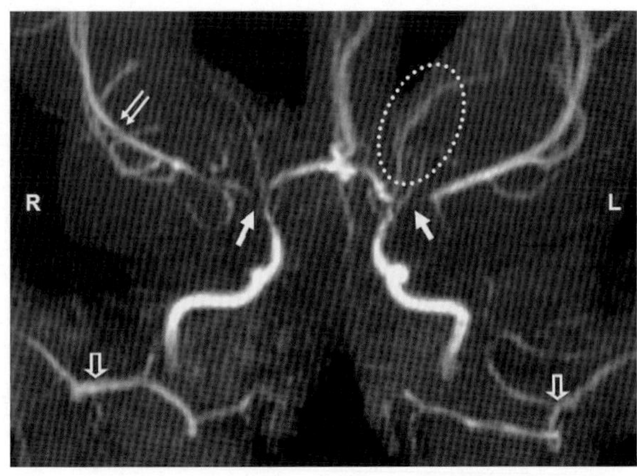

(A) In the AP view the aortic arch is left sided and there are four brachiocephalic vessels arising from the arch. The right subclavian artery (*R*) is the last branch; its origin is at the site of the isthmus, where there is a moderate narrowing (*white arrow*). **(B)** The LAO view of the aortic arch again shows discrete narrowing of the isthmus (*black arrow*). The abnormal branching pattern of the brachiocephalic arteries is shown in the axial view (*inset*) which shows the aberrant origin and course of the right subclavian artery (*R*), behind the trachea and esophagus. **(C)** A coronal oblique view of an intracranial three-dimensional time-of-flight magnetic resonance angiogram (MRA) reveals tapering of the distal internal carotid arteries, severe stenosis of the origins of the middle and anterior cerebral arteries (*white arrows*), enlarged lenticulostriate vessels (*dotted oval*), and decreased caliber of the distal branches of the middle cerebral artery (*double white arrows*). The external carotid branches are enlarged (*open white arrows*).

Differential Diagnosis

- ***Coarctation of the aorta, aberrant right subclavian artery, and moyamoya disease:*** Discrete narrowing of the aortic isthmus is diagnostic of coarctation, in this case associated with aberrant origin of the right subclavian artery. The intracranial MRA is diagnostic of moyamoya.
- *Arteritis:* The diagnosis of arteritis is an excellent consideration, as numerous vascular beds are involved.
- *Embolic arterial occlusion:* Given the history of new stroke symptoms, one must consider thrombotic, embolic, and other possibilities. However, the intracranial MRA findings are diagnostic and are known to have an association with some forms of congenital heart disease.

Essential Facts

- Coarctation of the aorta represents 5% of congenital heart defects and may be found in association with other structural defects of the heart, commonly ventricular septal defect.
- In coarctation of the aorta, numerous abnormalities of the aorta can be found, including bicuspid aortic valve, hypoplasia of the aortic arch, anomalous origin of the right subclavian artery, and stenosis of the left subclavian artery origin.
- Coarctation occurs at the site of the ductus arteriosus, presumably because ductal tissue, which narrows in the postnatal period as pulmonary resistance decreases, is to some degree incorporated in the wall of the aorta and occasionally the origin of the left subclavian artery.
- Moyamoya disease and intracranial aneurysms may be seen in these patients.
- Moyamoya has been found to be associated with congenital heart disease—namely, coarctation of the aorta and tetralogy of Fallot.
- Moyamoya has also been reported in association with Down syndrome, which is commonly associated with endocardial cushion defects.
- Moyamoya disease often presents with ischemic stroke, transient ischemic attacks, or seizure.
- Children with structural heart disease may also have cerebral vascular disease, such as moyamoya, arterial vascular malformations, and venous (vein of Galen) malformations.
- The most common complications after coarctation repair are recurrence of coarctation and formation of an aneurysm at the repair site.

Other Imaging Findings

- Collateral arteries develop in the intercostal, bronchial, paraspinal, and mesenteric vascular beds to bypass the level of coarctation.
- Coarctation of the left pulmonary artery can also occur as the ductus arteriosus closes.
- There may be an intimal "ridge" of tissue contributing to the luminal narrowing.

✔ Pearls & ✘ Pitfalls

✔ Coarctation of the aorta can be isolated or simple (i.e., not associated with other forms of congenital heart disease) or complex (i.e., found in association with structural congenital heart disease).

✔ Patients with complex congenital heart disease that includes coarctation of the aorta are much more likely to present in infancy or childhood than those with simple or isolated coarctation of the aorta, which may not be discovered until adulthood.

✘ The terms *preductal* (infantile) and *postductal* (adult), classically used to classify the type of coarctation, are confusing because the "location" of the coarctation is less important than the severity of the stenosis.

Case 63

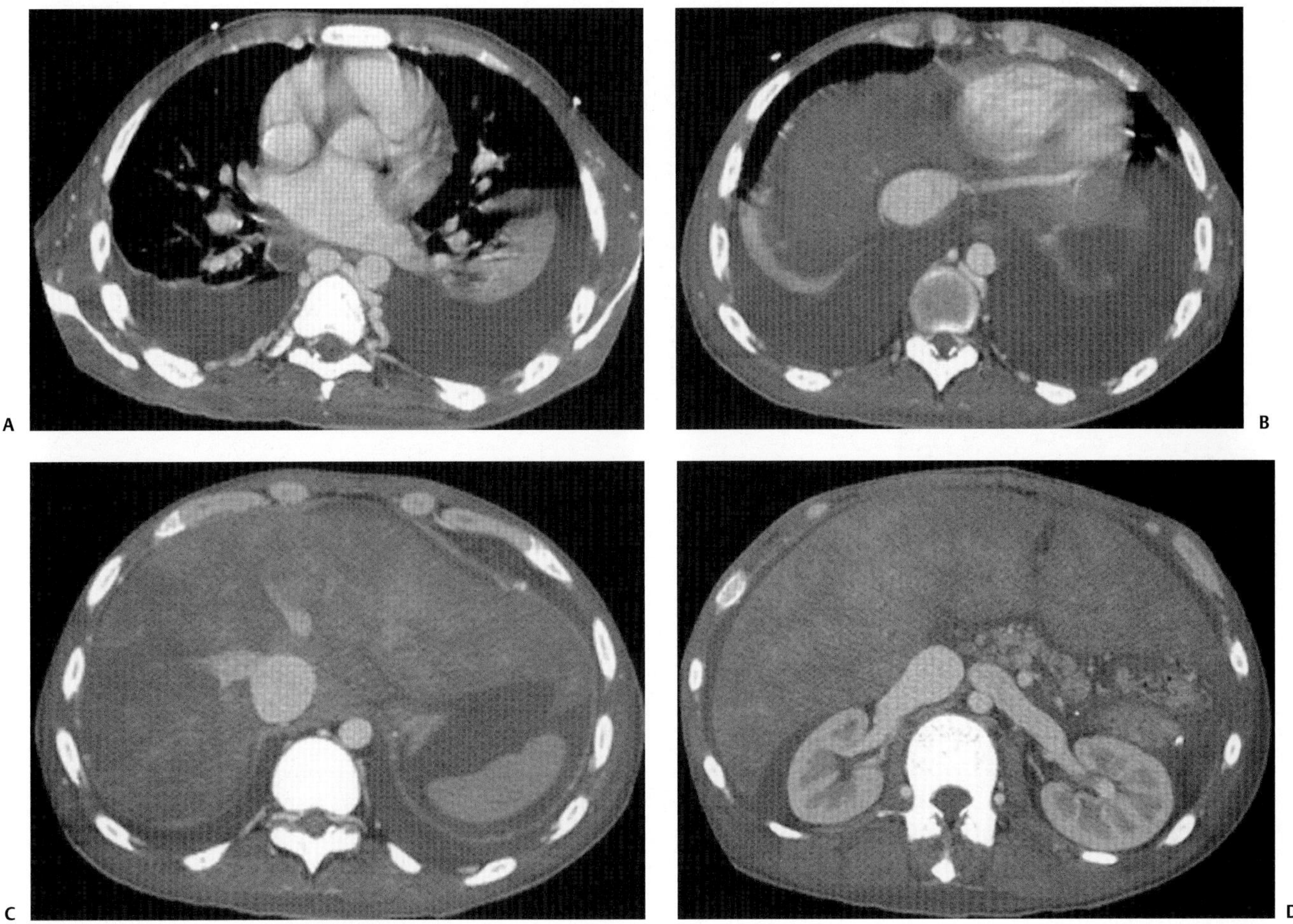

■ Clinical Presentation

Progressive shortness of breath, ascites, and lower extremity edema in a 24-year-old man

Imaging Findings

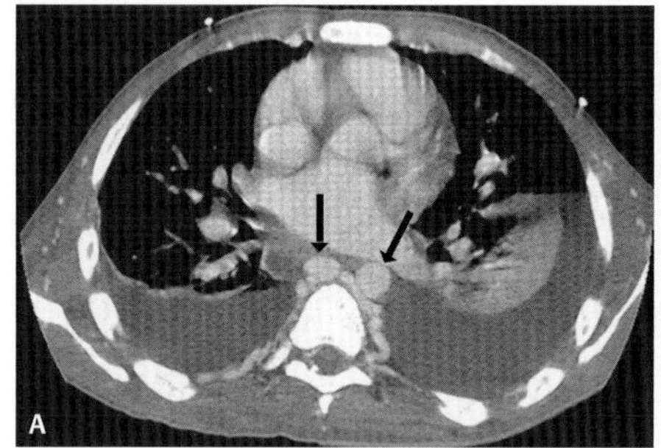

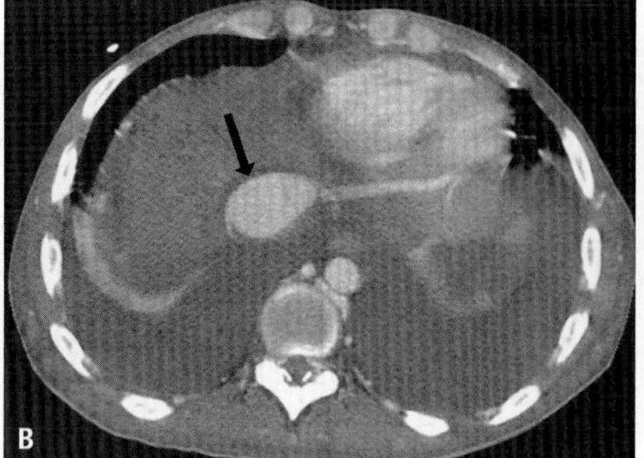

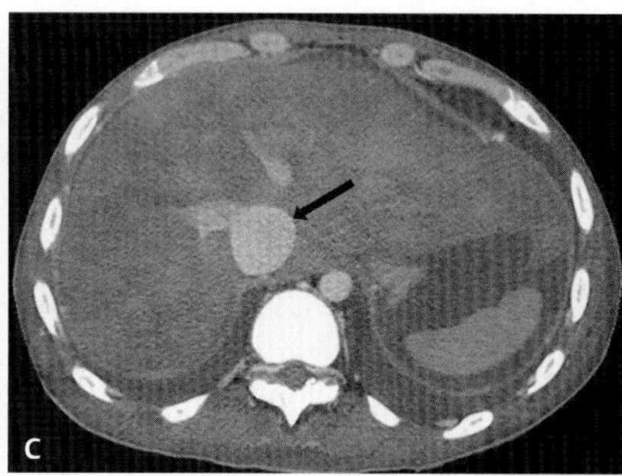

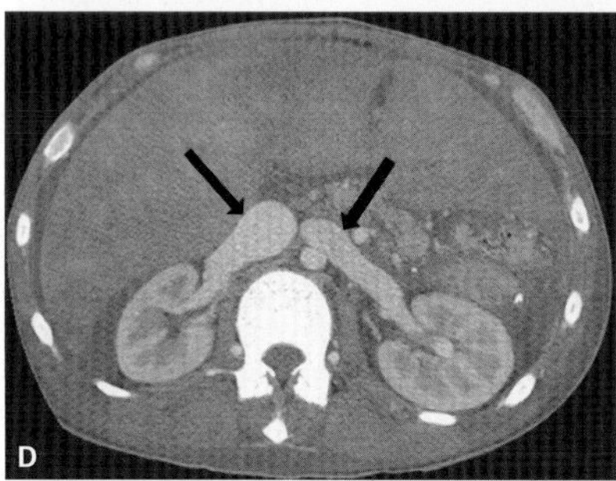

(A–D) Contrast-enhanced computed tomography (CT) images of the lower chest and upper abdomen reveal the abnormal prominence of dilated azygos and hemiazygos veins, phrenic veins, inferior vena cava, and renal veins. The heart is normal in size. Bilateral pleural effusions are noted, as well as ascites and congestive appearance of the liver.

Differential Diagnosis

- ***Restrictive cardiomyopathy (RCM):*** RCM is the least common of the three types of cardiomyopathies (dilated, hypertrophic, and restrictive). The World Health Organization defines it as a myocardial disease characterized by restrictive filling and reduced diastolic volume of either or both ventricles with normal or near-normal systolic function and wall thickness. Imaging findings show normal-size ventricles with some degree of atrial enlargement and normal appearance of the pericardium.
- *Constrictive pericarditis:* In constrictive pericarditis, there is abnormally increased systemic venous pressure and low cardiac output. The condition is also characterized by a thick, noncompliant, and often calcified pericardium that encases the heart, resulting in decreased diastolic filling and low systemic output.

Essential Facts

- RCM can be idiopathic (primary) or secondary to an infiltrative heart muscle disease that is the myocardial manifestation of a systemic disorder (e.g., amyloidosis, hemochromatosis, sarcoidosis, or scleroderma).
- RCMs are relatively rare disorders. The exact prevalence is not well-known and varies by region. In the United States, the most common form is idiopathic. In temperate and tropical regions of the world, Loeffler endocarditis (hypereosinophilic) and endomyocardial fibrosis are more common.
- The disease affects either or both ventricles, but often right side findings predominate.
- Patients present with gradually worsening fatigue, dyspnea, and right heart failure with progressive ascites and lower extremity edema.
- The natural history of RCM is generally poor, particularly in children. Affected patients typically have a long course of heart failure, which may be complicated by cirrhosis secondary to chronic hepatic congestion (cardiac cirrhosis), thromboembolism, arrhythmia, and progressive worsening of cardiac function.
- Echocardiography shows a nondilated, normally contracting left ventricle with normal wall thickness and dilated atria. In cases of an infiltrative disease like amyloidosis, an abnormal myocardial echotexture can also be appreciated.

Other Imaging Findings

- In patients with myocardial amyloidosis, contrast-enhanced magnetic resonance imaging shows widespread heterogeneous enhancement of the myocardium on delayed postcontrast inversion recovery T1-weighted gradient echo images.

✔ Pearls & ✘ Pitfalls

✔ When required, endomyocardial biopsy can be performed and is particularly useful to differentiate between endomyocardial fibrosis and infiltrative processes like amyloidosis.

✘ The clinical presentation of RCM and that of constrictive pericarditis can be very similar. Distinction between these two entities is crucial, as treatment and prognosis are entirely different.

Case 64

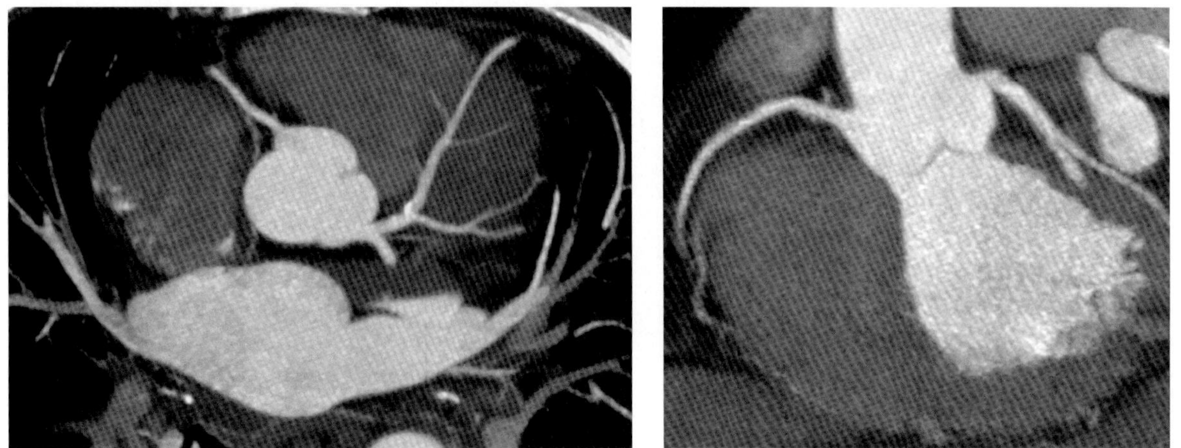

Clinical Presentation

A 73-year-old man presents with a history of hypertension, heart failure, and diabetes, as well as chronic atrial fibrillation.

Imaging Findings

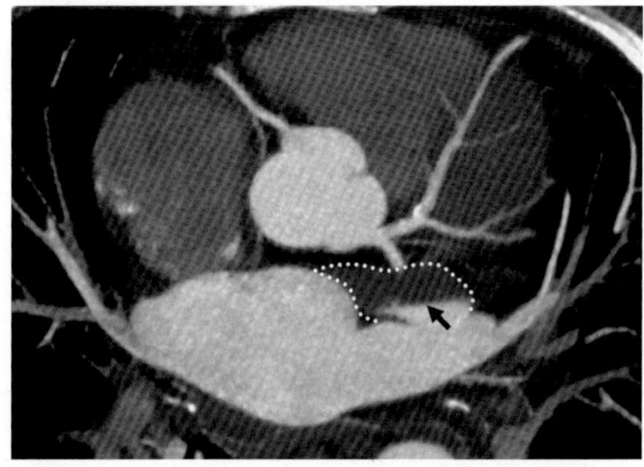

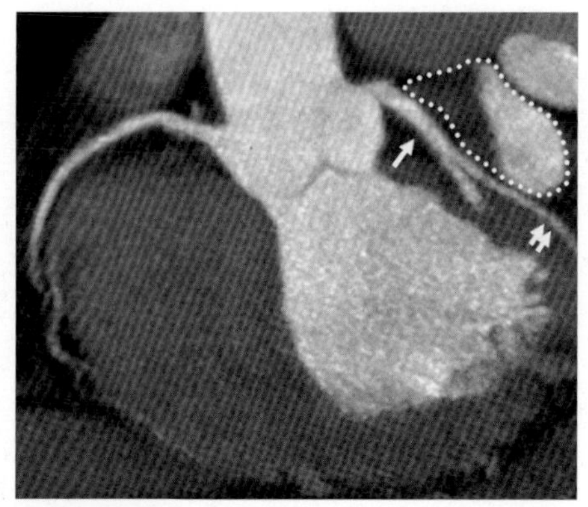

(A) In this axial maximum intensity projection image, the coronary anatomy is well seen, with only mild atherosclerotic disease in the left main and left anterior descending arteries. The left atrial appendage (LAA: *outlined with dotted white line*) does not fill completely with contrast, as it is partially filled with thrombus (*black arrow*). **(B)** In a coronal oblique image, the course of the left main (*white arrow*) and left circumflex (*double white arrow*) arteries and their relationship to the LAA (*dotted white line*) are seen. This relationship is important when a procedure to occlude the LAA is considered. Extrinsic compression of the coronary is theoretically possible if an LAA occlusion device expands the LAA.

Differential Diagnosis

- ***LAA thrombus:*** Soft-tissue-attenuation material in the distal LAA does not extend into the left atrial chamber. The tissue is well marginated.
- *LAA neoplasm:* The sharply defined tissue in the LAA is attached to a motionless (akinetic) wall; both are characteristic of chronic thrombus rather than neoplasm.
- *Left atrial thrombus:* The filling defect is clearly contained within the atrial appendage; it does not extend through the narrow mouth of the LAA into the atrial chamber.

Essential Facts

- The LAA, shaped like a windsock, has a narrow orifice.
- The LAA abuts the left pulmonary artery and overlies the bifurcation of the left main coronary artery.
- During atrial systole and during other periods when left atrial pressure is high, the LAA functions as a decompression chamber.
- Obliteration or amputation of the LAA may help to reduce the risk for thromboembolism, but it may result in undesirable physiologic sequelae such as reduced atrial compliance and a reduced capacity for atrial natriuretic factor secretion in response to pressure and volume overload.

Other Imaging Findings

- An echoic mass within the LAA on echo is helpful in the diagnosis but is frequently not detected with conventional two-dimensional transthoracic echocardiography (TTE).
- Transesophageal echocardiography is more sensitive than TTE in the detection of thrombus.
- Sensitivity of CT for detection of LAA thrombus can be increased by repeated contrast injection or delayed imaging.

✔ Pearls & ✘ Pitfalls

✔ Always look for LAA thrombus in patients with a history of atrial fibrillation.

✔ LAA thrombus can also be found in patients with a history of mitral valve disease or rheumatic valve disease.

✔ Specifically mention the presence or absence of LAA thrombus in reports of CT or magnetic resonance examinations performed to define pulmonary vein anatomy before ablation procedures.

✔ Cardiac thrombus develops on a motionless segment of the wall. A mass on a moving wall is a muscle bundle or neoplasm and is not thrombus.

✔ Chronic LAA thrombus is likely to be a smoothly marginated rather than an irregular filling defect.

✘ Stasis of blood in the LAA can appear similar to thrombus.

✘ Embolic disease from a cardiac source is more likely to be the presenting sign of an atrial mass (myxoma) rather than LAA thrombus.

Case 65

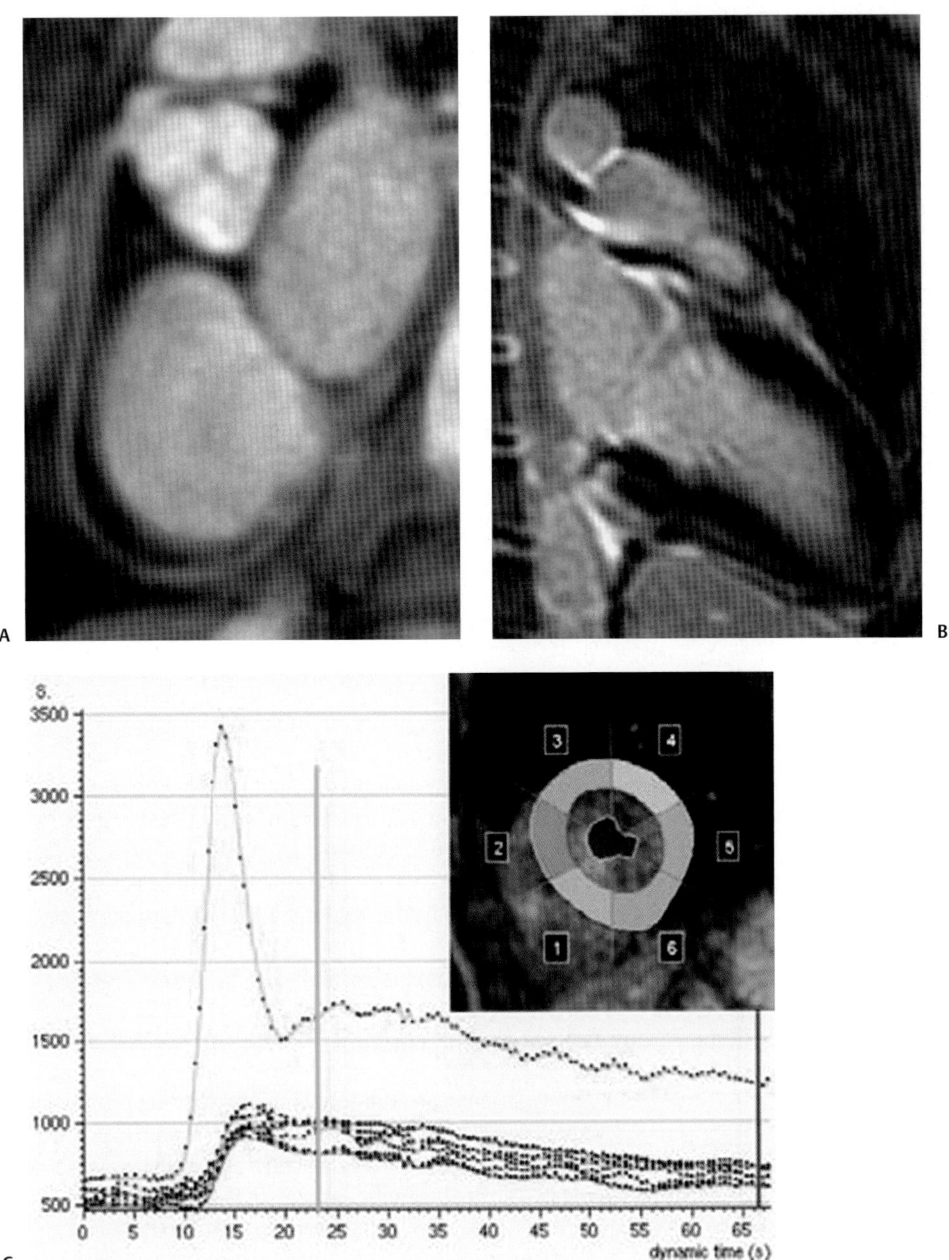

■ Clinical Presentation

A 15-year-old girl with a question of aortic valve stenosis as an infant but without heart-related symptoms underwent echocardiography for a school physical. The origin of the left coronary artery could not be found.

Imaging Findings

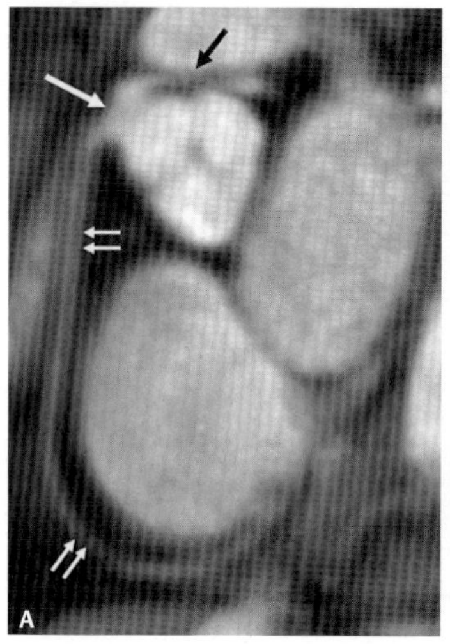
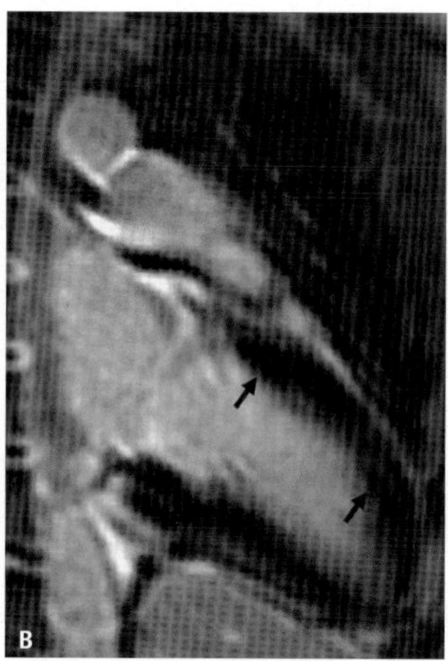
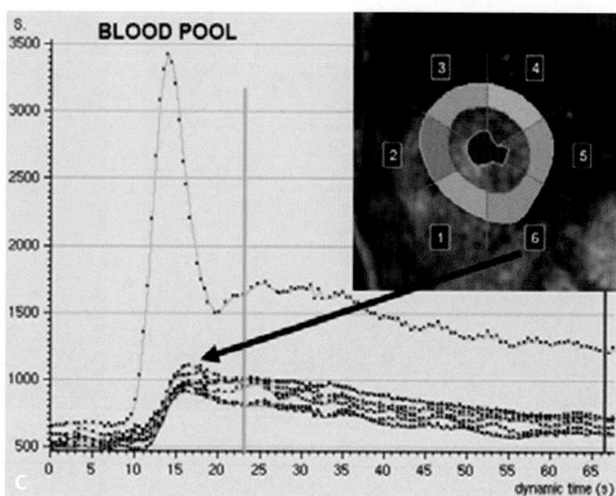

(A) The left main and right coronary arteries arise from the right sinus of Valsalva (*white arrow*). The left coronary (*black arrow*) is narrowed as it courses between the ascending aorta and main pulmonary artery. The course of the right coronary (*double white arrows*) is normal. **(B)** In a two-chamber view, the left ventricle (LV) myocardium is completely suppressed after gadolinium is given intravenously (*black arrows*). There is no abnormal enhancement to suggest this young girl has had an infarction. **(C)** The time–intensity curve shows the peak intensity and the washout of contrast in the blood pool (*blue curve*). A short-axis view of the middle LV (*inset*) shows segmental division of the myocardium (numbered *1–6*). In graphic form, the upslope of the signal change is equal between segments (*black arrow*), indicating a perfusion defect is not present. Although research is ongoing, there are currently no commercially available methods to quantify myocardial perfusion.

Differential Diagnosis

- There really is no differential diagnosis, given the clear depiction of the coronary artery origins. One must be confident in the normal position of each coronary sinus.
- Anomalous coronary artery origin is an uncommon finding. The combined incidence of anomalous origin of the right or left coronary artery from the left or right aortic cusps ranges from 0.17% in autopsies to 1.2% of patients undergoing cardiac catheterization.
- The incidence of the left main artery arising from the right coronary cusp is 0.15%.

Essential Facts

- Anomalous origin of a coronary artery is seen in < 1% of the general population.
- Coronary anomalies are implicated in chest pain, sudden death, syncope, myocardial infarction, and ventricular arrhythmia.
- The reason for the association with sudden death is controversial.
- "Malignant," potentially lethal forms of anomalous coronary artery origin include right coronary artery origin from the left and left main artery origin from the right, with the course of the artery between the main pulmonary artery and the ascending aorta.
- Given this course, there is presumably extrinsic compression of the proximal segment of the anomalous vessel during systole, as the caliber of the main pulmonary artery and aorta increase.
- Alternatively, the origin of the anomalous coronary artery may be at an acute angle from the anomalous orifice, resulting in narrowing of the vessel.
- The proximal course of the anomalous artery may be in the wall of the ascending aorta.
- The course of an anomalous coronary artery between the ascending aorta and the left atrium or over the conus is commonly referred to as "benign."
- Early diagnosis is made in children of school age as they become more involved in athletics, thus increasing physical activity.
- Prenatal development is normal.

Other Imaging Findings

- In young patients, an additional imaging finding is unlikely.
- Myocardial wall motion abnormalities may be seen in defined vascular distributions, correlating with the anomalous vessel.
- Adenosine stress magnetic resonance (MR) perfusion imaging may show myocardial perfusion defects.
- The noncoronary cusp and sinus of Valsalva lie adjacent to the interatrial septum.

✔ Pearls & ✘ Pitfalls

✔ Axial oblique two-dimensional images of the aortic valve and sinuses of Valsalva are essential for diagnosis.

✔ Multidetector computed tomography (CT) and three-dimensional MR images of the coronary arteries are diagnostic; the new gold standard is multidetector CT.

✔ MR is increasingly an excellent imaging modality as coil construction and gradients improve.

✘ It may be impossible to engage the origin of an anomalous coronary artery with standard catheters during cardiac catheterization. Therefore, cross-sectional imaging studies are essential in making the diagnosis.

Case 66

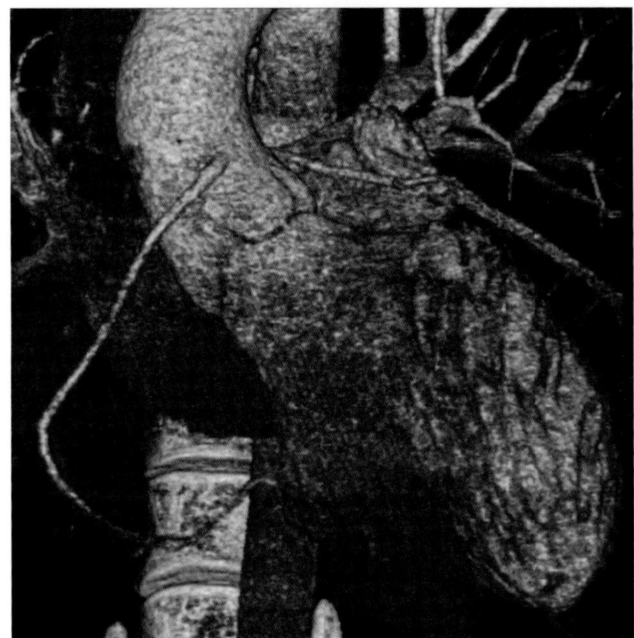
A

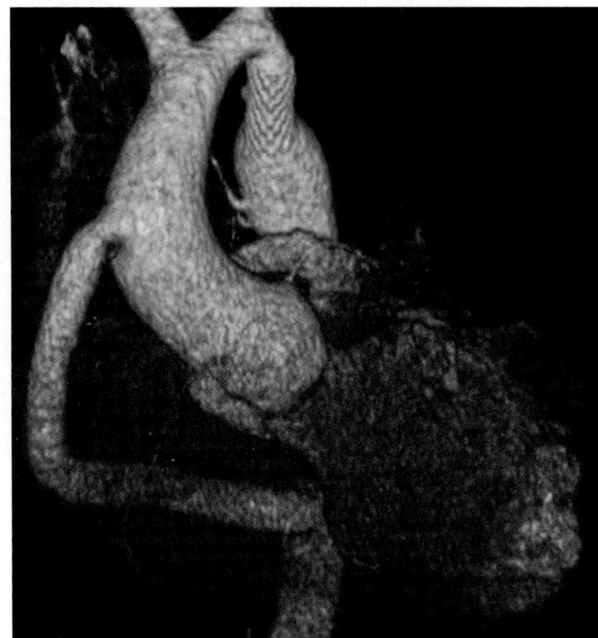
B

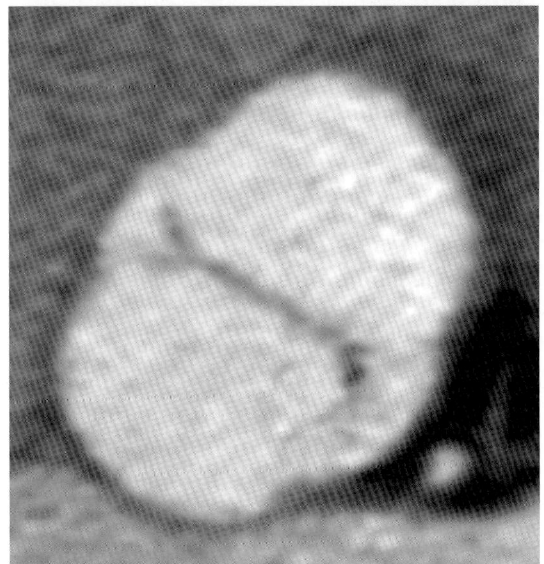
C

Clinical Presentation

A 15-year-old boy presents with a history of coarctation of the aorta, for which a stent was placed 9 years ago; the stent partially covers the origin of the left subclavian artery. A surgical procedure was performed recently to relieve the patient's persistent left upper extremity and lower extremity hypotension.

Imaging Findings

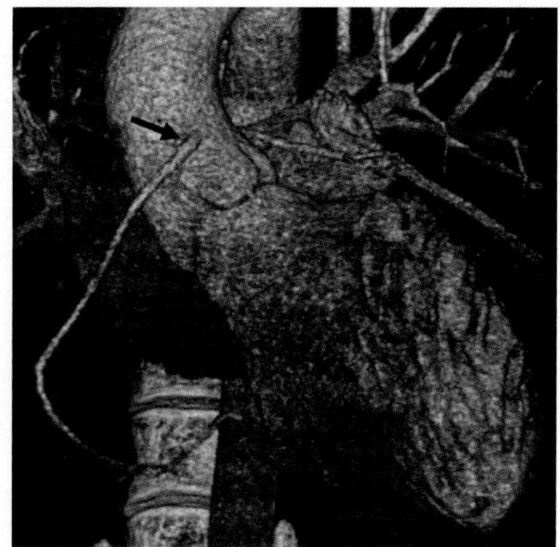
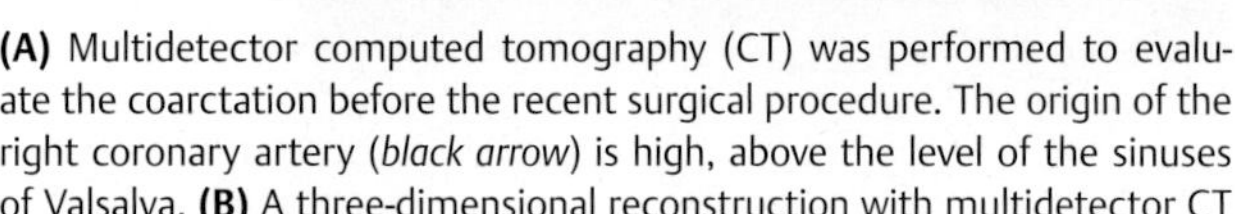
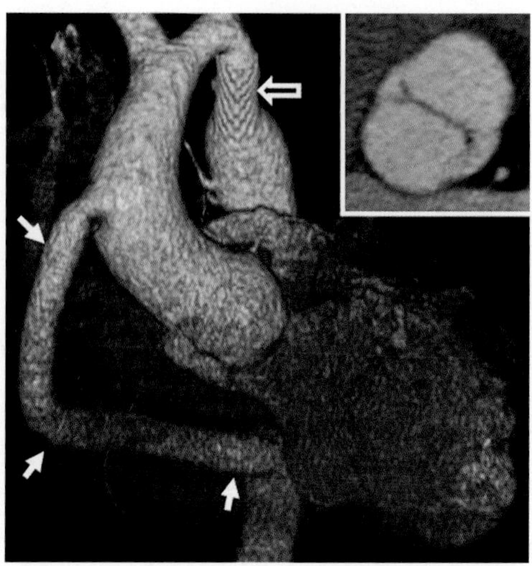

(A) Multidetector computed tomography (CT) was performed to evaluate the coarctation before the recent surgical procedure. The origin of the right coronary artery (*black arrow*) is high, above the level of the sinuses of Valsalva. **(B)** A three-dimensional reconstruction with multidetector CT data following surgery shows the patent newly placed aorta–aortic bypass graft (*white arrows*) and the stent (*open arrow*) at the site of the coarctation. Notice the diffuse hypoplasia of the aortic arch. The aortic valve is bicuspid (*inset*).

Differential Diagnosis

- ***Coarctation of the aorta, hypoplastic aortic arch, and aorta–aortic bypass:*** The patient has known coarctation of the aorta with persistent hypotension. The preoperative findings that relate to persistent hypertension are diffuse hypoplasia of the aortic arch and partial obstruction of the left subclavian artery origin by the stent at the site of the coarctation. An aorta–aortic graft bypasses these areas to supply increased visceral and lower extremity blood flow.
- *Interruption of the aortic arch:* Although the aortic arch is of small caliber, there is no interruption.
- *Aortic dissection related to stent placement:* Although it is possible to see dissection of the aorta as a complication of stent placement and angioplasty, the diffuse narrowing of the aortic arch and the absence of a false lumen indicate other diagnoses.

Essential Facts

- Coarctation of the aorta may be either a focal or a diffuse segmental narrowing of the aortic lumen.
- There may be a posterior "shelf" of medial tissue on the posterior wall of the aorta that acts as the focal point of obstruction.
- When diffuse, the coarctation is more likely associated with other cardiac malformations.
- As the ductus arteriosus closes and ductal tissue shrinks, the severity of the coarctation may increase.
- Aortic obstruction causes increased afterload of the left ventricle, leading to hypertension in the upper extremities; hypotension is found in the lower extremities.
- Coarctation of the aorta is found in up to 36% of girls with Turner syndrome.

Other Imaging Findings

- Aortic arch hypoplasia and a bicuspid aortic valve are sometimes seen.
- Premature atherosclerosis is seen in the coronary arteries.
- Dilatation of the left subclavian artery and the intercostal arteries occurs in 5% of patients.

✔ Pearls & ✘ Pitfalls

✔ The description of coarctation as "preductal" versus "postductal" is outdated. Currently, the term *juxtaductal* is used to more accurately describe the anatomical pathology.

✘ Patent ductus arteriosus may lessen the degree of coarctation.

✘ A patent ductus arteriosus may allow perfusion of organs distal to the level of coarctation.

Case 67

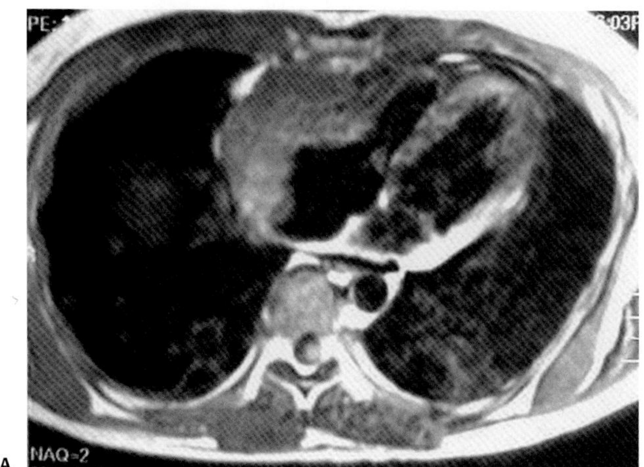

A

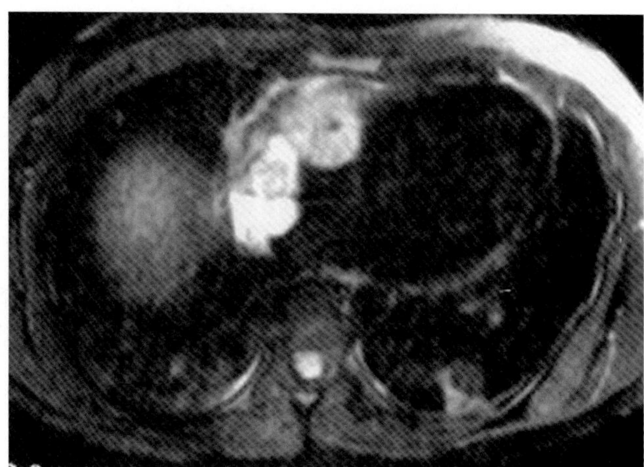
B

Clinical Presentation

Dyspnea and chest pain in a 42-year-old woman

Imaging Findings

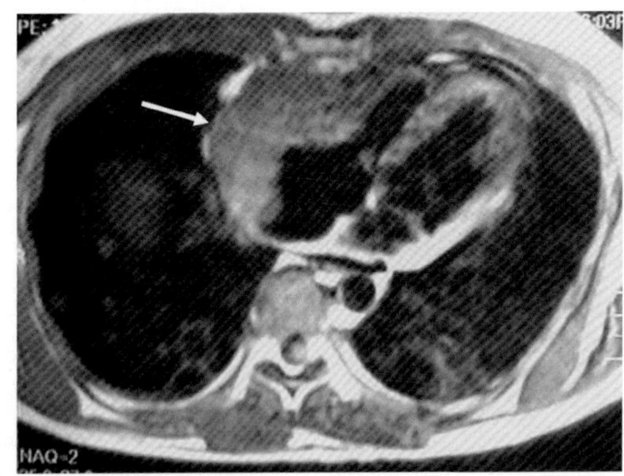

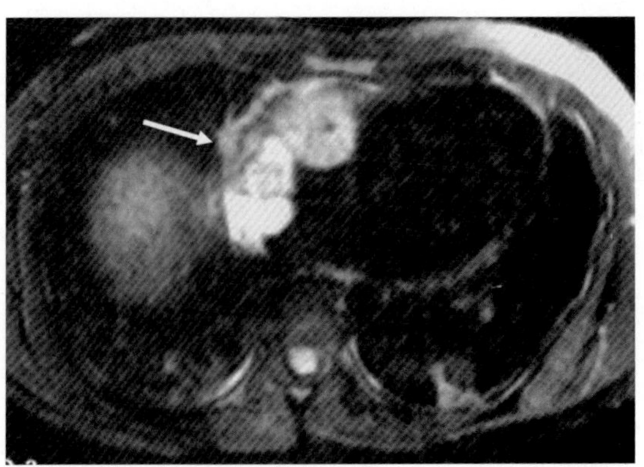

(A) Axial and **(B)** fat-suppressed T1-weighted magnetic resonance (MR) images after gadolinium injection show an abnormal, irregularly enhancing soft-tissue mass infiltrating the lateral wall of the right atrium and right ventricle. No pericardial effusion is noted. Incidental notice is made of bibasilar pulmonary parenchymal opacities.

Differential Diagnosis

- ***Angiosarcoma of the right atrium:*** This is one of the most prevalent primary cardiac malignant tumors, with 80% of cardiac angiosarcomas occurring in the right atrium.
- *Cardiac lymphoma:* Primary cardiac lymphomas (typically large B-cell lymphoma) present in immunocompromised patients and middle-aged men. In most cases, multiple masses are present, invading multiple chambers in addition to the pericardium.
- *Cardiac metastasis:* Cardiac metastases are the most common malignant tumors. They are often associated with pericardial metastasis, so the association of a soft-tissue mass and a pericardial mass or effusion is common.

Essential Facts

- Primary cardiac angiosarcomas are highly aggressive tumors that are almost always fatal.
- At the time of diagnosis, 66 to 89% of patients have distant metastases.
- The most commonly affected patients are adult men, with the average age at diagnosis 41 years.
- The most common imaging findings are cardiomegaly, pericardial effusion, and an infiltrative soft-tissue mass.
- The soft-tissue mass is broad-based and exhibits heterogeneous enhancement, with nonenhancing areas that represent necrosis.

Other Imaging Findings

- Cardiac angiosarcomas are vascularized tumors that exhibit variable degrees of enhancement and hypervascularity on contrast-enhanced computed tomography and MR images.

✔ Pearls & ✘ Pitfalls

✔ Cardiac angiosarcomas typically affect the right atrium; in contrast, undifferentiated cardiac sarcomas more often arise in the ventricles.

✘ Affected patients may present with symptoms of cardiac valve obstruction, acute chest pain, or congestive heart failure with dyspnea and orthopnea. Clinical diagnosis is difficult, and imaging techniques are required for correct diagnosis and tumor identification.

Case 68

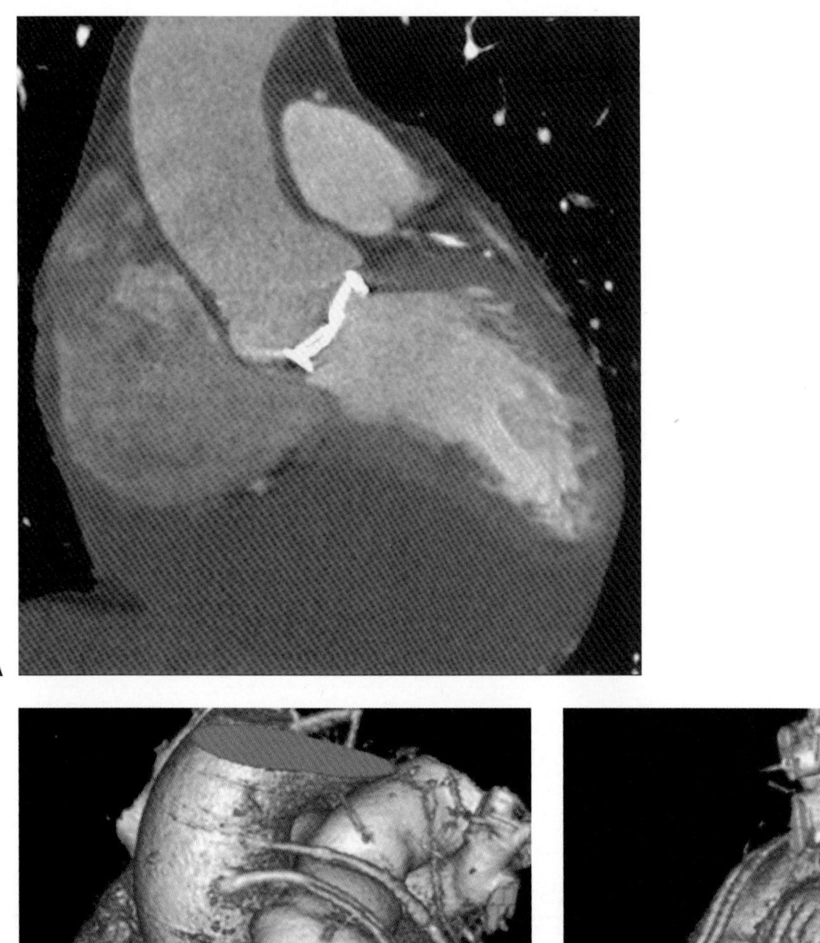
A

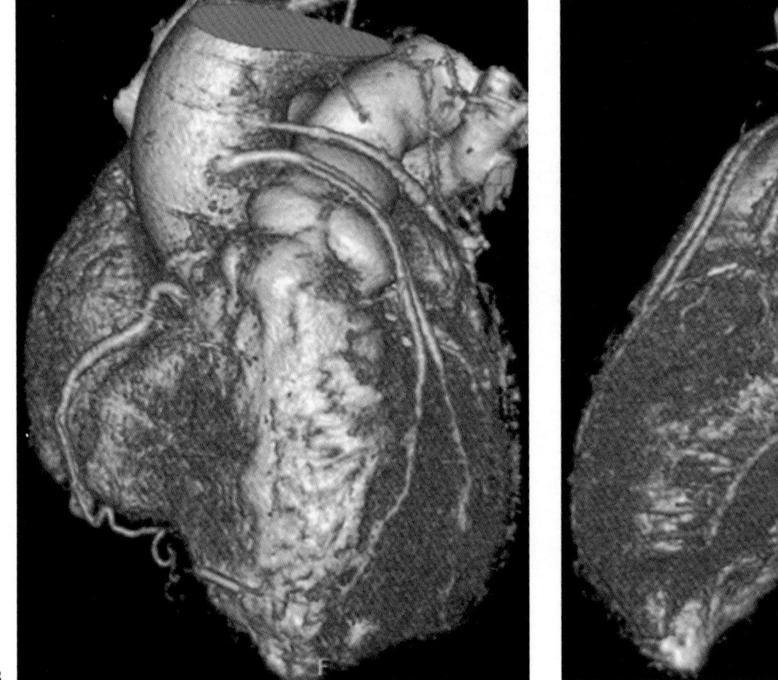
B

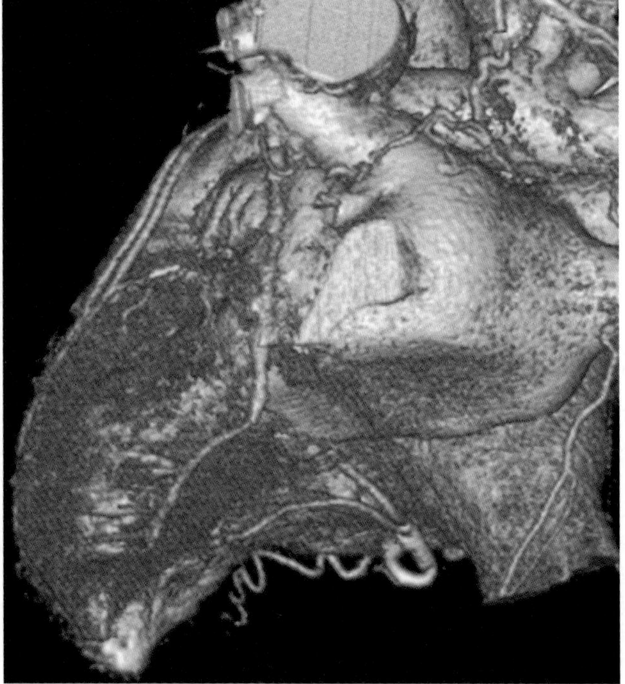
C

Clinical Presentation

A 67-year-old man with a history of a coronary artery bypass graft (CABG) and aortic valve replacement now presents with exercise intolerance and abnormal but limited echocardiographic findings.

Imaging Findings

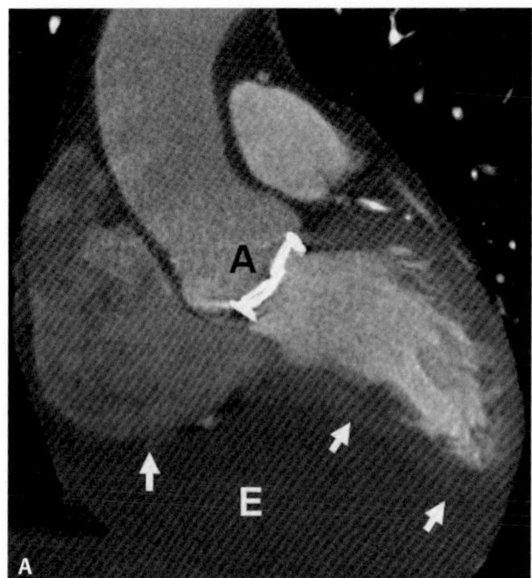

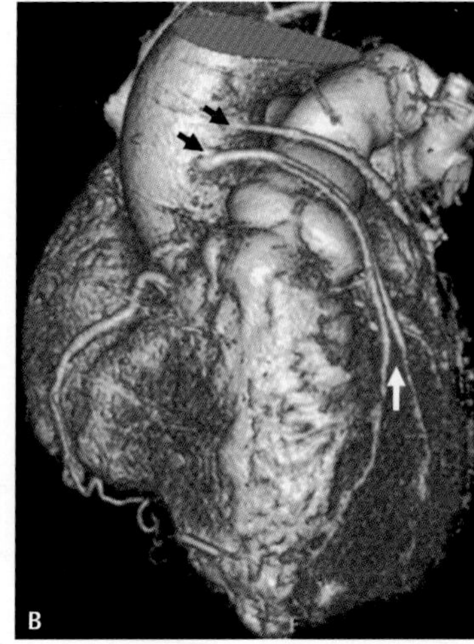

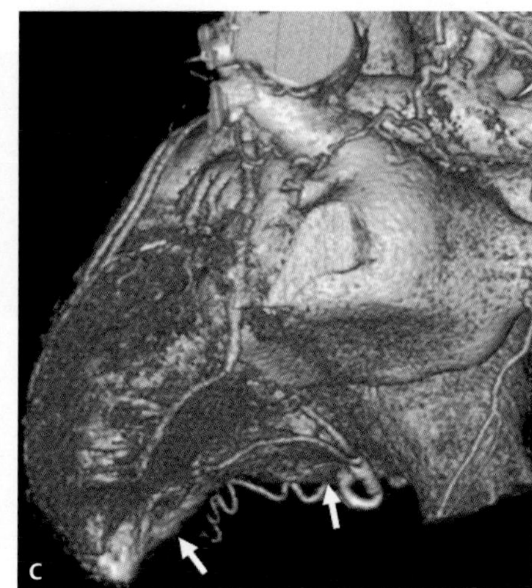

(A) In the coronal plane, the prosthetic aortic valve (*A*) is seen. A low-attenuation pericardial fluid collection (*E*) is under the heart, resulting in distortion of the shape of the heart. **(B)** Saphenous vein grafts arise from the anterior surface of the ascending aorta (*black arrows*) and extend to the left anterior descending artery and a diagonal branch (*white arrow*) and the LCx. **(C)** The distorted shape of the heart is clearly seen in this three-dimensional view of its undersurface (*white arrows*).

Differential Diagnosis

- ***Loculated postoperative pericardial effusion:*** Distortion of the shape of the heart implies the fluid collection is within the pericardial sac.
- *Pericardial cyst:* Pericardial cysts rarely cause a mass effect on the heart and are most often located in the right costophrenic angle.
- *Pericardial abscess:* The patient does not have symptoms typical of abscess such as fever and is not ill-appearing. The walls of the collection do not enhance.

Essential Facts

- The incidence of pericardial effusion after cardiac surgery ranges from 50 to 85%.
- The incidence of pericardial tamponade due to postoperative pericardial effusion is unknown.
- Postoperative pericardial effusions are more common following CABG than after valve replacement surgery.
- Postoperative pericardial effusion is likely due to disruption of venous or lymphatic drainage from the heart.
- Loculated effusions and those that are anterior may be difficult to evaluate completely with echocardiography.

Other Imaging Findings

- Echocardiography was limited in the diagnosis of this large-volume pericardial effusion because the acoustic window was restricted.
- Magnetic resonance (MR) and computed tomography (CT) allow imaging of the entire chest and pericardial fluid collections and masses.
- Fluid signal and attenuation should be that of fluid. Hemorrhage, infection, and neoplasm can alter the attenuation and signal of pericardial fluid.
- Pericardial thickening may be detected with MR or electrocardiography-gated multidetector CT.

✔ Pearls & ✘ Pitfalls

✔ Normally, ~15 to 50 mL of pericardial fluid is present.

✘ Hemorrhage, infection, and neoplasm can alter the attenuation and signal of pericardial fluid.

Case 69

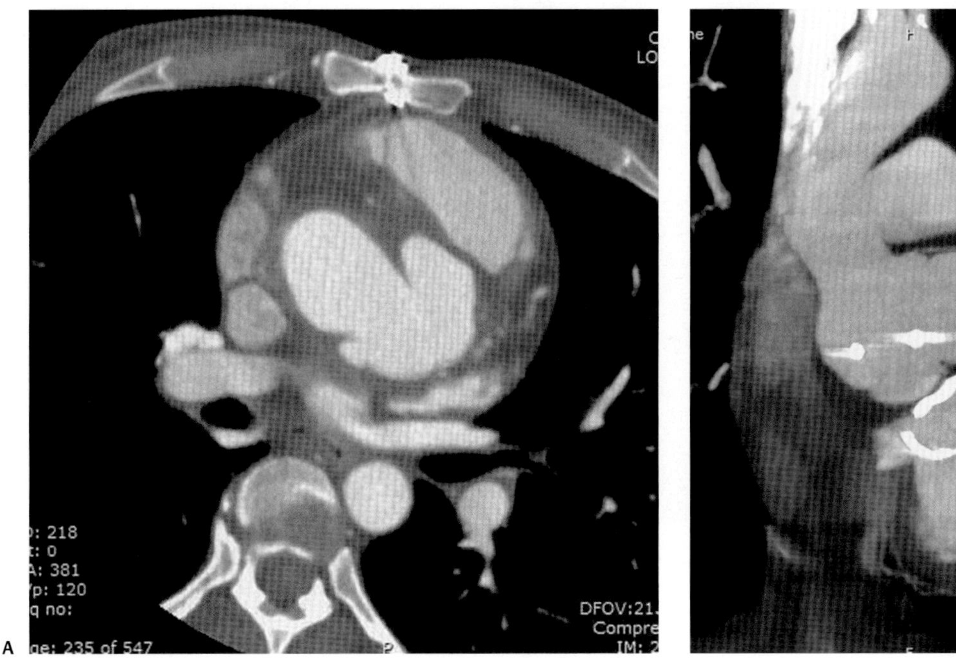

A B

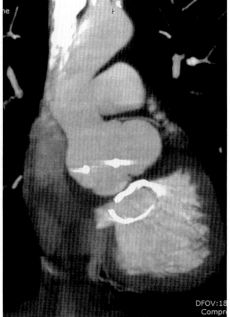

■ Clinical Presentation

A 44-year-old woman with a history of intravenous drug abuse presents with fever and chest pain. The patient has had an aortic valve replacement.

Imaging Findings

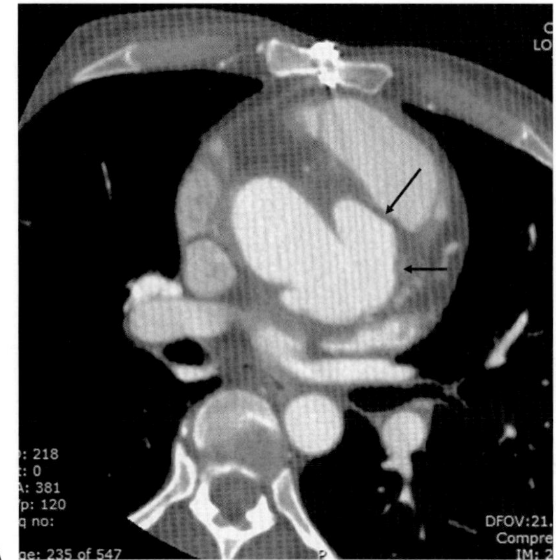

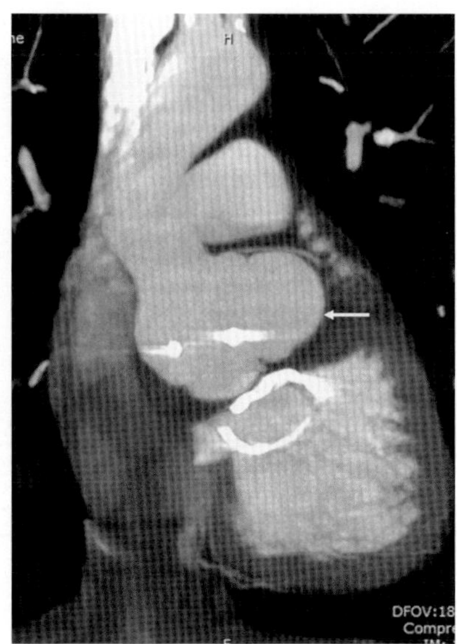

(A) Axial and **(B)** coronal cardiac-gated multislice computed tomography angiography images demonstrate the presence of an abnormal outpouching, as well as dilatation of the aortic root and mass effect on the left main coronary artery. More pronounced dilatation is seen affecting the left sinus of Valsalva.

Differential Diagnosis

- ***Mycotic pseudoaneurysm of the aortic root, complicating an aortic valve endocarditis:*** Acquired pseudoaneurysm of the aortic root or mycotic pseudoaneurysm of the sinus of Valsalva results from weakening of the media from diverse causes, such as syphilis, trauma, and endocarditis. In the latter case, the infection may progress to the intima and media of the aortic wall, weakening the wall and causing a pseudoaneurysm.
- *Congenital sinus of Valsalva aneurysm:* This results from structural weakness of the lamina elastica of the media at the base of the aorta and typically grows within the cardiac silhouette. When ruptured, it presents with an intracardiac shunt and congestive heart failure.
- *Traumatic pseudoaneurysm of the ascending aorta:* The most common traumatic pseudoaneurysm of the aorta involves the aortic isthmus at the level of the ligamentum arteriosum. Ascending aorta involvement is rare (1%). A clinical history of trauma and the presence of a mediastinal hematoma are important clues for this diagnosis.

Essential Facts

- Pseudoaneurysm of the aortic root is an infrequent complication of infective endocarditis.
- Pseudoaneuryms are most frequently associated with prosthetic valve endocarditis.
- Whereas congenital aneurysms of the sinus of Valsalva more often involve the right coronary sinus, infective pseudoaneurysms involve all sinuses with equal frequency.
- *Staphylococcus aureus* and *Streptococcus viridans* are the most frequently responsible infective organisms.
- The clinical prognosis is grave, with heart failure, sepsis, renal failure, stroke, and peripheral embolization seen in a significant number of cases.

Other Imaging Findings

- Magnetic resonance with its multiplanar capability may show the ascending aorta perivalvular pseudoaneurysm as an abnormal cavity contiguous with the aortic root, with free flow between the aortic lumen and the cavity.

✔ Pearls & ✘ Pitfalls

✔ In patients with a history of aortic valve replacement surgery, a pseudoaneurysm of the aortic root or sinus of Valsalva favors the diagnosis of a mycotic pseudoaneurysm. This can be associated with an aortic para-annular abscess.

✘ Pseudoaneurysms of the aortic root are commonly mistaken for abscesses on transthoracic and transesophageal echocardiograms.

Case 70

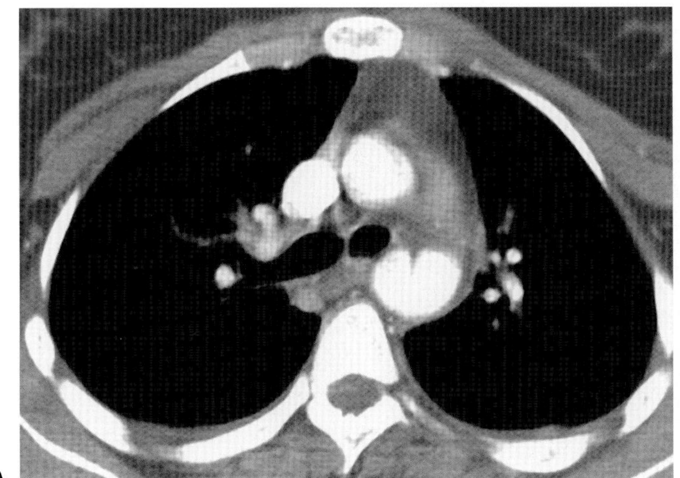

A

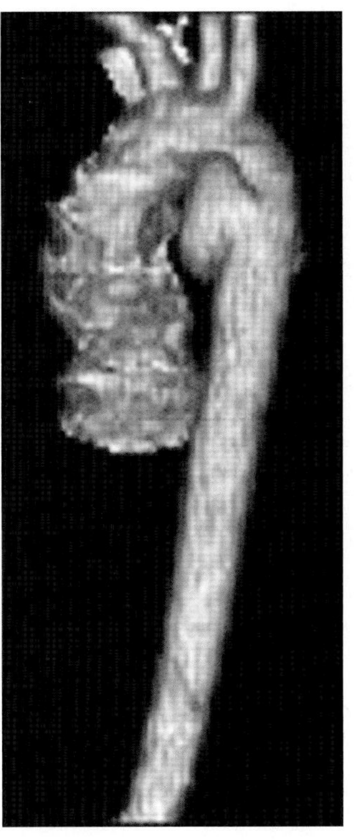

B

Clinical Presentation

A 21-year-old man presents with chest pain after a motor vehicle accident.

Imaging Findings

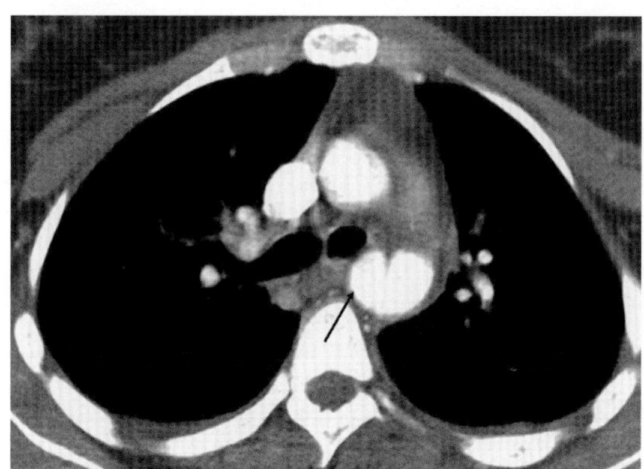
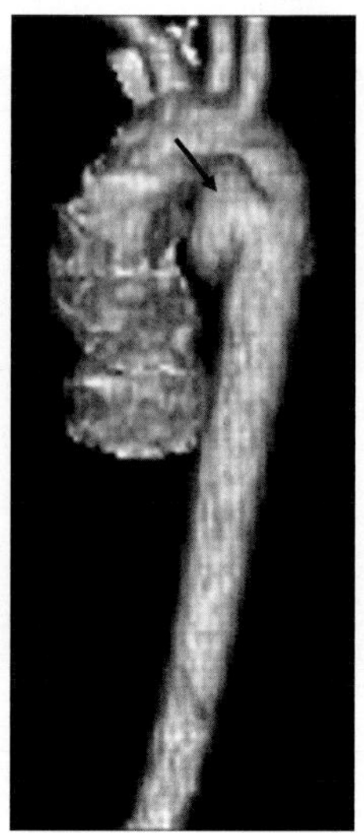

Contrast-enhanced computed tomography (CT) axial image **(A)** and three-dimensional volume-rendering reconstruction **(B)** demonstrate a deformity of the aorta with an abnormal saccular formation at the level of the ligamentum arteriosum. Minimal mediastinal hematoma is present.

Differential Diagnosis

- ***Traumatic aortic injury (TAI):*** Approximately 90% of TAIs occur in the region of the aortic isthmus, just distal to the origin of the left subclavian artery. The association of a mediastinal hematoma in contact with the aorta at the level of the aortic arch and an irregularity of the aortic wall with a pseudoaneurysm confirms this diagnosis.
- *Nonaortic bleeding and hematoma:* In ~80% of trauma patients with mediastinal hematomas, the bleeding is nonaortic in nature. When the hematoma is confined to the anterior mediastinum, a sternal fracture is usually responsible; when the hematoma is in the posterior mediastinum, a vertebral fracture is usually the source of bleeding.
- *Atherosclerotic saccular aneurysm of the aorta:* In such case, the aortic contour is abnormal because of the aneurysm, but typically no periaortic hematoma is present, except if there is leaking. Calcium at the level of the aneurysm favors an atherosclerotic chronic lesion.

Essential Facts

- A wide mediastinum in a trauma victim should raise concern for a mediastinal hematoma. In a victim of a motor vehicle accident or someone with a penetrating thoracic injury, the possibility of a vascular injury should always be the first consideration.
- At least 70% of TAIs are fatal at the scene of trauma.
- A rapid deceleration or blunt chest trauma should arouse suspicion of aortic injury.
- The fixed aortic isthmus that corresponds to the portion of the descending thoracic aorta between the origin of the left subclavian artery and the site of attachment of the ligamentum arteriosum is where the majority of TAIs occur.
- Mediastinal hemorrhage is highly sensitive but less specific for the diagnosis of TAI.
- The association of a mediastinal hematoma in contact with the aortic wall with a contour deformity of the aorta (e.g., pseudoaneurysm, intimal tear, or pseudocoarctation) is the most reliable combination of signs to make this diagnosis.

Other Imaging Findings

- Catheter aortography may be needed if helical CT of the aorta is indeterminate or inadequate to exclude injury or to confirm and define the extent of injury before surgery or endovascular repair.

✔ Pearls & ✘ Pitfalls

✔ Contrast-enhanced CT has 100% sensitivity and 100% negative predictive value for the detection of TAI.

✘ Diagnostic pitfalls may result from residual thymic tissue or atelectasis mimicking a mediastinal hematoma, from streak or pulsation artifacts, or from a patent ductus arteriosus that may mimic an abnormal aortic wall.

Case 71

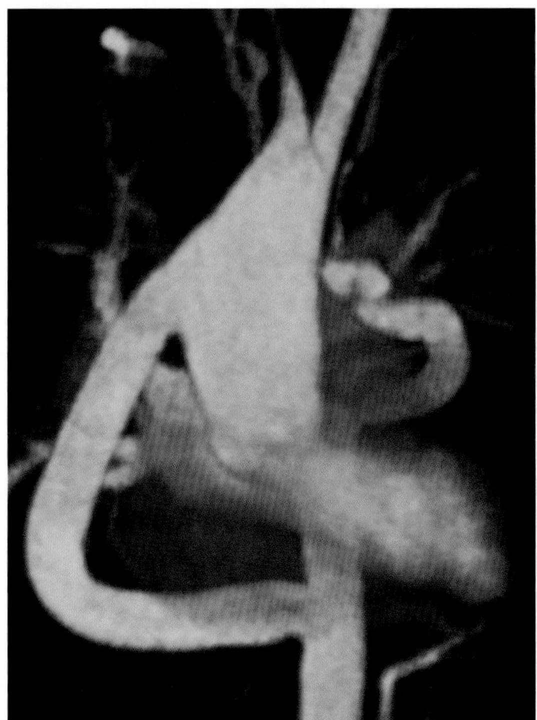
A

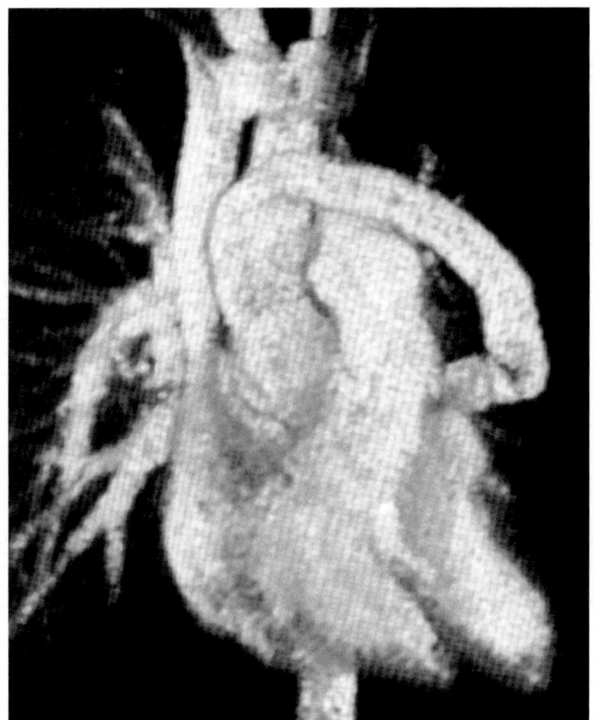
B

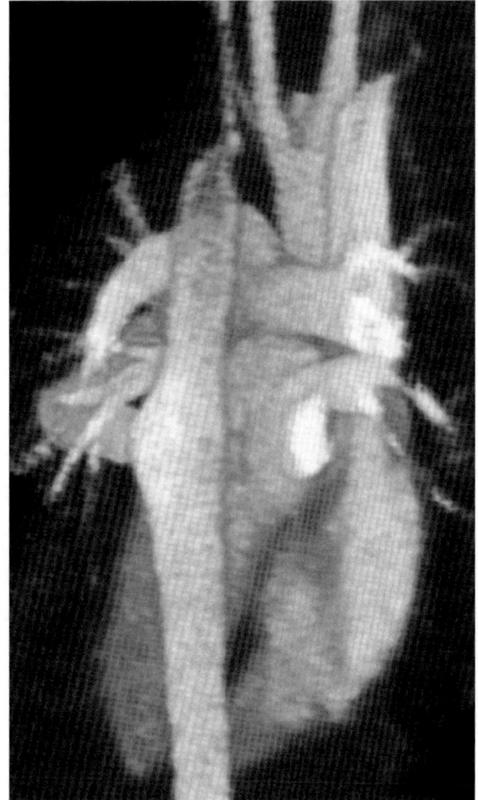
C

■ Clinical Presentation

Two young adult patients are shown. Each has the same form of congenital heart disease and has undergone surgical palliation, one as a neonate, the other as an adolescent.

Imaging Findings

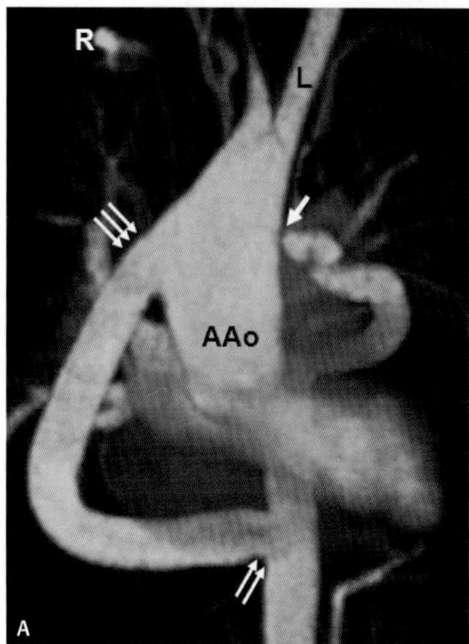

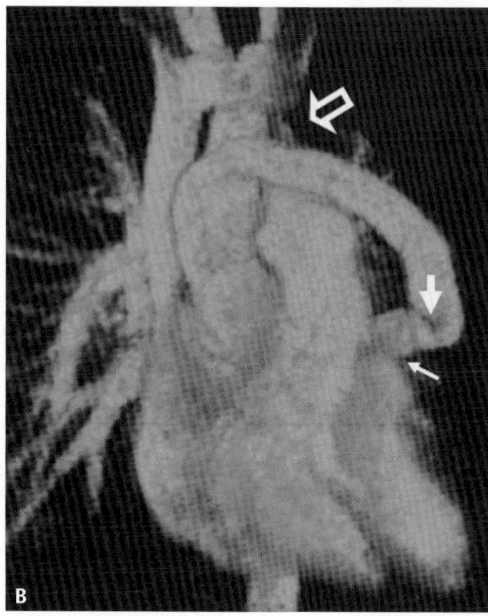

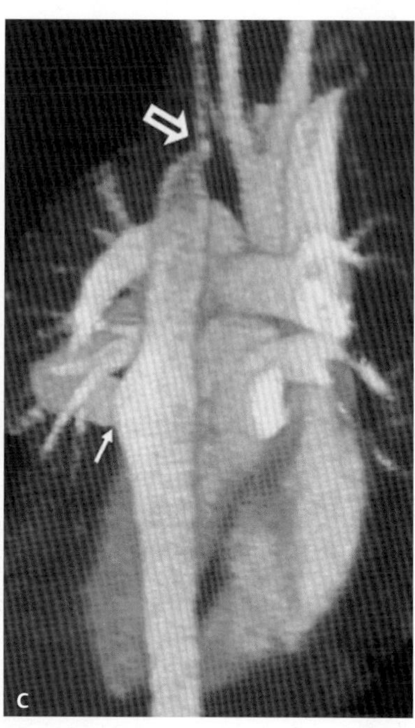

(A) A gadolinium-enhanced three-dimensional time-of-flight (TOF) magnetic resonance angiogram (MRA) image shows the normal-caliber ascending aorta (*AAo*), which tapers as the left common carotid artery (*L*) branches from the proximal arch; note the marked tapering of the adjacent right common carotid artery. The right subclavian artery (*R*) is of small caliber and arises from a collateral or distal branch of the aorta. There are two aorta–aortic bypass grafts. The one placed in infancy is stenosed at the proximal end (*white arrow*). The graft constructed more recently is patent, extending from the ascending aorta (*triple white arrows*) to the descending aorta (*double white arrows*). **(B)** In the second patient, an anteroposterior three-dimensional gadolinium-enhanced TOF MIP image reveals the absence of the aortic arch (*open arrow*) and a patent aorta–aortic bypass graft. In the graft there is a kink (*large white arrow*) resulting in stenosis, but normal caliber in the graft distally (*white arrow*). **(C)** In the posteroanterior view, the MRA shows the interruption of the aortic arch and the origin of the left vertebral artery (*open arrow*). The distal anastomosis of the graft is patent (*white arrow*).

Differential Diagnosis

- ***Interruption of the aortic arch (IAA):*** In both patients, the aortic arch is discontinuous, interrupted between the origins of the left common carotid and left subclavian arteries. The first patient also has an aberrant origin of the right subclavian artery.
- *Coarctation of the aorta:* The etiology and location of coarctation are distinctly different from the findings of IAA. The aortic narrowing occurs at the level of the ductus arteriosus in coarctation.
- *Aortic arch hypoplasia:* Hypoplasia of the aortic arch is often associated with coarctation, but this diagnosis means the aortic arch remains patent.

Essential Facts

- IAA is classified as follows:
  - Type A: IAA distal to the left subclavian artery
  - Type B: IAA between the left common carotid and left subclavian arteries (commonly associated with DiGeorge syndrome and thymic agenesis)
  - Type C: IAA between the innominate and left common carotid arteries
- IAA is discontinuity of the aortic arch, which may represent the most extreme form of coarctation of the aortic arch, but it usually affects the transverse arch rather than the isthmus.
- A patent ductus arteriosus (PDA) and ventricular septal defect (VSD) are present.
- When the PDA closes, upper versus lower body differential cyanosis is seen.
- Surgical correction is directed toward reestablishing flow to the distal arch vessels and systemic circulation.

Other Imaging Findings

- Aberrant origin of the right subclavian artery may occur as a branch of the aorta, distal to the interruption.

✔ Pearls & ✘ Pitfalls

✔ Determination of the type of IAA is made based on the location of the interruption.

✘ VSD, a necessary shunt to decompress the LV, is due to posterior malalignment of the conal septum and is not an unrelated structural component of congenital heart disease.

Case 72

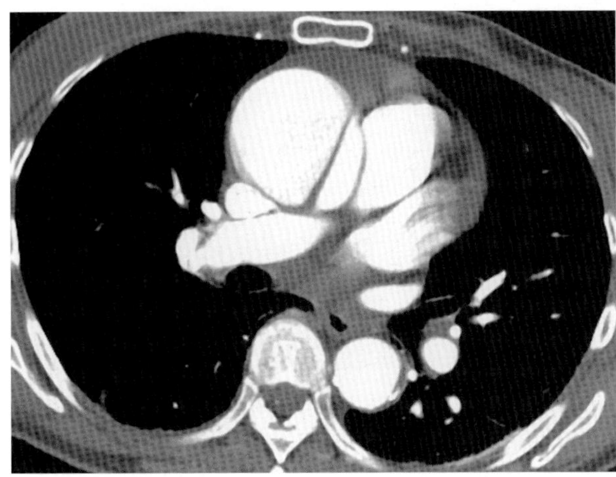
A

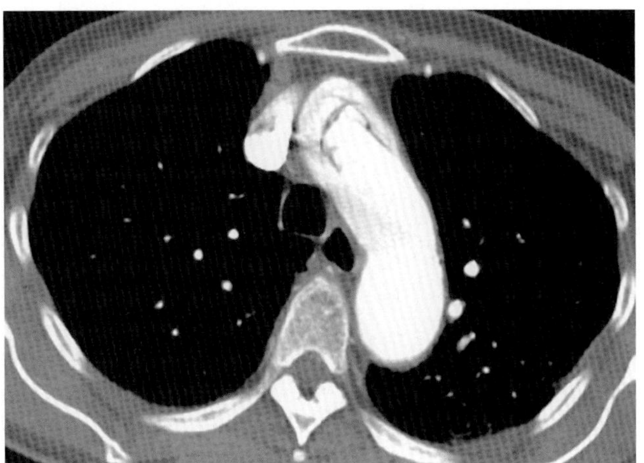
B

Clinical Presentation

Acute chest pain and hemiparesis on the left side in a 65-year-old woman

Imaging Findings

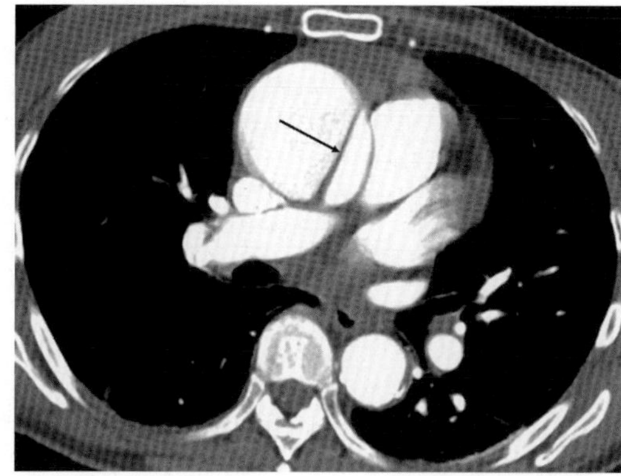

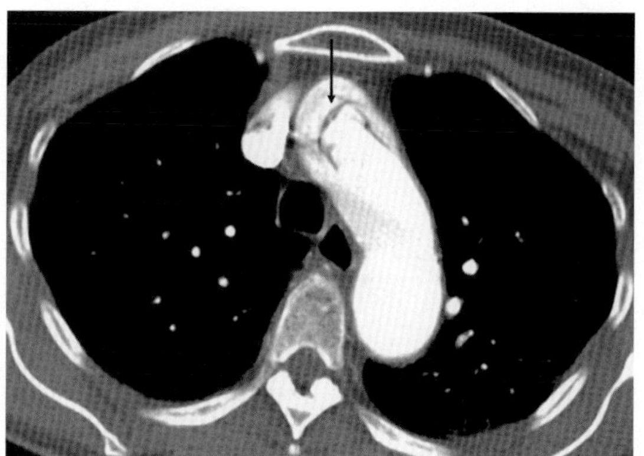

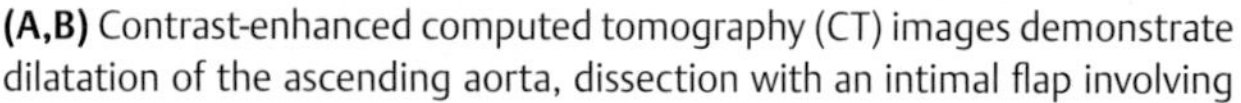

(A,B) Contrast-enhanced computed tomography (CT) images demonstrate dilatation of the ascending aorta, dissection with an intimal flap involving the dilated segment and the aortic arch, and a moderate amount of pericardial fluid.

Differential Diagnosis

- ***Aortic dissection:*** Contrast-enhanced CT angiography of the thoracic aorta demonstrates an intimal flap (aortic media) extending from the ascending aorta and aortic root to the horizontal segment of the aortic arch resulting from a Stanford type A aortic dissection.
- *Aortic motion artifact:* Older CT scanners with long gantry rotation time, as well as tachycardia, can cause pulsation artifact that produces linear densities in the aortic lumen. This artifact is rarely a diagnostic problem given current technology with multidetector CT, in which gantry rotation is faster.

Essential Facts

- An aortic dissection usually begins from a laceration of the aortic intima and inner layer of the aortic media, which creates a communication between the aortic lumen and the splitting media.
- The true lumen is usually smaller with faster flow.
- The false lumen is usually larger with slower and more turbulent flow.
- According to the Stanford classification, all dissections involving the ascending aorta are designated as type A (60%). This is a surgical emergency with a higher rate of complications, including rupture into the pericardium and extension to the coronary arteries or to the carotid arteries, producing stroke.
- Dissections involving any part of the aorta distal to the left subclavian artery are designated type B (40%) and are treated medically.
- Multidetector CT has nearly 100% sensitivity, specificity, and accuracy for the diagnosis of acute aortic disorders, including aortic dissection.

Other Imaging Findings

- Multidetector CT is now the preferred imaging modality for suspected acute aortic dissection. In patients with poor renal function or allergy to iodine contrast, multiplanar transesophageal echocardiography and magnetic resonance imaging are excellent alternative imaging modalities, with a sensitivity and specificity between 90 and 99%.

✔ Pearls & ✘ Pitfalls

✔ The so-called intimal flap really represents the aortic media detached from the other layers of the aortic wall.

✘ Slow injection rates (< 3 mL/s) or inappropriate timing may produce poor enhancement of the aortic lumen and may fail to demonstrate the aortic flap.

Case 73

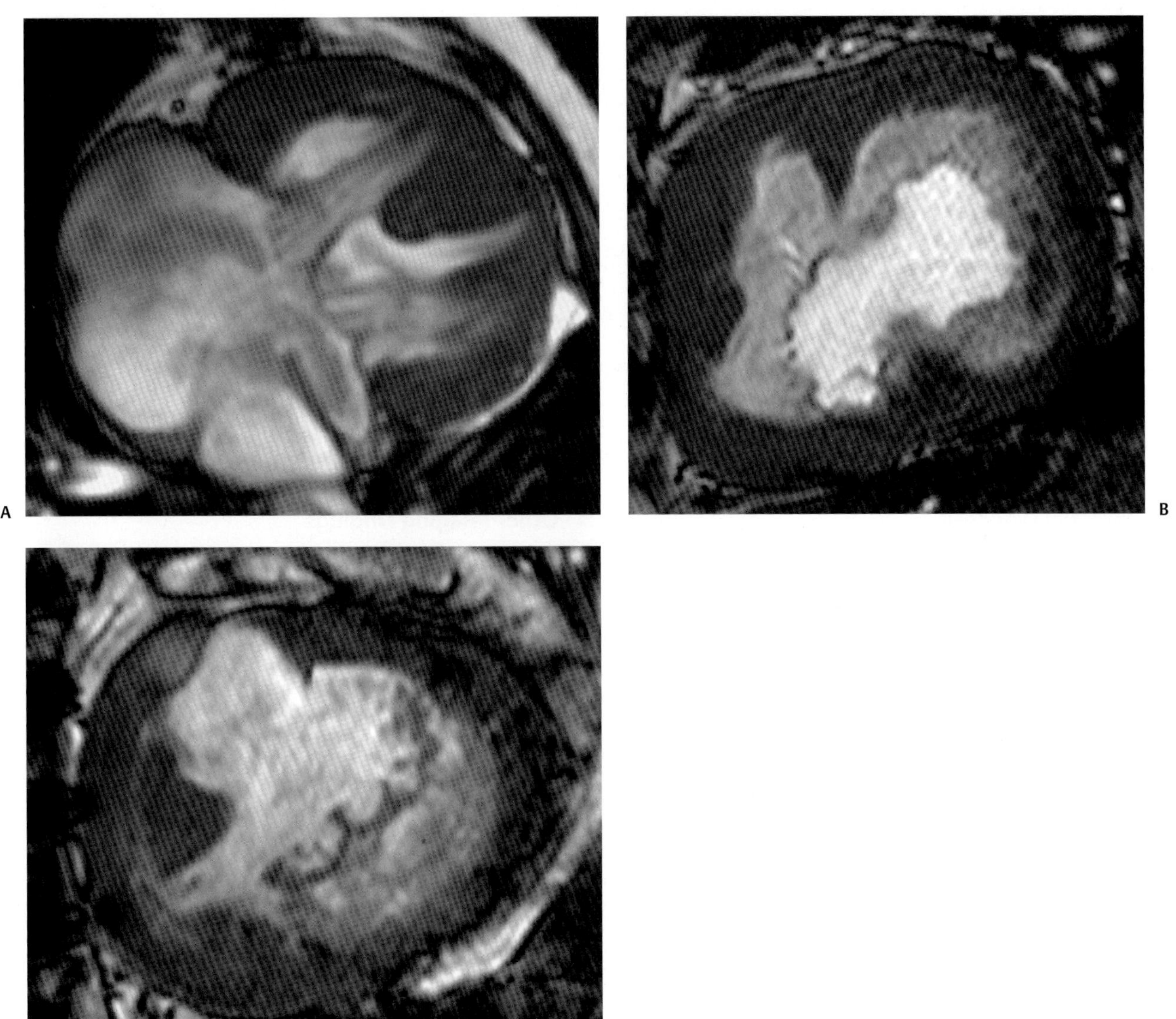

Clinical Presentation

A 12-year-old girl with known congenital heart disease presents with shortness of breath and abnormal findings on a transthoracic echocardiogram.

Imaging Findings

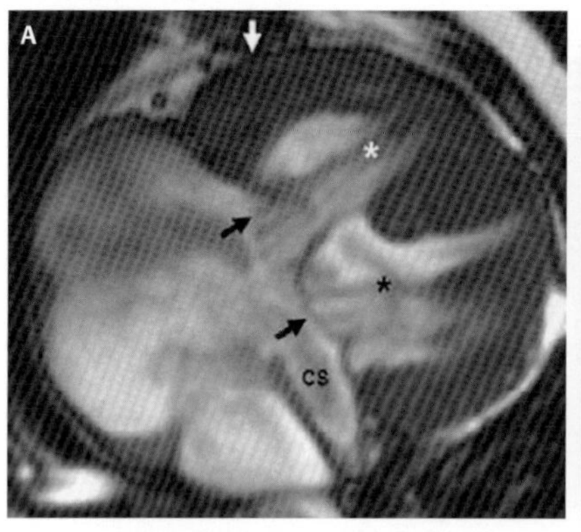

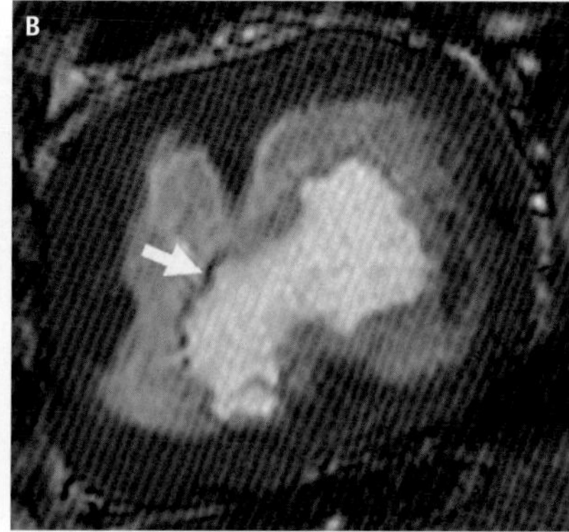

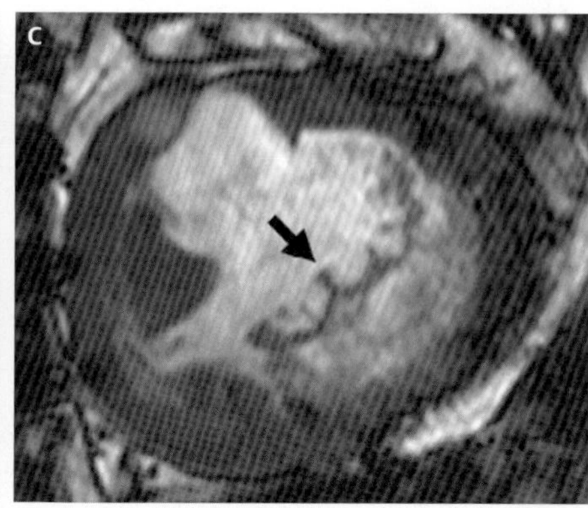

(A) A four-chamber view of the heart shows continuity of the atrioventricular valves (*black arrows*) and a large ventricular septal defect (VSD). The coronary sinus (*CS*) empties into the left side of the common atrium. Chordae tendineae extend through the right ventricle (*white asterisk*) and left ventricle (*black asterisk*) to the leaflets of the common valve. The wall of the right ventricle is thickened (*white arrow*). **(B,C)** In the short-axis view, at the base of the heart, the common atrioventricular valve is open (*white arrow*) and closed (*black arrow*).

Differential Diagnosis

- ***Complete atrioventricular septal defect (AVSD):*** The atrioventricular valves are completely contiguous, separating the common atrium from the ventricles and a large VSD.
- *Partial AVSD:* In a partial AVSD, the atrioventricular valves are partially contiguous across defects of the interatrial and interventricular septa.
- *VSD:* The interventricular septum is made of membranous and muscular tissue. VSD is the most common type of congenital heart disease.

Essential Facts

- AVSD is also referred to as an endocardial cushion defect.
- Most children will have symptomatic congestive heart failure.
- The majority (75%) of patients with complete AVSDs also have Down syndrome.
- First-degree atrioventricular block is common.
- The endocardial cushion includes both atrioventricular valves, the inlet portion of the ventricular septum, and the atrial septum primum.

Other Imaging Findings

- Hypertrophy of the right ventricular myocardium
- Dilatation of the right ventricle
- Valve leaflets bridged across the atrioventricular defect

✔ Pearls & ✘ Pitfalls

✔ The ventricular structure may appear to be a single ventricle, with equal right and left ventricle chamber size and minimal septal tissue.

✔ If the common valve is more developed on either the right or the left, the contralateral ventricular chamber will be underdeveloped.

✘ AVSD can be associated with a double-outlet right ventricle, subaortic stenosis, and tetralogy of Fallot.

Case 74

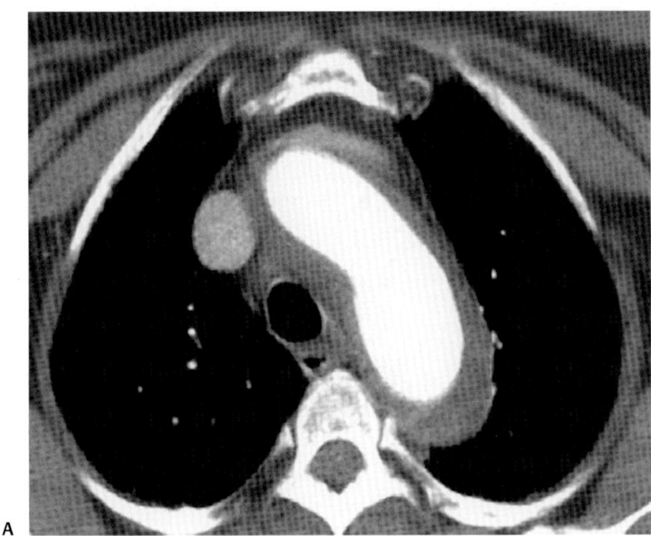

A

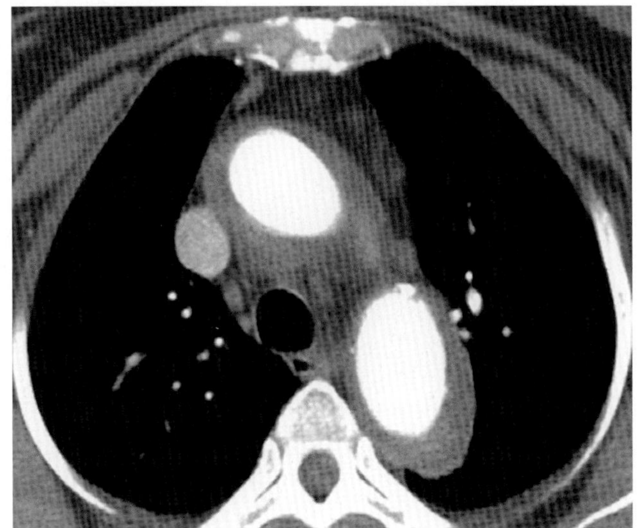

B

Clinical Presentation

Severe acute back pain in a 72-year-old woman

Imaging Findings

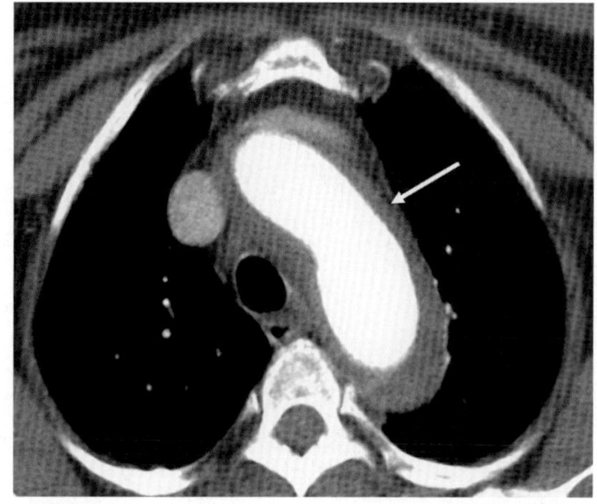

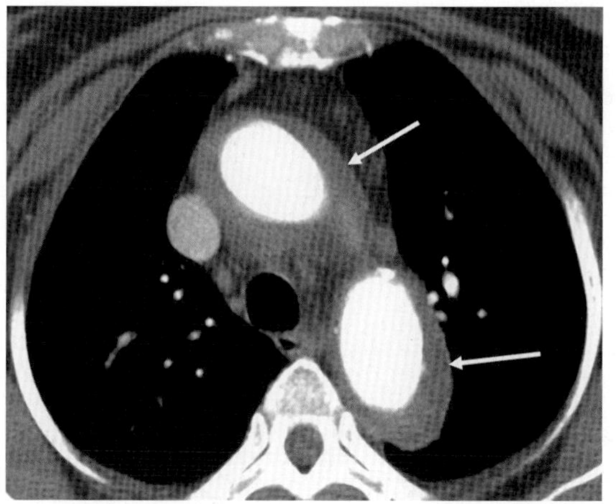

(A,B) Contrast-enhanced computed tomography of the thoracic aorta: axial images at the level of the aortic arch and aortopulmonary window show high-density tissue concentrically surrounding and thickening the aortic wall.

Differential Diagnosis

- ***Intramural hematoma of the aorta:*** The relatively high-density tissue concentrically surrounding the aortic wall is consistent with an intramural hematoma.
- *Aortic dissection:* Intramural hematoma of the aorta has been considered a variant of aortic dissection with no entry or false lumen. In the images shown, there is no flow, which is in favor of an intramural hematoma, in which there is no intimal tear and no communication between the hematoma and the true lumen.
- *Thrombosed aortic aneurysm:* Thrombosed aneurysms tend to be less diffuse and lower in density than an acute intramural hematoma. The thrombus may be concentric or eccentric with a crescent shape and may present with internal calcification.
- *Aortitis:* Inflammatory diseases may produce abnormal thickening of the aortic wall with focal or diffuse involvement, also with a soft-tissue-density rim surrounding the vessel wall.

Essential Facts

- Intramural hematoma of the aorta is characterized by abnormal bleeding of the vasa vasorum of the aortic wall into the media, creating a hematoma that propagates along the media layer.
- This weakens the aortic wall, which may evolve to either outward aortic wall rupture or inward rupture through the media, creating a communicating dissection. Progression of the intramural hematoma occurs in ~60% of cases, including 16% developing overt dissection.
- The overall mortality rate of intramural hematoma of the aorta is similar to that of classic aortic dissection (21% vs. 24%).
- Intramural hematoma of the aorta may present as a primary event in patients with arterial hypertension or as a secondary event due to a penetrating atherosclerotic ulcer.
- Stable disease may represent gradual regression of the hematoma.
- Patients with type A intramural hematomas (ascending aorta and arch) are more likely than those with type B (distal to the left subclavian artery) to develop complications such as double-barreled dissection (80% vs. 12%).

Other Imaging Findings

- Magnetic resonance imaging can be used to determine the age of an intramural hematoma based on changes in signal intensity. An acute intramural hematoma of the aorta presents an intermediate signal intensity on T1-weighted images because of the presence of oxyhemoglobin. In the subacute stage (> 8 days), the presence of methemoglobin produces high signal intensity.

✔ Pearls & ✘ Pitfalls

✔ Intramural hematoma of the aorta is a potentially lethal condition, with frequent progression to aortic rupture, dissection, or aneurysm formation.

✘ An intramural hematoma of the aorta should not be confused with an aortic thrombus, which is a more benign and stable condition. A hematoma is subintimal, in contrast to a mural thrombus, which is in the luminal side of the intima and may be calcified.

Case 75

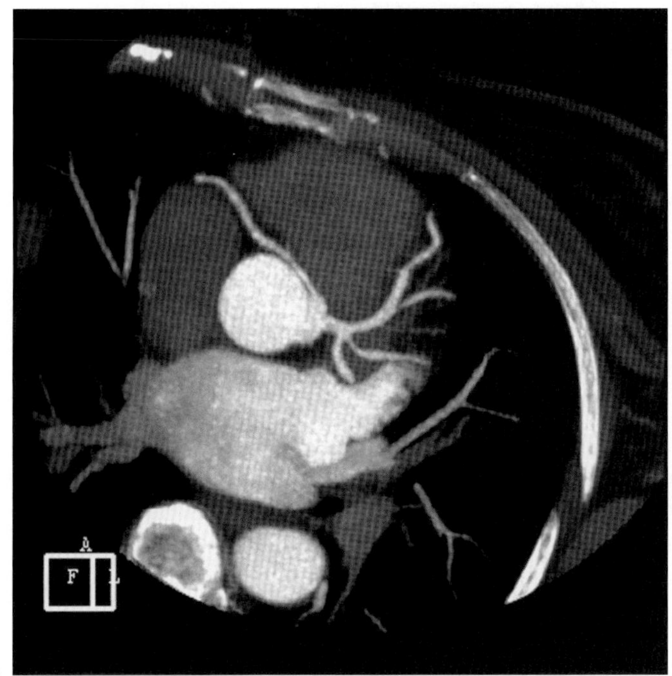

A

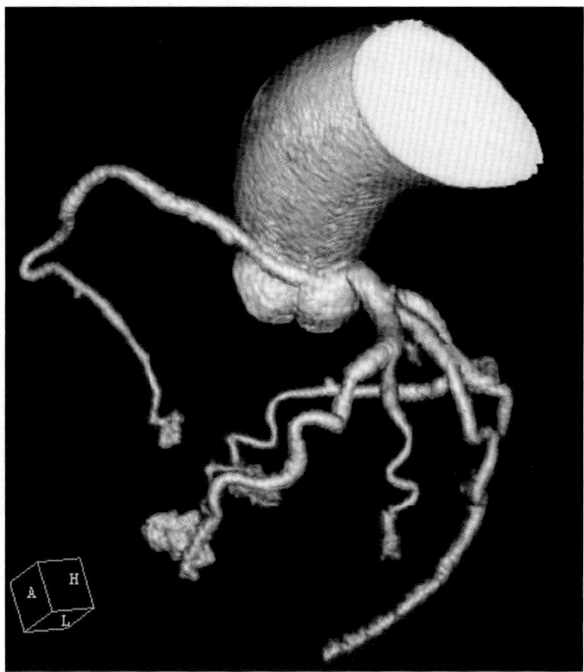

B

Clinical Presentation

Atypical chest pain in a 28-year-old woman

Imaging Findings

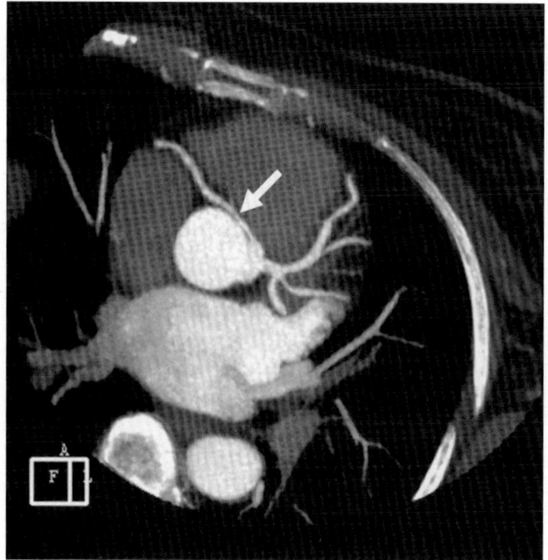

A

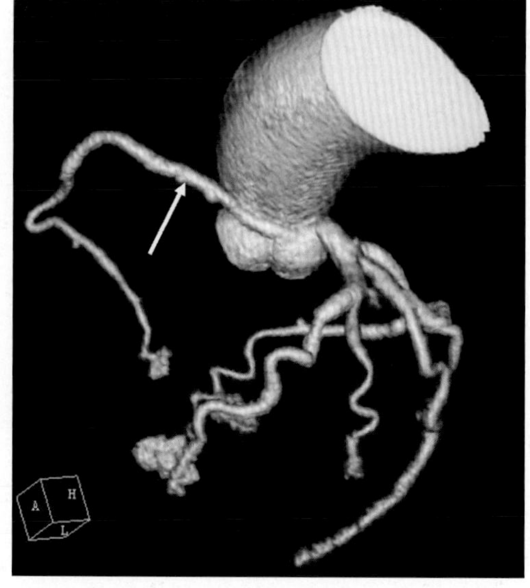

B

Contrast-enhanced cardiac-gated computed tomography angiography (CTA): Axial maximum intensity projection **(A)** and three-dimensional volume-rendering **(B)** images depict an abnormal pattern of origin and distribution of the coronary arteries, with the right coronary artery (RCA) arising from the left coronary sinus. The vessel, which is abnormal in origin, is seen going to the right between the aorta and the outflow tract of the right ventricle.

Differential Diagnosis

- ***Aberrant origin of the RCA from the left aortic sinus:*** An aberrant RCA from the left coronary sinus may present from the same ostium or from an independent ostium. In this case, the aberrant RCA has an interarterial course, between the proximal pulmonary artery trunk (anterior) and the aorta (posterior).
- *Normal origin of the RCA, left main coronary artery (LMCA), and its branches:* The normal anatomy of the coronary artery system consists of independent origin of the right and left coronary arteries, each one arising from its corresponding coronary sinus. The images shown do not follow this rule.

Essential Facts

- The prevalence of anomalous origin of the coronary arteries is between 0.2 and 2.5% (average, ~1.0%).
- Even though relatively rare, aberrant coronary arteries have been implicated in premature cardiac mortality. This is the most common cardiac abnormality (61%) found in nontraumatic sudden death in young adults.
- Other clinical manifestations are arrhythmias, syncope, angina, and myocardial infarction.
- Anomalies of the origin of the RCA are among the most commonly reported (30–50%).
- There are three subtypes of anomalous origin of the RCA from the left sinus of Valsalva based on the course of the anomalous artery: interarterial, retroaortic, and prepulmonic.
- The most common course of an anomalous RCA arising from the left sinus of Valsalva is interarterial, with the aberrant artery passing between the pulmonary artery (or outflow tract of the right ventricle) and the aorta ("malignant" type).
- This anomaly can be associated with sudden cardiac death, particularly during exercise, because of compression or ostial narrowing of the dilated aorta.

Other Imaging Findings

- CTA with dynamic images during the different phases of the cardiac cycle with cardiac-gated multidetector CT can show caliber changes of the aberrant vessel when present.

✔ Pearls & ✘ Pitfalls

✔ The prevalence of coronary artery anomalies in patients with congenital heart disease is much higher (3–36%, depending on the type of congenital cardiopathy) than in the general population (1%).

✘ CTA outperforms invasive catheter angiography in the identification of anomalous coronary arteries (100% sensitivity, 97% specificity) and in defining the anatomical course of the anomalous vessel. Catheter angiography is less sensitive (50%) and less specific for this purpose.

Case 76

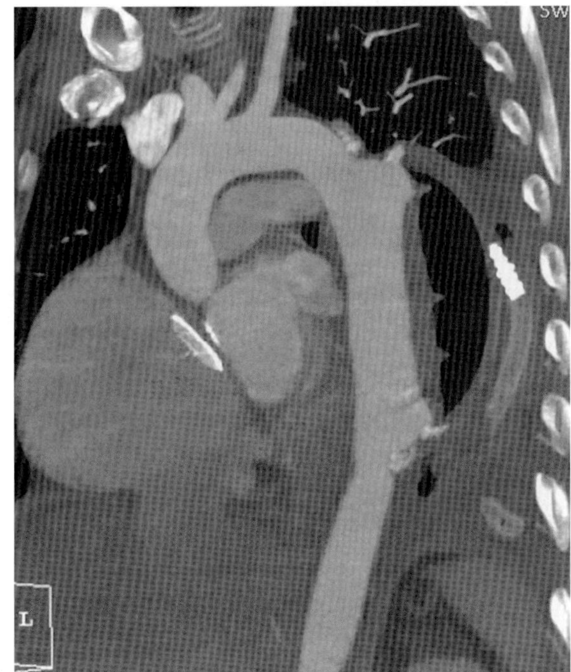

A

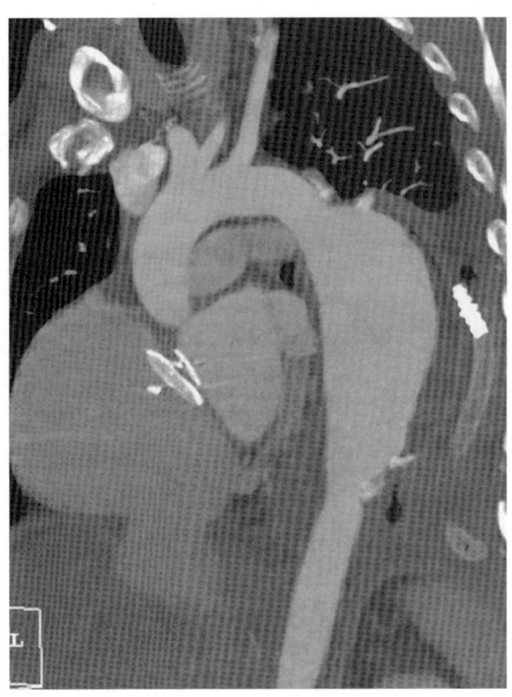

B

Clinical Presentation

A 49-year-old man presents with severe heart failure and a history of percutaneous closure of an atrial septal defect. The patient has had another surgical procedure, implantation of a device in the thoracic aorta.

Imaging Findings

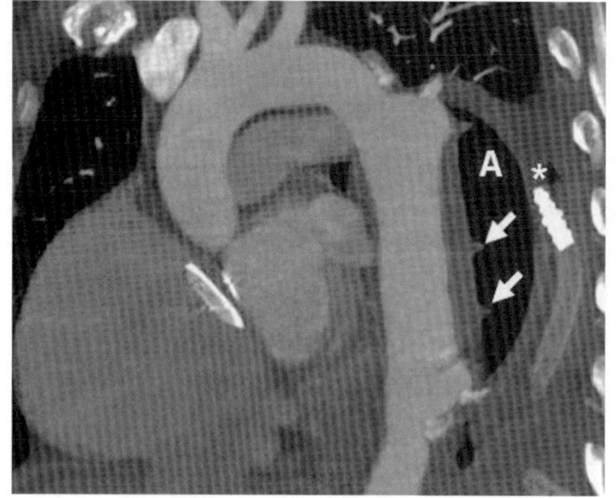

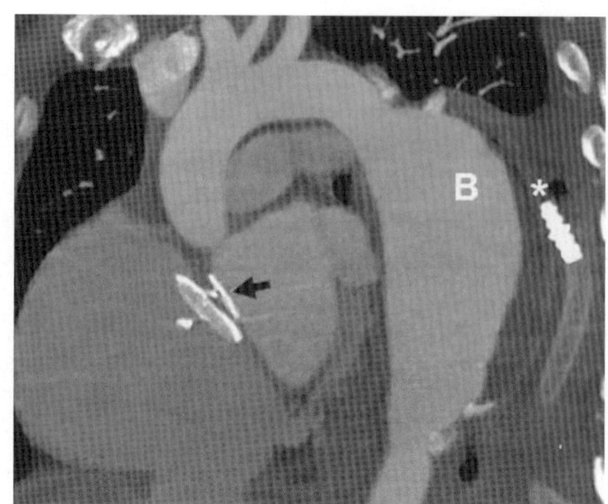

Sagittal oblique two dimensional reconstruction images of the aorta show an aortic assist device sewn into the lumen of the proximal descending thoracic aorta. **(A)** During systole a balloon is expanded by a pump via a catether (*asterisk*), propelling blood into systemic arteries. The balloon is partially filled with air (*A*) (*asterisk*). Kinks in the wall of the balloon are evident as it is inflated (*white arrow*). **(B)** In diastole, the assist device (*asterisk*) is deflated, and the aorta is filled with blood (*B*). The atrial septal defect closure device is also visualized (*black arrow*).

Differential Diagnosis

- ***Aortic assist device:*** Various devices are used to augment function of the left ventricle (LV) in patients with heart failure.
- *Intra-aortic balloon pump (IABP):* This type of aortic assist device is contained within the aortic lumen and is a short-term method of decreasing the workload required from the LV.
- *Aortobronchial fistula:* Air could be found in the aorta with this type of fistula, but more likely, the bronchial tree would fill with blood.

Essential Facts

- This device is sewn into the thoracic aorta and functions to augment the systolic effect of the LV.
- Right ventricular and LV assist devices are used in some patients with heart failure. These devices are connected to either or both ventricles; the devices are commonly placed in the upper abdomen.
- An artificial heart is another method of "assisting" the native heart, by entirely taking over the cardiac pumping function.
- Each of the available assist devices is used on a short- or long-term basis as a "bridge" or method to maintain adequate cardiac output, either until the heart function can recover (IABP) or until cardiac transplant.
- Use of cardiac assist devices has been reported in patients with congenital heart disease.

Other Imaging Findings

- The wall of this assist device has several creases, a sign of wear.

✔ Pearls & ✘ Pitfalls

✔ As part of inpatient treatment, the aortic assist device remains filled with saline.

✔ Upon discharge of the patient from the hospital, it is impossible to keep the balloon filled with saline. Consequently, the balloon begins to fill with air.

✔ Electrocardiography-gated multidetector computed tomography is required to visualize the pumping action of the balloon.

✘ Creases form in the balloon wall as the balloon is inflated and deflated.

✘ Each crease becomes a site of weakening of the balloon wall, which can lead to rupture of the balloon.

✘ Balloon rupture is likely to be catastrophic, especially if rupture occurs when the balloon contains air, causing fatal air embolism to the brain or embolism to abdominal viscera.

Case 77

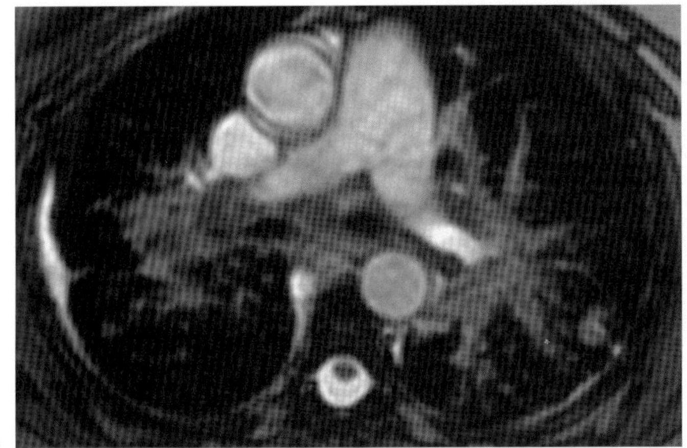
A

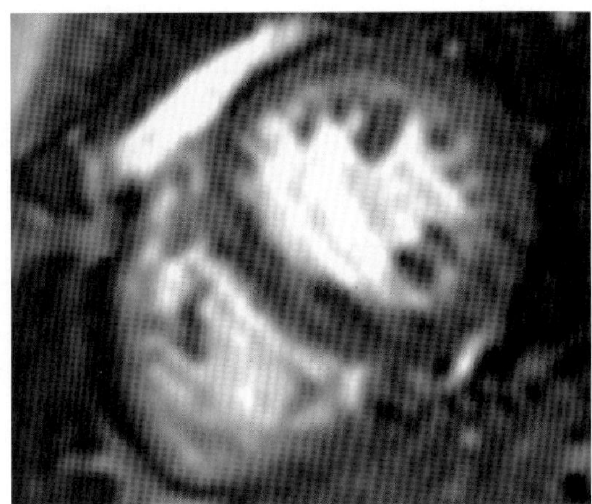
B

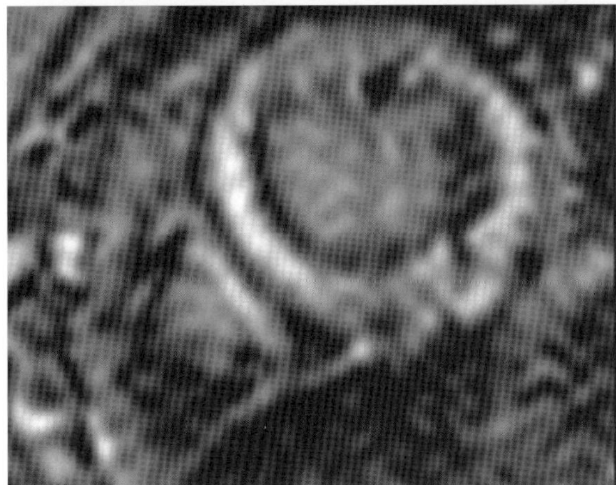
C

Clinical Presentation

A 49-year-old African American woman presents with a history of hypertension and mild exertional dyspnea. She was recently diagnosed with pulmonary disease and underwent cardiac magnetic resonance imaging (MRI) for further evaluation after referral from cardiac electrophysiology.

Imaging Findings

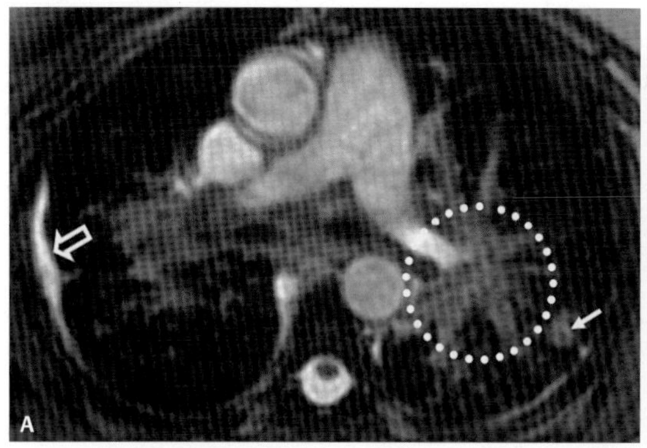

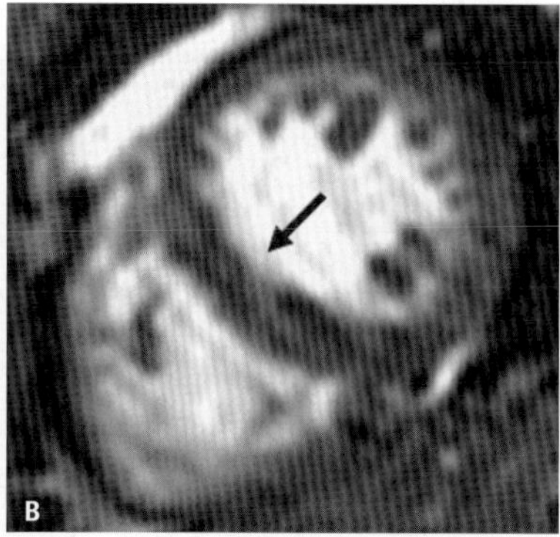

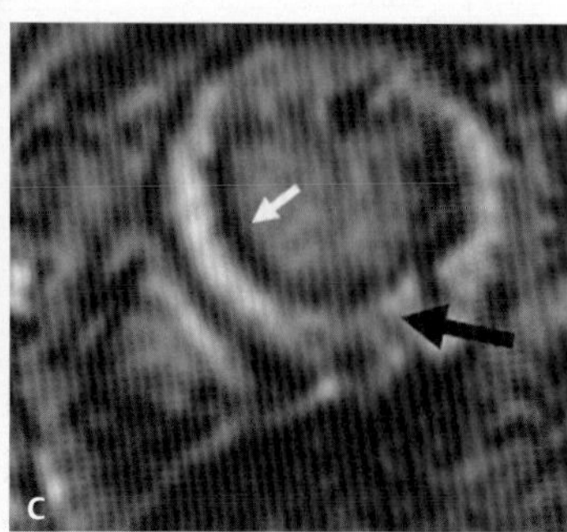

(A) An axial image at the level of the pulmonary hila shows several abnormalities: hilar lymph nodes (*dotted white circle*), a pulmonary nodule (*white arrow*) and pleural thickening (*open white arrow*). **(B)** In the short axis, the myocardial thickness is normal and signal is heterogeneous (*black arrow*). Delayed gadolinium enhancement of the myocardium is intense (*larger black arrow*) but spares the endocardium (*white arrow*). **(C)** Delayed gadolinium enhancement of the mid myocardium is intense (*black arrow*) but spares the endocardium (*white arrow*).

Differential Diagnosis

- ***Pulmonary and cardiac sarcoidosis:*** Sarcoidosis is an idiopathic granulomatous disease that initially affects pulmonary tissues and subsequently may involve cardiac and neural tissues.
- *Lung cancer:* The combination of hilar lymphadenopathy, a pulmonary nodule, and pleural thickening raises concern for lung cancer, but the clinical history does not support the diagnosis of neoplasm.
- *Infectious myocarditis:* Enhancement of the mid myocardium of the left ventricle (LV) can be seen in patients with myocarditis, but hilar lymphadenopathy and pulmonary nodules indicate another etiology.

Essential Facts

- Cardiac sarcoidosis produces symptoms in only 5% of patients.
- Histologic findings of cardiac sarcoidosis have been found at autopsy in 20 to 50% of patients with pulmonary sarcoidosis.
- The clinical sequelae of sarcoid granulomas within the myocardium range from asymptomatic conduction abnormalities to fatal ventricular arrhythmias.
- Chronic sarcoid infiltration may demonstrate primarily midmyocardial and epicardial delayed enhancement in a noncoronary distribution.
- Myocardial inflammation in sarcoidosis often involves the septum and sometimes the LV wall, whereas the papillary muscle and the right ventricular wall are rarely affected.

Other Imaging Findings

- Sarcoid infiltrates are visible on MRI as intramyocardial focal zones with increased signal intensity on both black blood and early enhanced images because of edema associated with inflammation.
- In the acute phase, first-pass perfusion studies do not show segmental ischemic defects but range from normal to early increased segmental enhancement.
- Cine MRI functional images in patients with cardiac sarcoidosis may exhibit segmental contraction abnormalities.
- With severe cardiac involvement, massive infiltration may sometimes lead to diffuse myocardial thickening and marked contraction abnormalities.
- In severe disease, congestive cardiomyopathy and heart failure develop secondary to conduction and contraction abnormalities.
- On echo sequences of advanced sarcoidosis, septal wall thinning, systolic and diastolic LV dysfunction, regional wall motion abnormalities, and pericardial effusion are noted.
- Early cardiac sarcoidosis is difficult to diagnose; enhancement diminishes after steroid therapy.
- Thallium 201 shows segmental defects in areas of myocardial deposits.

✔ Pearls & ✘ Pitfalls

✔ Correlate cardiac findings with chest radiography and computed tomography (CT).

✔ Secondary imaging findings on MRI—mediastinal and hilar lymphadenopathy, pulmonary fibrosis and nodules, and pleural disease—are primary findings on CT.

✘ Imaging findings are not specific for the diagnosis of cardiac sarcoidosis.

✘ Myocardial biopsy is the only known method for definitive diagnosis.

Case 78

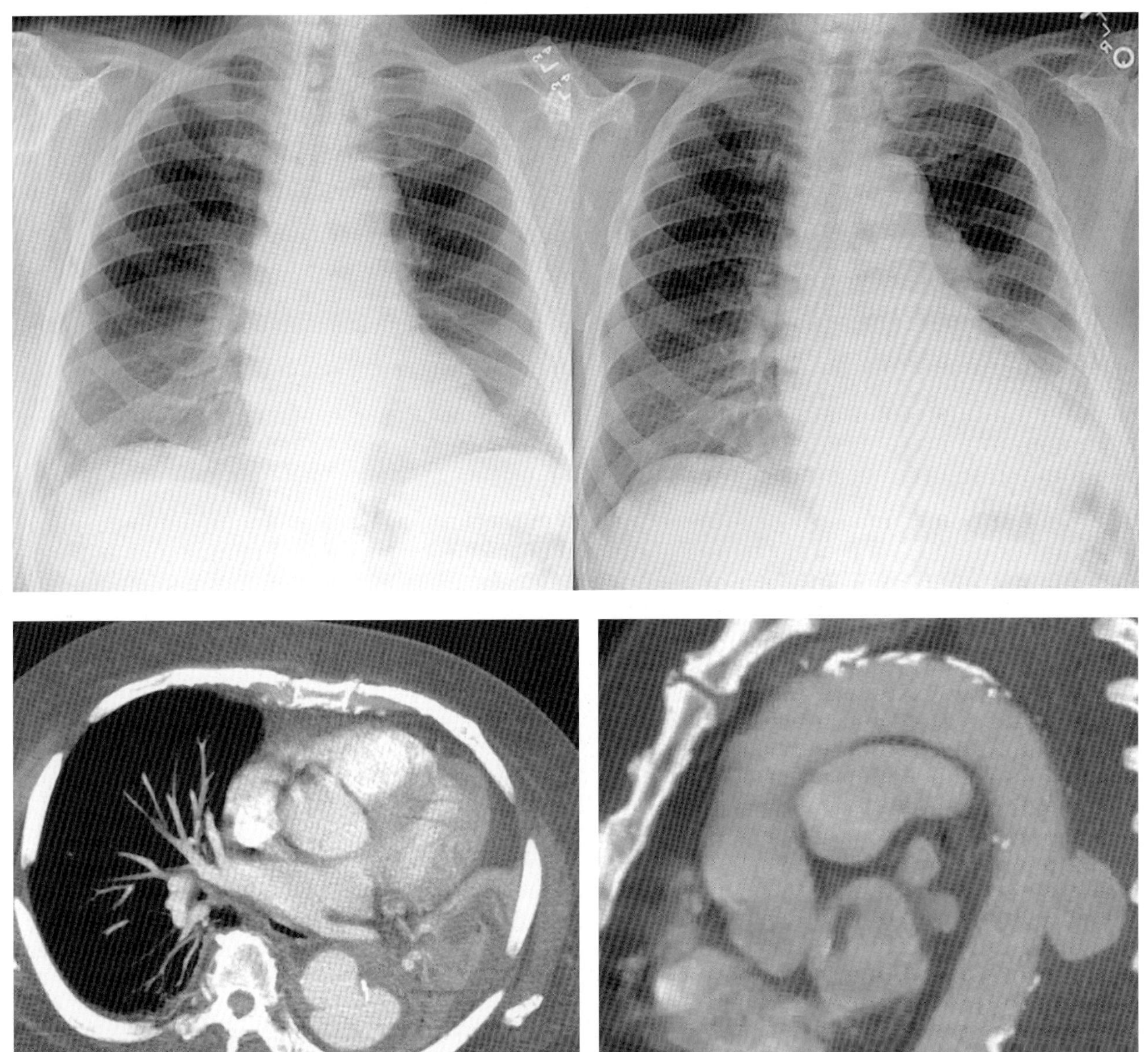

A

B

C

Clinical Presentation

A 95-year-old man presents with a new finding on chest radiographs.

Imaging Findings

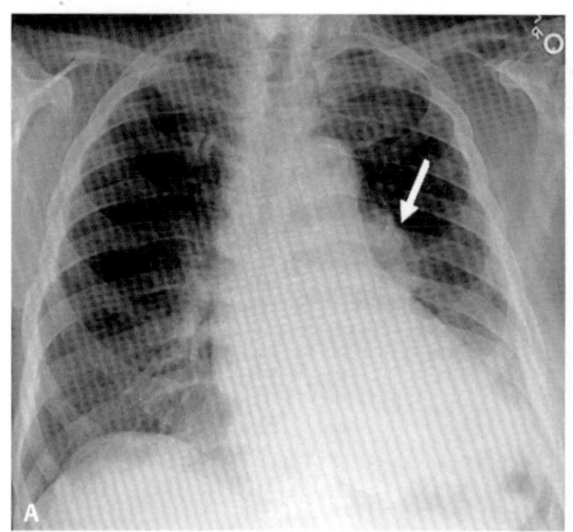

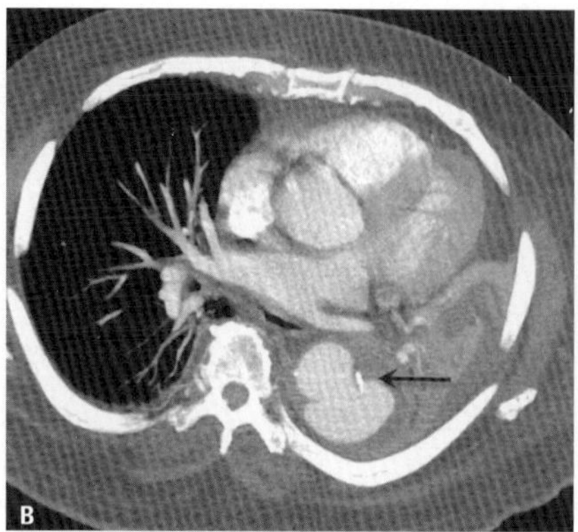

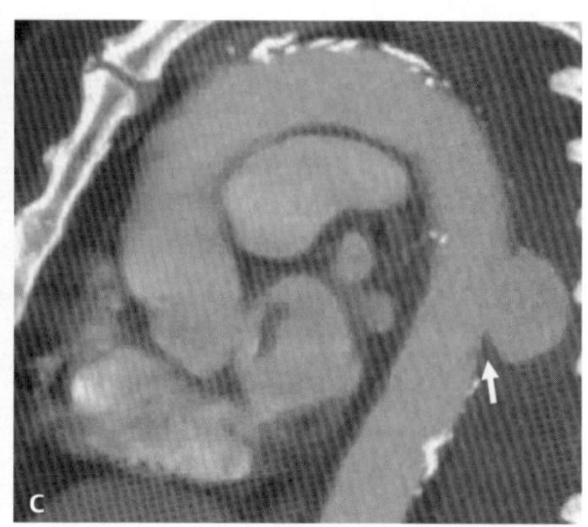

(A) The second chest radiograph, taken one month after the first seen in the case presentation, reveals a new mass at the level of the left hilum (*white arrow*). **(B)** A contrast enhanced CT angiogram (CTA) of the chest shows a focal outpouching of the posterolateral aortic lumen/wall (*black arrow*). The left lower lobe of the lung is collapsed and there is a high attenuation hemorrhagic pleural effusion. **(C)** The saggittal oblique reconstructed CTA image of the aorta shows the aortic lesion forms an acute angle with the normal descending thoracic aorta (*white arrow*).

Differential Diagnosis

- ***Pseudoaneurysm of the thoracic aorta:*** The focal, saccular outpouching of the aorta in this patient has a narrow neck, a finding typical of pseudoaneurysm rather than a true aneurysm.
- *True aneurysm of the thoracic aorta:* True aneurysms usually have a broad neck or are fusiform with circumferential dilatation of the aorta.
- *Aortic rupture:* The presence of the hemorrhagic pleural effusion indicates that blood may be leaking from the site of the pseudoaneurysm, but the aorta has not yet ruptured.

Essential Facts

- A pseudoaneurysm is formed when the intima of the aorta is disrupted; the other layers of the aorta remain intact.
- A true aneurysm involves all layers of the aorta.
- Atherosclerotic disease, trauma, and potentially infection are commonly associated with pseudoaneurysms of the aorta.
- Atherosclerotic disease is most common in the transverse aortic arch and descending aorta.
- Focal disruption of the intima or plaque ulceration can be caused by atherosclerotic disease. If high arterial pressure causes the outer layers of the aortic wall to expand in a focal manner, a pseudoaneurysm is formed.
- Traumatic pseudoaneurysms occur at the point of attachment or tethering, such as at the site of the ductus ligament.
- In patients who develop pseudoaneurysm following aortic grafting, up to 50% of pseudoaneurysms will not have clinical findings of infection but are culture-positive.
- The most common organism is *Staphylococcus epidermidis.*

Other Imaging Findings

- The short-term change in the mediastinum should raise immediate concern for an aneurysm rather than a mass.
- Hemorrhagic pleural effusion indicates leakage of blood from the pseudoaneurysm, possibly a precursor to aortic rupture.

✔ Pearls & ✘ Pitfalls

✔ Saccular shape and a narrow neck are imaging hallmarks of pseudoaneurysm.

✘ Intramural hematoma may have a crescent shape or result in fusiform enlargement of the aorta.

✘ Abdominal aortic pseudoaneurysms are often diagnosed late or following disastrous complications.

Case 79

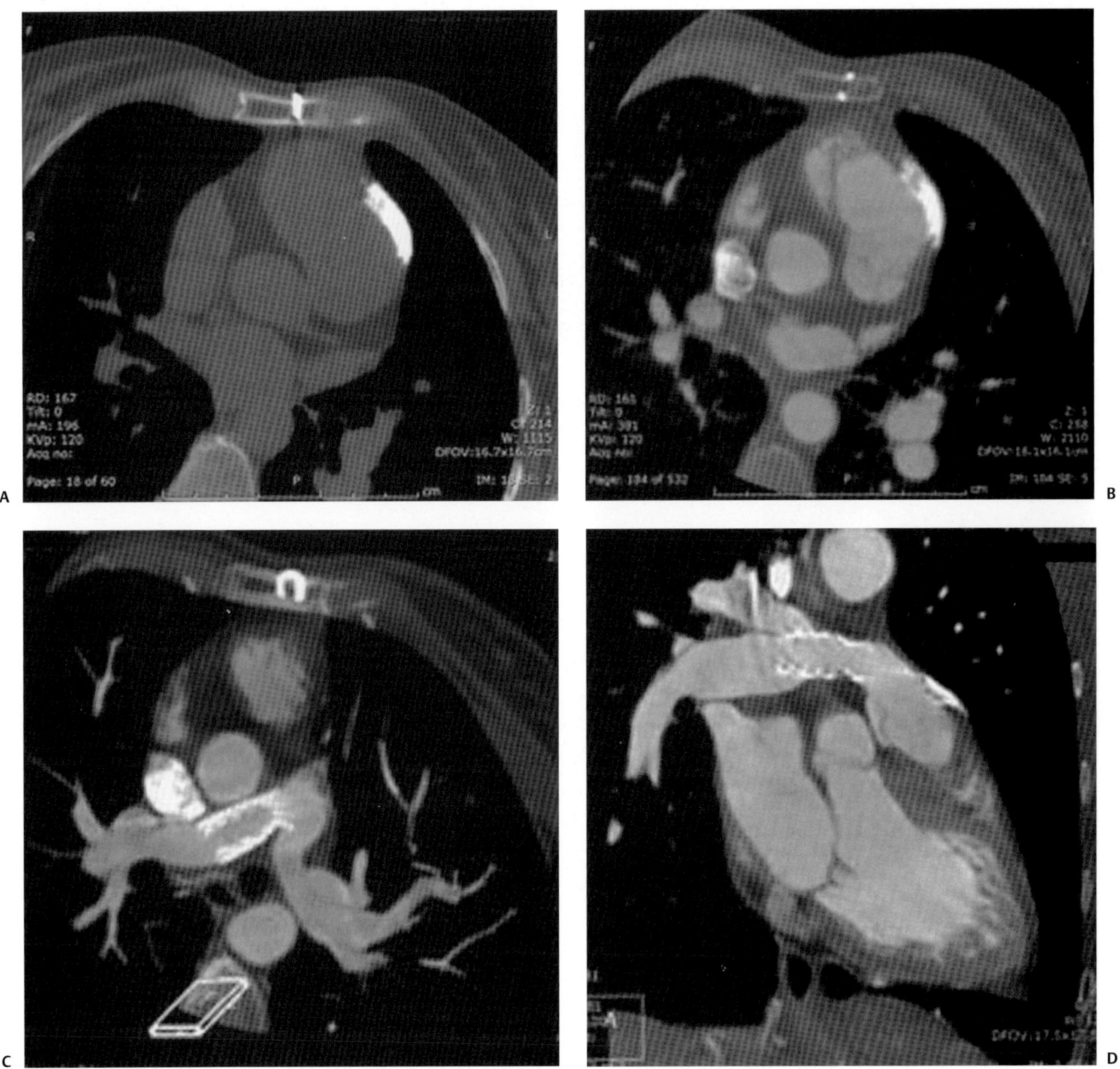

■ Clinical Presentation

A 41-year-old woman presents with a history of fatigue, cardiac surgery in infancy, and prenatal maternal rubella.

Imaging Findings

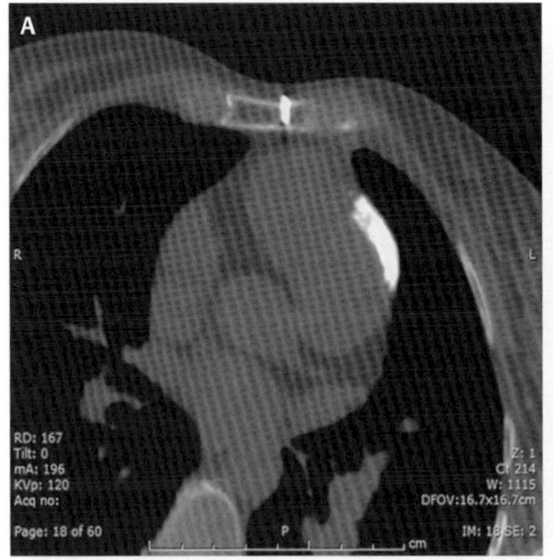
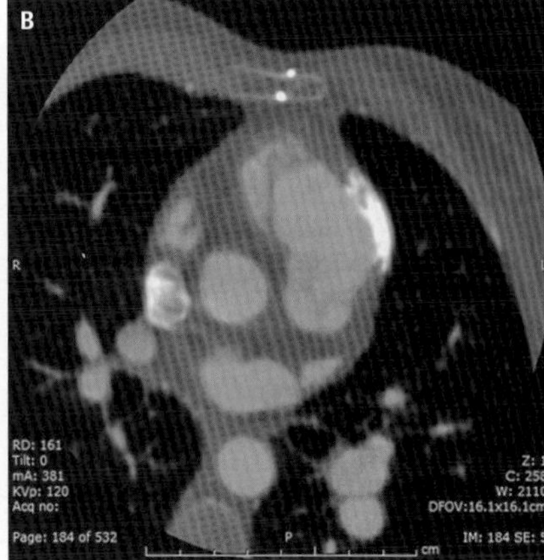
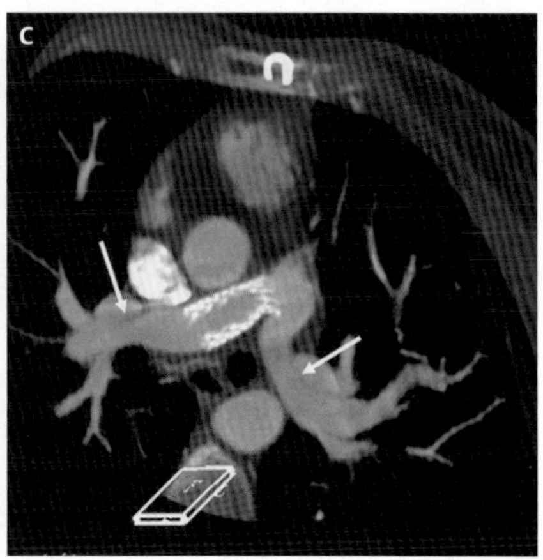
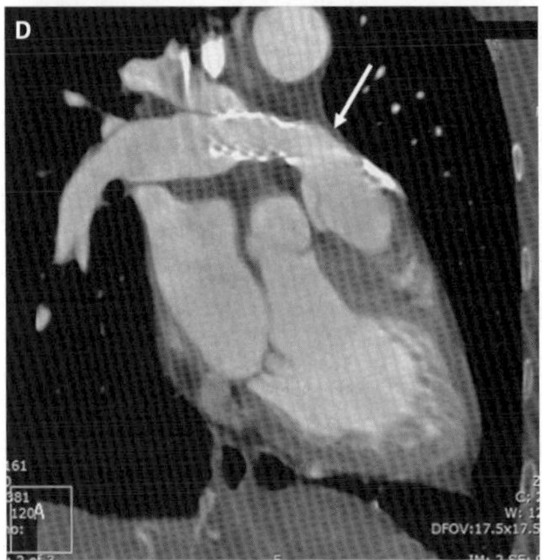

(A) Non–contrast- and contrast-enhanced cardiac-gated computed tomography images in **(B)** axial, **(C)** axial oblique maximum intensity projection, and **(D)** coronal oblique imaging planes showing pulmonary artery stenosis bilaterally. The right pulmonary artery stenosis was previously treated with an intravascular stent. Postoperative changes with a calcified graft from remote surgical correction of stenosis of the main pulmonary artery are also noted.

Differential Diagnosis

- ***Pulmonary artery stenosis (PAS):*** PAS is a valvular, subvalvular, or supravalvular obstruction to the normal emptying of the right ventricle.
- *Pulmonary arterial hypertension:* Abnormal calcification of the pulmonary artery may result from severe chronic pulmonary hypertension. In such cases, the diameter of the central pulmonary arteries is typically enlarged.

Essential Facts

- Obstruction at a supravalvular level is the most common type (60%) of PAS and may affect the main trunk of the pulmonary artery, central arteries, or more peripheral branches either as single or multiple strictures.
- Childhood PAS is frequently seen in association with other congenital heart defects (e.g., tetralogy of Fallot, Williams syndrome, and Noonan syndrome) or with congenital/maternal rubella, carcinoid syndrome, cutis laxa, and Ehlers–Danlos syndrome.
- In adults, PAS may be secondary to a congenital anomaly (rubella) or acquired, resulting from surgery (lung transplant and systemic-to-pulmonary shunt), vasculitis (Takayasu disease and Behçet syndrome), chronic thromboembolism, fibrosing mediastinitis, tumor, or silicosis.
- It has been proposed that more centrally located segmental PAS is more commonly congenital, whereas more peripheral segmental PAS is more commonly from other diseases.
- Gay's classification of supravalvular PAS includes four types. Type 1 is a single stenosis of the main, right, or left pulmonary artery. Type 2 is stenosis at the bifurcation of the main trunk extending to the right and left arteries. Type 3 involves multiple stenoses of the peripheral pulmonary branches. Type 4 consists of a combination of central and peripheral pulmonary artery stenoses.
- Microscopic evaluation of the narrow segment reveals primarily fibrous intimal proliferation, medial hypoplasia, and loss of elastic fibers.

Other Imaging Findings

- There may be post-stenotic dilatation of the affected pulmonary artery.

✔ Pearls & ✘ Pitfalls

✔ Williams syndrome is characterized by elfin fascies, abnormal dentition, supravalvular aortic stenosis, mental retardation, hypercalcemia, and sometimes pulmonary artery stenosis.

✔ Noonan syndrome is characterized by short stature, pectus excavatum, ventricular septal defect, and multiple PAS.

✘ The presence of an unmatched segmental lung perfusion defect on a ventilation/perfusion scan in a patient with PAS has frequently led to the mistaken diagnosis of pulmonary thromboembolic disease.

Case 80

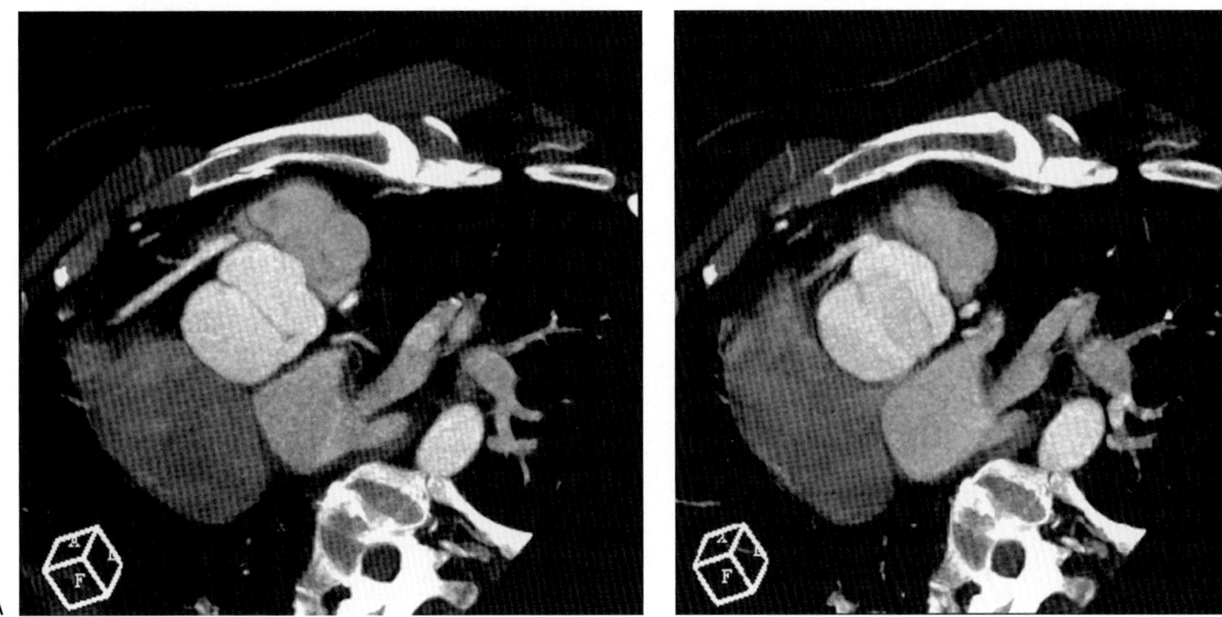

A B

Clinical Presentation

Murmur in a 38-year-old man with a history of ventricular septal defect (VSD) repaired in infancy

Imaging Findings

A 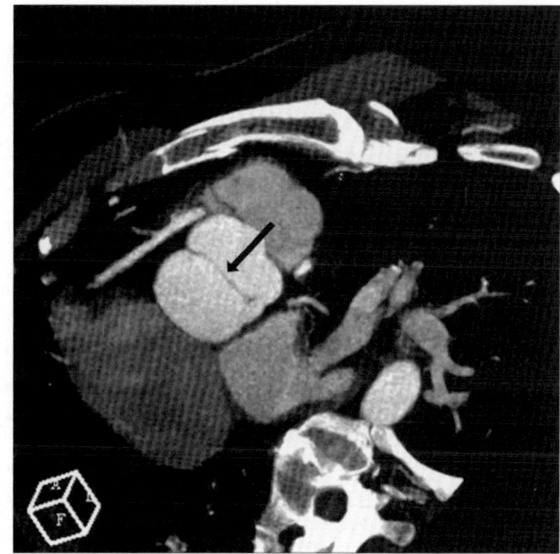

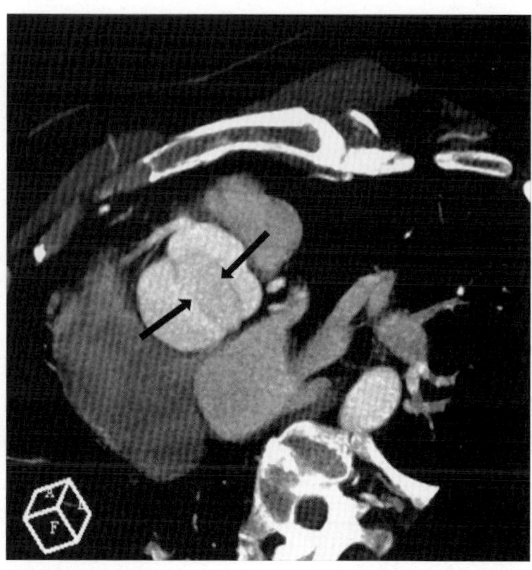 B

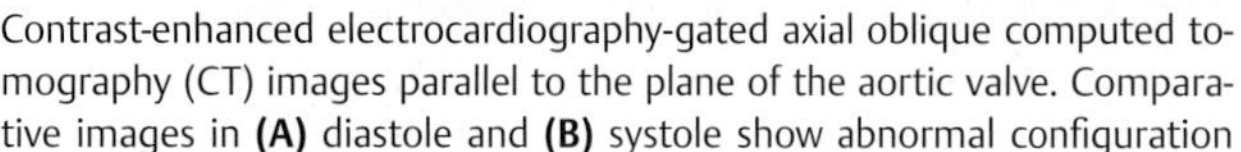
Contrast-enhanced electrocardiography-gated axial oblique computed tomography (CT) images parallel to the plane of the aortic valve. Comparative images in **(A)** diastole and **(B)** systole show abnormal configuration of the aortic valve, with only two leaflets and a single coaptation line in diastole and two commissures visualized in systole.

Differential Diagnosis

- ***Bicuspid aortic valve (BAV):*** A BAV has two instead of the typical three leaflets and one commissure instead of three.
- *Normal aortic valve:* The normal aortic valve has three leaflets that during diastole coapt in the midline, producing a “Mercedes-Benz” star configuration, and fully open during ventricular systole.
- *Unicuspid aortic valve:* In this uncommon anomaly, the abnormal valve is intrinsically stenotic and occasionally also incompetent. It appears as a diaphragm with a central opening or as a raphe with one lateral attachment.

Essential Facts

- Among all congenital cardiac malformations, the BAV is the most common.
- It affects 1 to 2% of the general population, with a higher prevalence in men than in women.
- Common complications associated with BAV include aortic stenosis (50%), aortic regurgitation (2%), infective endocarditis (30%), aortic dilatation, aneurysm formation, dissection (5%), and rupture.
- BAV may be associated with other congenital cardiovascular abnormalities, in particular aortic coarctation (50–80%). Other common associations are interruption of the aorta (36%) and VSD (20%).
- Patients with BAV often have a more generalized disorder of vascular connective tissue that causes a loss of elastic tissue (e.g., Marfan and Turner syndromes).
- A BAV typically presents with unequal cusp size, due to fusion of two of the cusps, and one central raphe.
- An anomalous origin of the coronary arteries is rarely present.
- Most cases of BAV are sporadic, but familial occurrence has been reported in > 10% of affected individuals.
- Treatment of BAV is mainly surgical.
- Surgery to repair the aortic root or replace the ascending aorta in patients with BAV is recommended if the diameter of the aortic root is > 5 cm or expands by ≥ 0.5 cm per year.

Other Imaging Findings

- Echocardiography is the imaging modality of choice for the evaluation of the aortic valve. Cardiac magnetic resonance imaging (MRI) and cardiac CT angiography are excellent imaging modalities for the evaluation of the aortic arch, which is often required in these patients.

✔ Pearls & ✘ Pitfalls

✔ Patients with BAV and dilatation of the aortic root or ascending aorta (diameter > 4 cm) should undergo annual evaluation of the aortic root/ascending aorta size and morphology evaluation of echocardiography, MRI, or contrast-enhanced CT.

✘ The bicuspid morphology of a BAV may be obscured by severe calcification and fibrosis.

Case 81

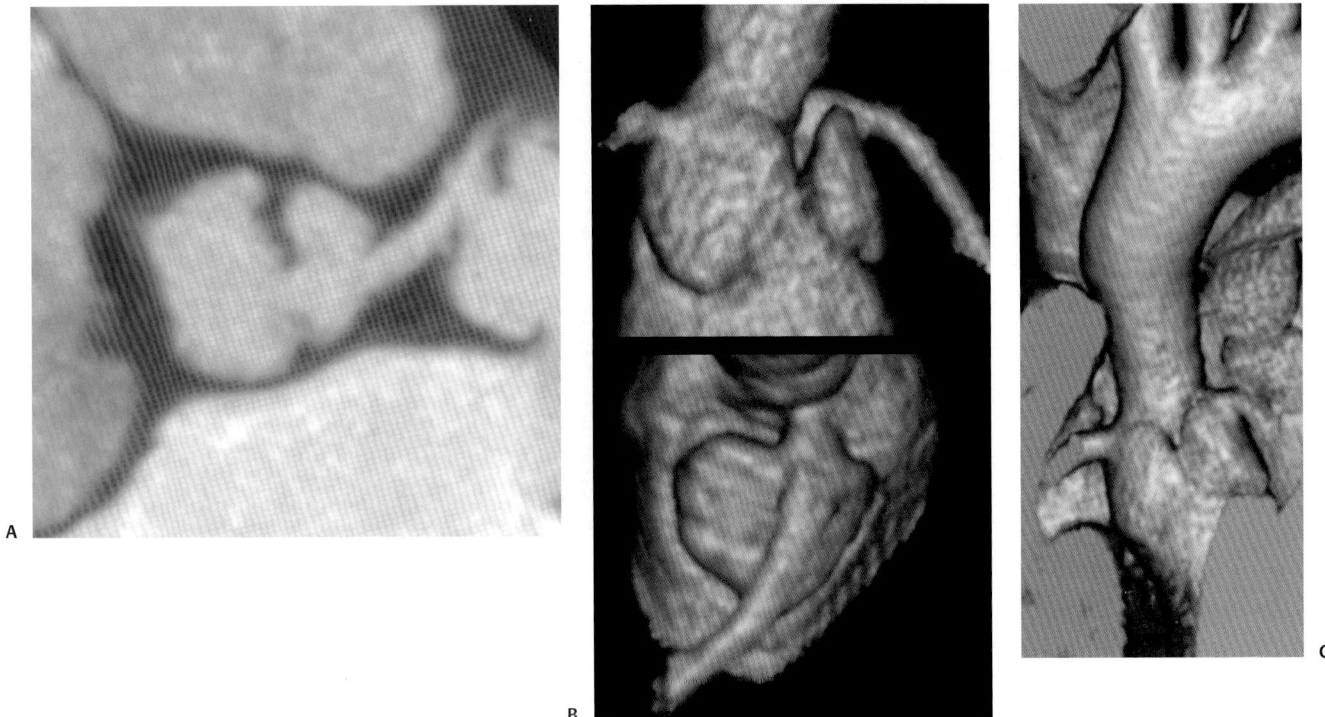

Clinical Presentation

A 10-year-old boy presents with a history of William syndrome and supravalvular aortic stenosis (SVAS).

Imaging Findings

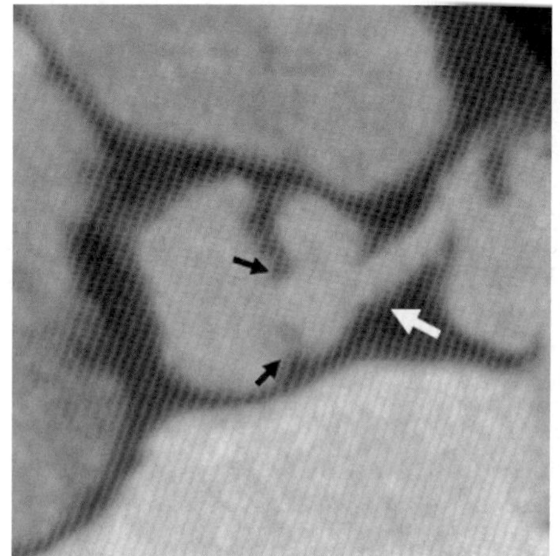

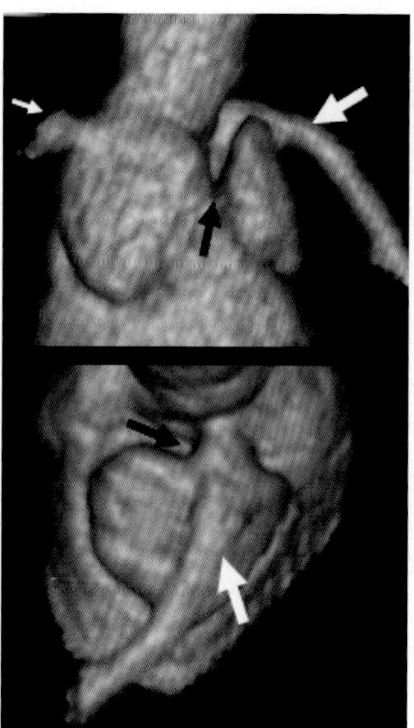

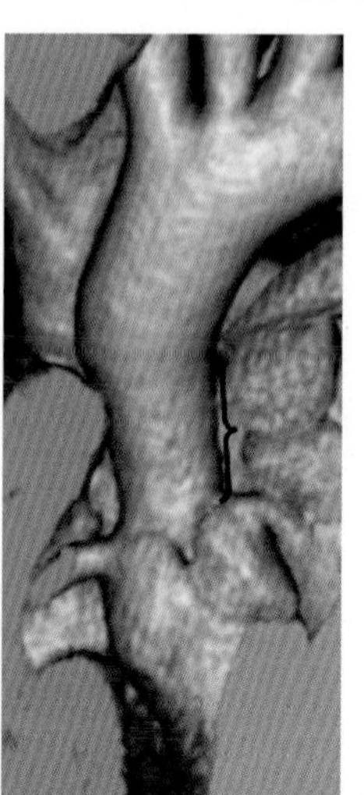

(A) At the superior margin of the sinuses of valsalva prominent, abnormal aortic leaflet commissural fusion is asymmetric (*black arrows*). The origin of the left main coronary artery (*white arrow*) is almost isolated from the lumen of the ascending aorta. **(B)** Three-dimensional volume-rendered views of the sinuses of Valsalva show the origin and proximal course of the left main coronary artery (*large white arrows*), the origin of the right coronary artery (*small white arrow*), and the deep crevices caused by the valve commissures (*black arrows*). **(C)** A three-dimensional volume-rendered view of the sinotubular junction shows mild tubular hypoplasia of the proximal ascending aorta (*bracket*).

Differential Diagnosis

- ***Isolation of the left coronary artery ostium and supravalvular aortic stenosis (SVAS):*** In patients with Williams syndrome, there may be numerous congenital abnormalities or malformations of the aortic subvalvular, valvular, and supravalvular regions.
- *Bicuspid aortic valve:* The appearance of the partially fused commissures at the sinotubular junction raises suspicion for bicuspid morphology of the aortic valve, but at the level of the valve annulus, the trileaflet valve was seen.
- *Anomalous origin of the left main coronary artery:* The left and right coronary arteries arise from the left and right coronary sinuses, respectively. There is no coronary artery arising from the noncoronary cusp or abnormally from the right or left cusp.

Essential Facts

- Williams syndrome is a rare (1 in 7500 births) genetic syndrome that manifests as cardiac and developmental problems.
- Patients have characteristic facial features, such as a small upturned nose, a wide mouth with full lips, a small chin, and puffiness around the eyes.
- Hypertension and hypercalcemia are also found in patients with Williams syndrome.
- In addition to the aorta and aortic valve, the pulmonary arteries may be narrowed.
- When isolated, the ostium of the left main coronary artery may be completely occluded.
- Ischemia and infarction may result, depending on the degree of isolation.
- Aortic valve replacement is the optimal method of repair, as repair of the native valve is usually impossible.

Other Imaging Findings

- When the left coronary ostium is isolated, a segment of the left main coronary artery may be tunneled within the ascending aorta.
- The valve may be tricuspid, but the aortic leaflet may be small and immobile and perhaps partially adherent to the aortic wall.
- Aortic valve insufficiency is a commonly associated finding.

✔ Pearls & ✘ Pitfalls

✔ Aortic and pulmonary artery findings may progress over time, so monitoring with echocardiography and other imaging modalities, such as magnetic resonance imaging (MRI) and computed tomography (CT), is required.

✔ Choose MRI as the initial and preferred follow-up imaging modality when needed, as there is no radiation dose.

✔ CT can be essential, as in this case, to reveal the anatomy of the aortic valve and coronary artery ostia.

✘ Coronary artery catheterization can fail, as it may be impossible to catheterize the left main coronary artery.

Case 82

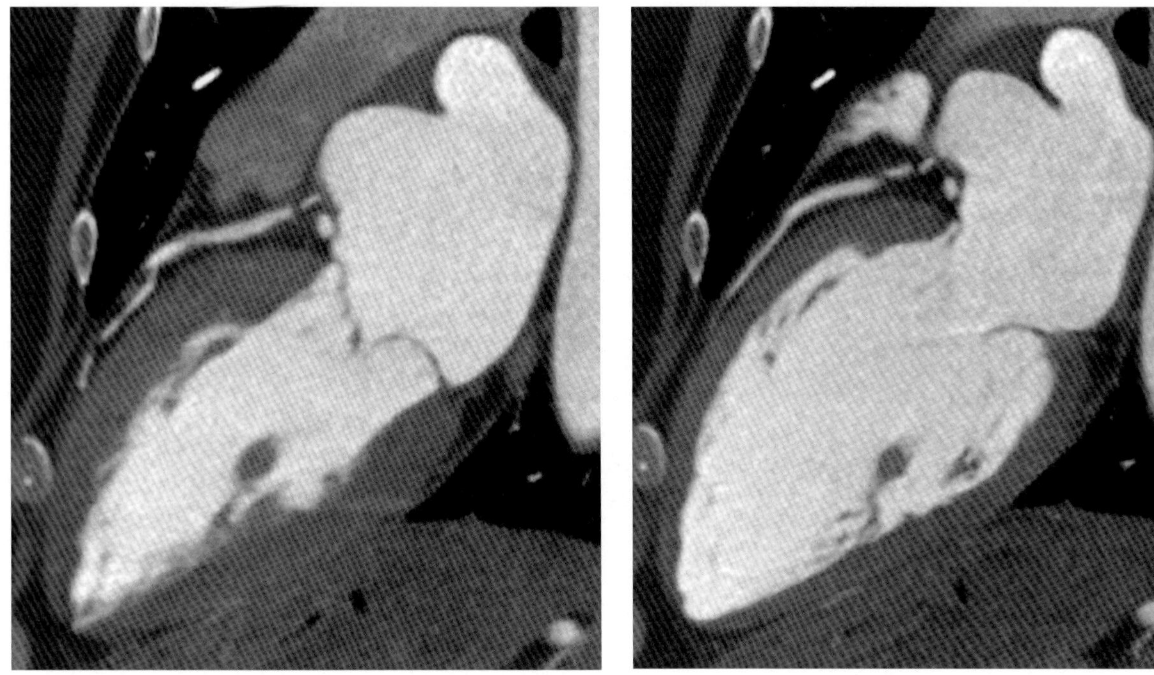

Clinical Presentation

A 53-year-old woman presents with a history of chest pain.

Imaging Findings

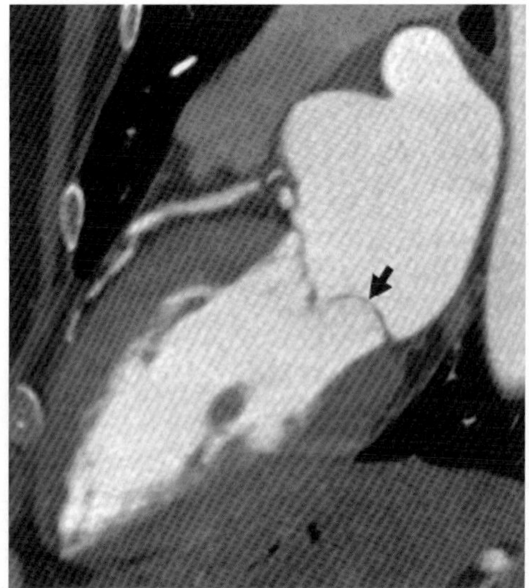

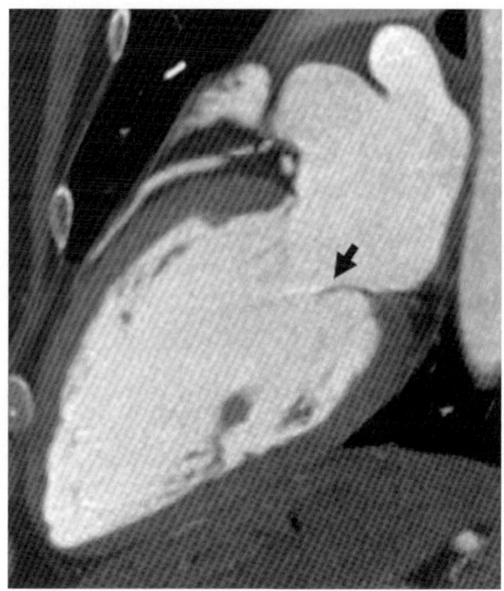

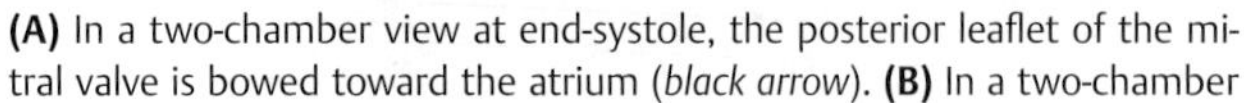

(A) In a two-chamber view at end-systole, the posterior leaflet of the mitral valve is bowed toward the atrium (*black arrow*). **(B)** In a two-chamber view at end-diastole, the mitral valve is open and has a normal appearance (*black arrow*).

Differential Diagnosis

- ***Mitral valve prolapse:*** Bowing of the mitral valve toward the atrium occurs in some patients with structural abnormalities of the valve, as pressure in the left ventricle is increased during systole.
- *Mitral valve stenosis:* The mitral valve opens normally during diastole.
- *Mitral valve regurgitation:* Functional parameters such as valve regurgitation are not typically assessed by multidetector computed tomography, even when retrospective electrocardiography gating is used. The left atrium is not enlarged, a finding commonly seen in mitral valve regurgitation.

Essential Facts

- Structural abnormalities of the mitral valve that can be seen in patients with mitral valve prolapse include increased size, valve leaflet asymmetry, elongation of the leaflets, posterior leaflet scalloping, and focal thickening of the anterior leaflet.
- Although most often a benign finding, mitral valve regurgitation may be present.
- A "click" may be heard during auscultation.

Other Imaging Findings

- Hypertrophic cardiomyopathy
- Papillary muscle anomalies (both muscles may attach directly to the anterior leaflet)
- Thrombus attached to the mitral leaflets
- Embolic cerebral vascular accident

✔ Pearls & ✘ Pitfalls

✔ Patients should be monitored for the development of mitral regurgitation, usually with echocardiography.

✔ Cardiac magnetic resonance imaging can be useful for better visualization of the mitral valve and to assess for hypertrophic cardiomyopathy, which is associated with prolapse in some patients.

✘ The valsalva maneuver, which decreases ventricular preload, can induce mitral valve prolapse.

Case 83

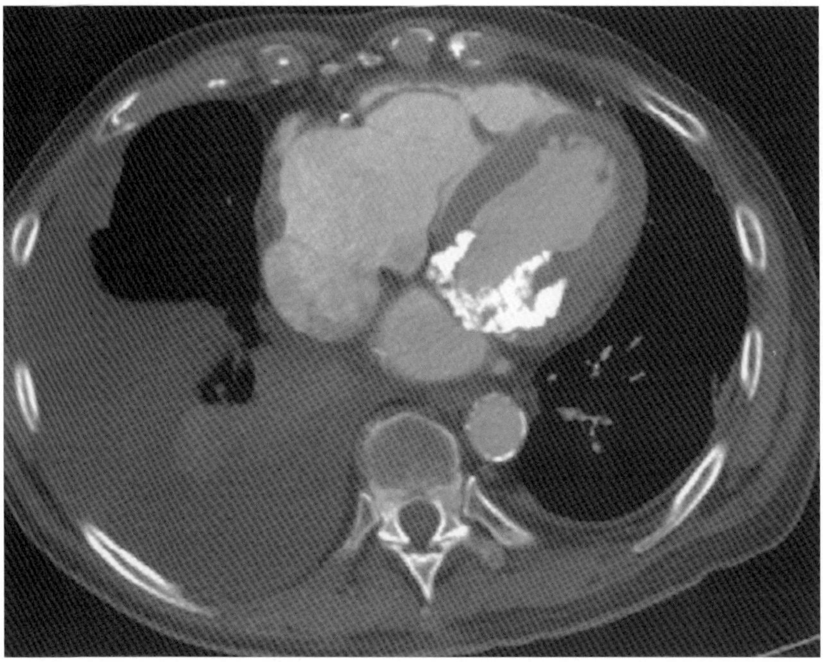

■ Clinical Presentation

A 55-year-old woman presents with a history of mitral valve replacement.

Imaging Findings

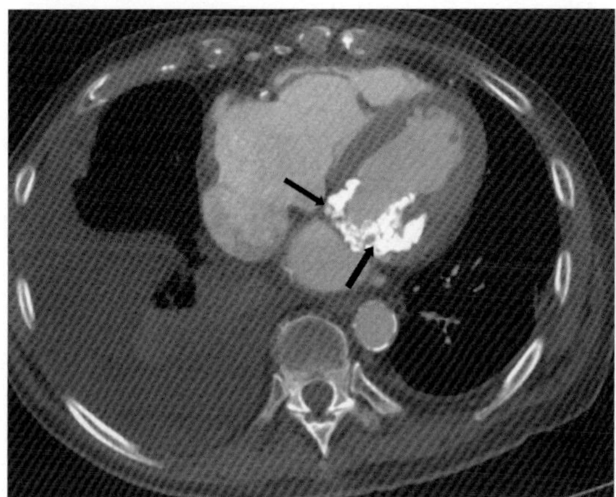

Contrast-enhanced chest computed tomography image shows an extensive calcification of the mitral valve annulus extending to the adjacent myocardium. A large pleural effusion on the right side is also appreciated.

Differential Diagnosis

- ***Mitral annulus calcification:*** Mitral valve calcification can be centered in the valve itself or extend to the mitral annulus and even to the adjacent myocardium. It can be an incidental finding with no significant valvular dysfunction, but when present, dysfunction is more often insufficiency than stenosis.
- *Dystrophic calcification:* Dystrophic myocardial calcification is characteristic of remote ischemic heart disease or an old and healed infarcted myocardium and is typically in the anterior wall of the left ventricle.
- *Metastatic calcification:* Hypercalcemia and hyperphosphatemia in patients with hyperparathyroidism, such as those with chronic renal insufficiency undergoing long-term hemodialysis, can induce metastatic calcification of the myocardium. In such cases, the calcium deposits can affect the mitral valve annulus but also tend to involve other areas of the myocardium.

Essential Facts

- There is a close association between mitral valve calcification and rheumatic heart disease.
- When the calcified valve function is affected, stenosis is more common than regurgitation.
- Mitral annulus calcification is more commonly a degenerative process that tends to affect elderly women.
- Calcification of the mitral annulus is generally associated with mitral valve disease.
- Patients with extensive mitral annulus calcification are at higher risk for peripheral embolization and stroke.
- An association between mitral annular calcification, coronary artery calcification, and severe coronary artery disease has been documented.

Other Imaging Findings

- On conventional radiographs of the thorax, mitral annulus calcification has a C-shaped appearance at the expected position of the valve.

✔ Pearls & ✘ Pitfalls

✔ Mitral annulus calcification has minimal impact on the global function of the mitral valve but is a marker of increased cardiovascular risk.

✘ Mitral valve calcification and mitral annulus calcification can coexist, but their pathophysiology and functional and clinical significance are different.

Case 84

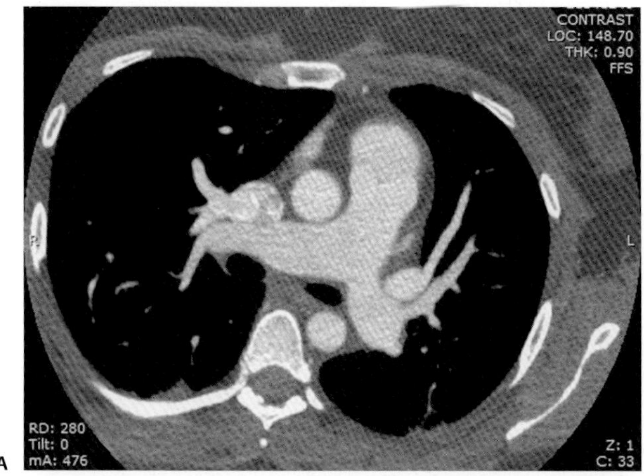

A

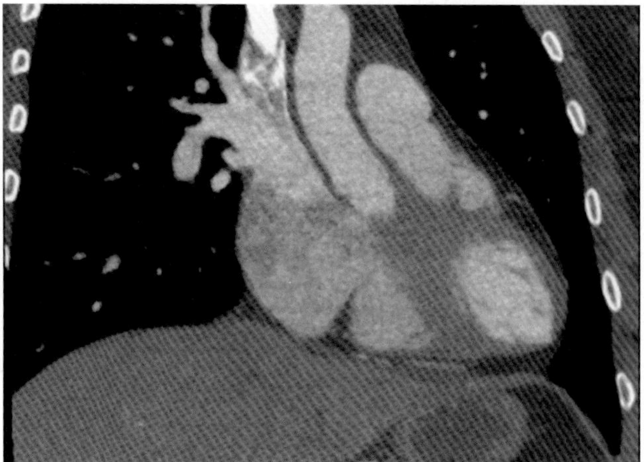
B

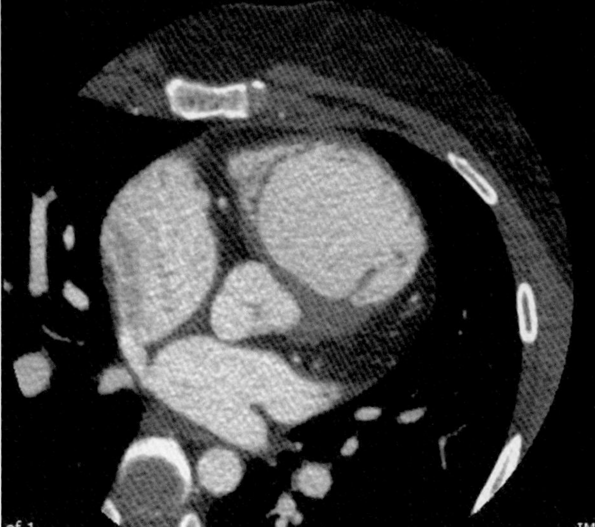

C

Clinical Presentation

A 34-year-old woman presents with a murmur on physical examination, and an echocardiogram reveals an enlarged right atrium and ventricle.

Imaging Findings

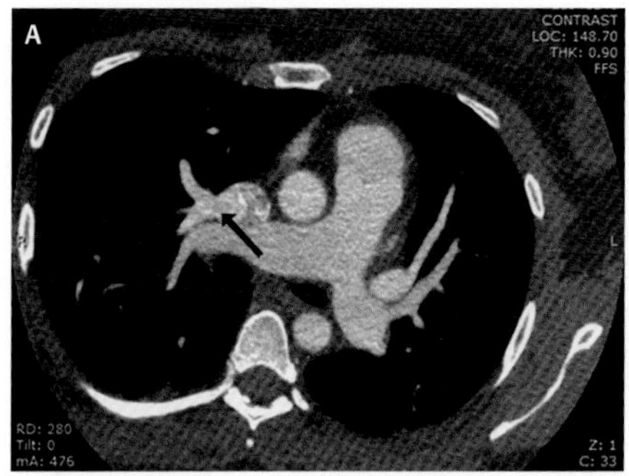

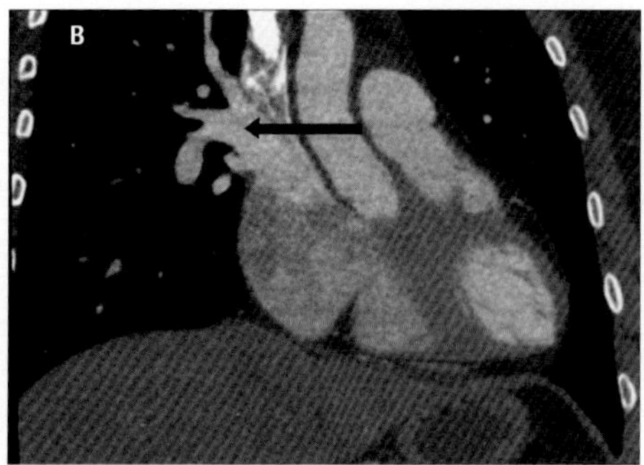

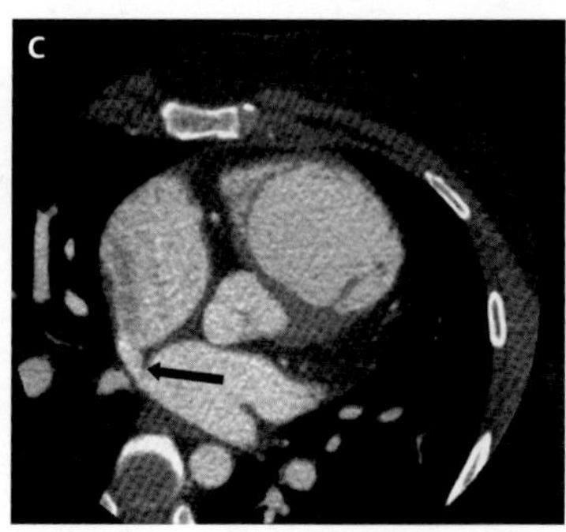

Contrast-enhanced cardiac-gated computed tomography angiography (CTA): Axial **(A)** and coronal **(B)** images show abnormal drainage of the right upper lobe pulmonary veins to the superior vena cava. **(C)** Axial image at the level of the cardiac atria shows abnormal communication between the right and left atria.

Differential Diagnosis

- ***Sinus venosus atrial septal defect (ASD) with partial anomalous pulmonary venous return (PAPVR):*** Sinus venosus ASDs are typically seen in the superior aspect of the interatrial septum and are commonly associated with PAPVR.
- *Ostium secundum ASD:* Ostium secundum interatrial defect is a true defect of the atrial septum and involves the region of the fossa ovalis. It is not associated with PAPVR.
- *Ostium primum ASD:* Ostium primum interatrial defects are within the spectrum of ASDs, atrioventricular septal defects, and endocardial cushion defects. They are commonly associated with large ventricular septal defects. They are not commonly associated with PAPVR.

Essential Facts

- The sinus venosus defect is typically located posterior to the junction of the right atrium and superior vena cava.
- Sinus venosus ASD is almost always (> 90%) associated with PAPVR of some or all of the right upper lobe to the superior vena cava.
- Sinus venosus ASDs constitute 5 to 10% of all interatrial defects.
- There is increased flow into the right atrium and ventricle so that the right-sided cardiac chambers are enlarged.
- Diagnosis of this condition may be difficult by transthoracic echocardiography, and additional imaging with transesophageal echocardiography, CTA, or magnetic resonance imaging is usually needed.
- Endovascular closure is not possible, so surgery is the treatment of choice.
- The most common complications after surgery are sinus node dysfunction (secondary to injury of the sinoatrial node), superior vena cava obstruction, and residual shunt.

Other Imaging Findings

- Sixteen percent of these patients present with a persistent left superior vena cava draining into the left coronary sinus.

✔ Pearls & ✘ Pitfalls

✔ A sinus venosus ASD should be suspected in patients with unexplained right atrial and right ventricular enlargement.

✘ Sinus venosus ASD can be wrongly diagnosed as ostium secundum ASD. Identification of the associated PAPVR is key for the correct diagnosis.

Case 85

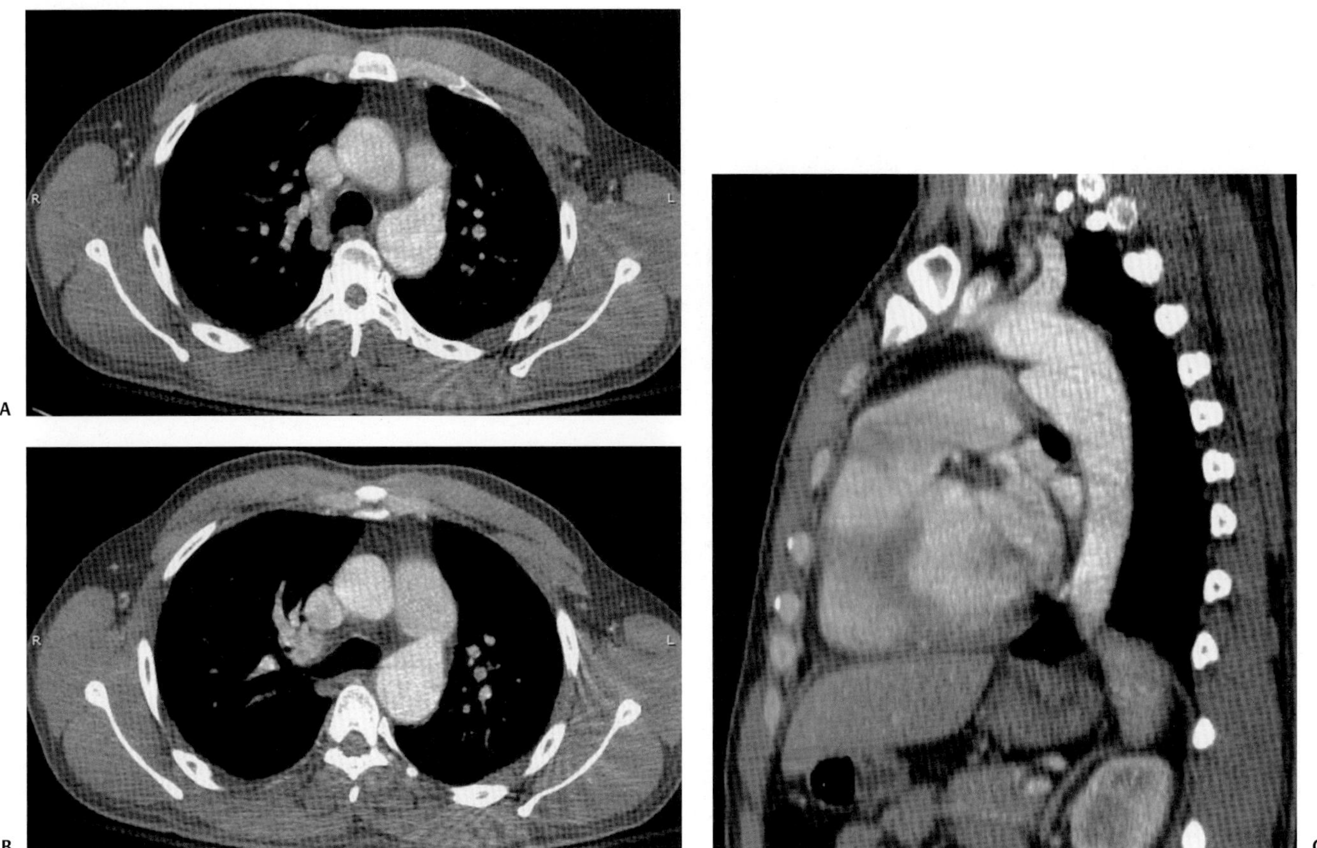

A B C

Clinical Presentation

A 28-year-old man presents with dyspnea on exertion and heart murmur on a physical examination.

Imaging Findings

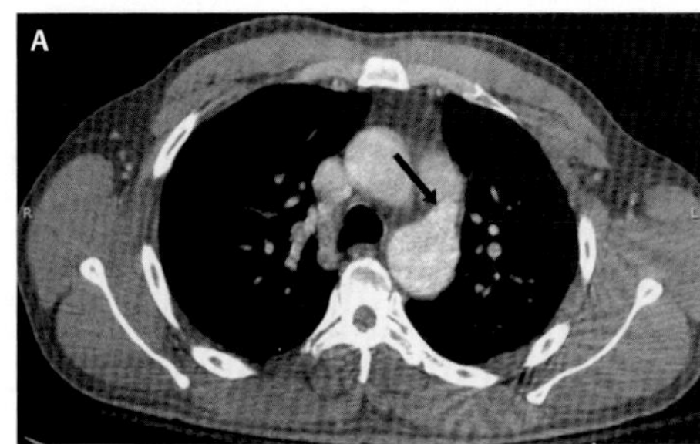

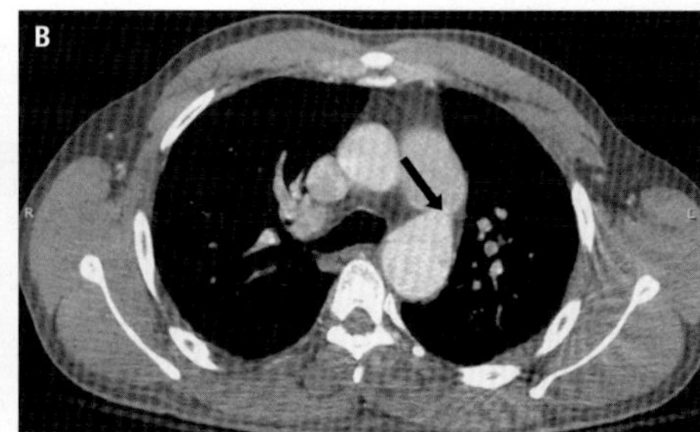

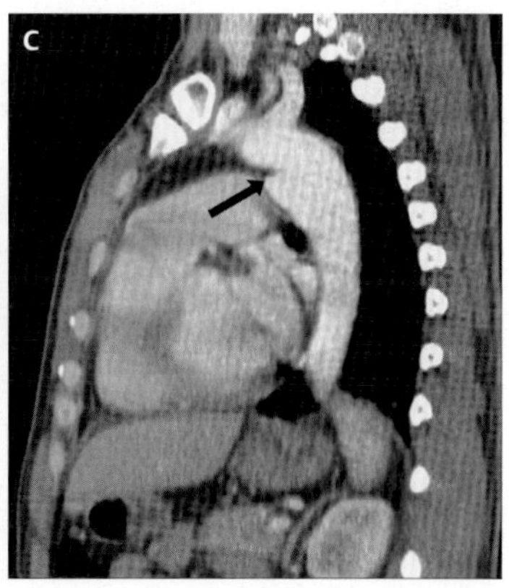

(A,B) Axial and **(C)** sagittal contrast-enhanced thoracic computed tomography (CT) images demonstrate a funnel-shaped deformity of the inferior aspect of the aortic arch projecting toward the left pulmonary artery.

Differential Diagnosis

- ***Patent ductus arteriosus (PDA):*** A vascular structure between the aortic arch and the left pulmonary artery is consistent with a PDA.
- *Ductus diverticulum:* The ductus diverticulum is a smooth focal bulge along the inferior and anteromedial aspects of the aortic isthmus, in the region of the ligamentum arteriosum. On CT, magnetic resonance imaging, or catheter angiography, it can be seen as a "bump" in the contour of the aortic arch in normal subjects.
- *Aortic pseudoaneurysm:* In trauma patients, a focal bulge of the aortic wall at the level of the ligamentum arteriosum can have a similar appearance. It typically is more irregular, more oval or rounded in shape, less tubular, and almost always associated with a mediastinal hematoma.

Essential Facts

- The ductus arteriosus is an essential fetal vascular structure that normally closes at birth or shortly after (24–48 hours); it permits right ventricular flow to be diverted away from the high-resistance pulmonary circulation into the systemic circulation.
- The resulting fibrous band after the ductus closes is the ligamentum arteriosum.
- Persistence after the first few weeks of life is abnormal.
- The hemodynamic and clinical impact of a PDA depends on its size, the magnitude of the shunting, the underlying cardiovascular status, and the presence of associated anomalies.
- A PDA results in left-to-right shunting with increased volume to the pulmonary circulation, increased flow returning to the left chambers, and left-heart volume overload.
- The incidence of PDA in children born at term is 1 in 2000 births; it accounts for 10% of all cases of congenital heart disease.
- In the normal heart, a PDA is found between the proximal left coronary artery, near its origin, and the descending thoracic aorta just distal to the left subclavian artery.

Other Imaging Findings

- Conventional chest radiograph findings vary depending on the size and magnitude of the shunting. When significant shunting occurs, cardiomegaly with left atrial and left ventricular enlargement, increased pulmonary vasculature, and prominent central pulmonary arteries can be seen.

✔ Pearls & ✘ Pitfalls

✔ Conclusive diagnosis of a PDA on CT relies on the ability to prove anatomical continuity and flow between the aorta and the pulmonary artery to differentiate it from a small diverticulum, which can have a similar appearance on axial images.

✘ Color Doppler is a very sensitive imaging modality for the detection of a PDA and is commonly used for the quantification of the resulting shunt; however, in patients with pulmonary hypertension and low-velocity ductus flow, demonstration of the patent ductus may be very difficult.

Case 86

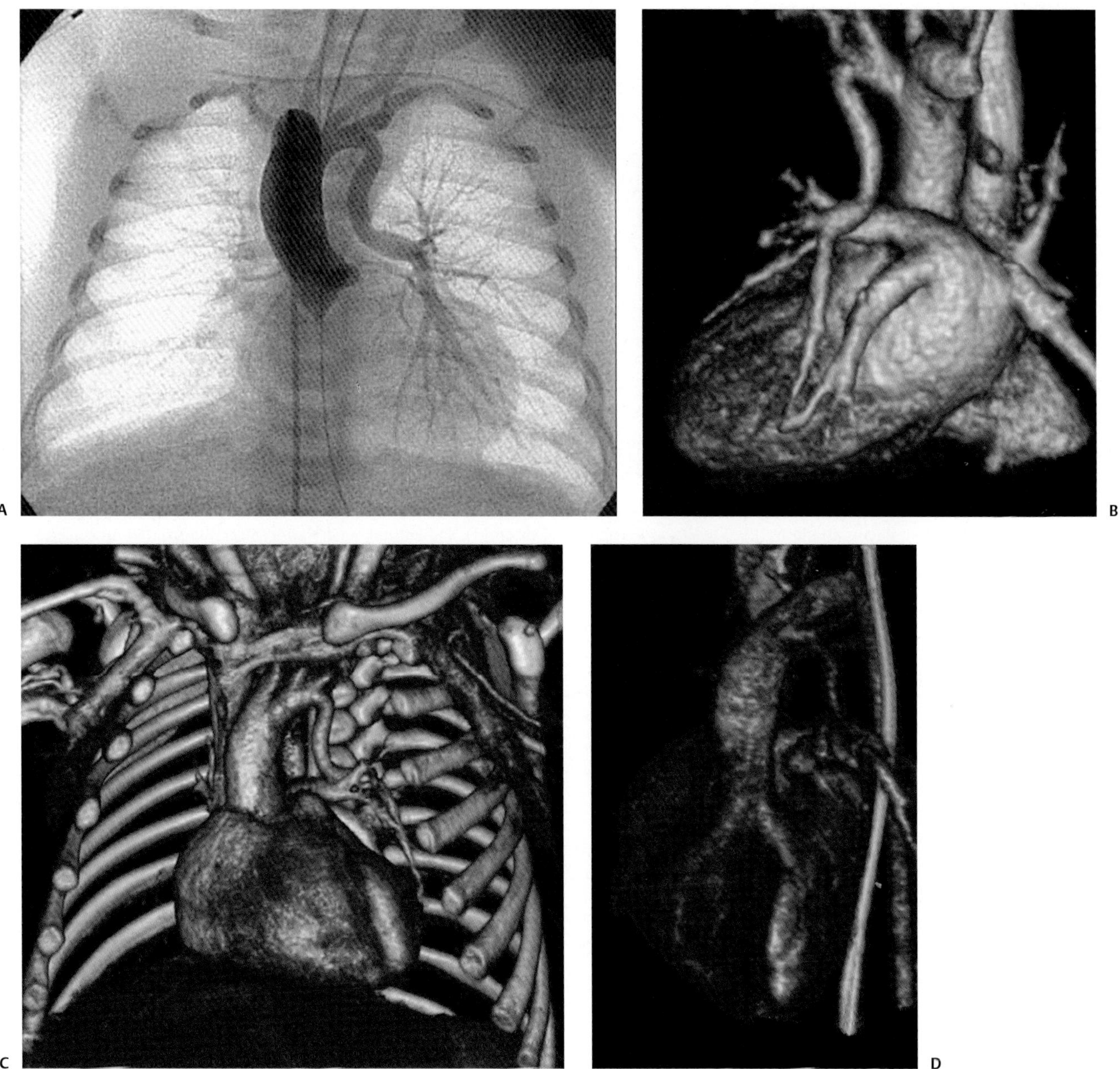

Clinical Presentation

A 6-day-old boy presents with cyanotic congenital heart disease.

Imaging Findings

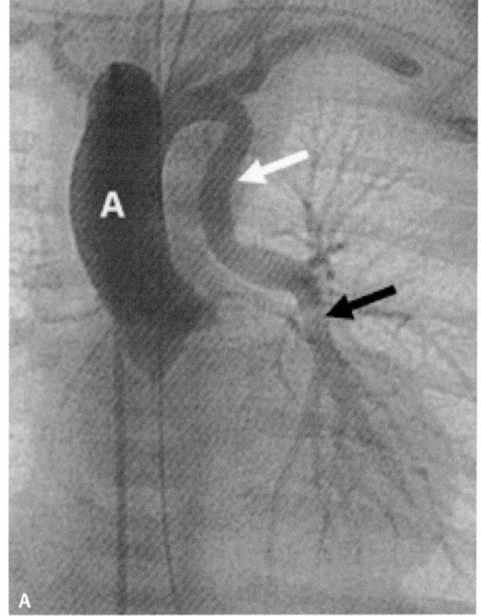

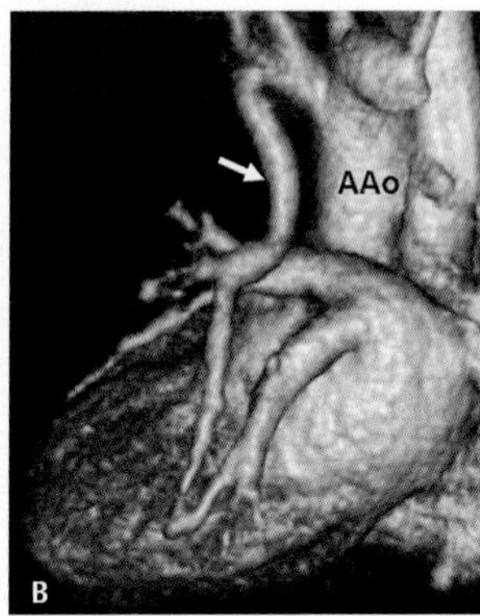

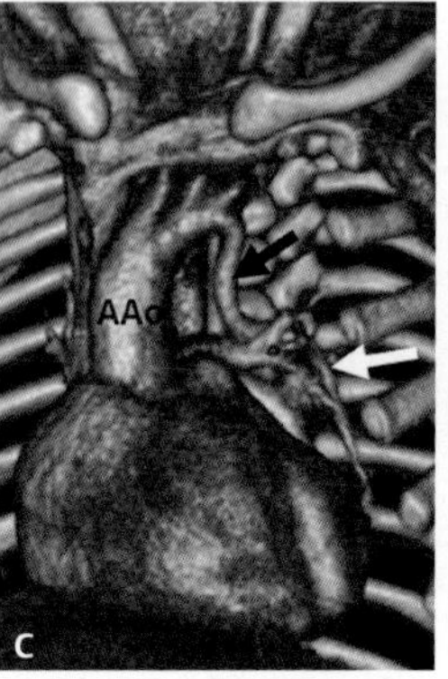

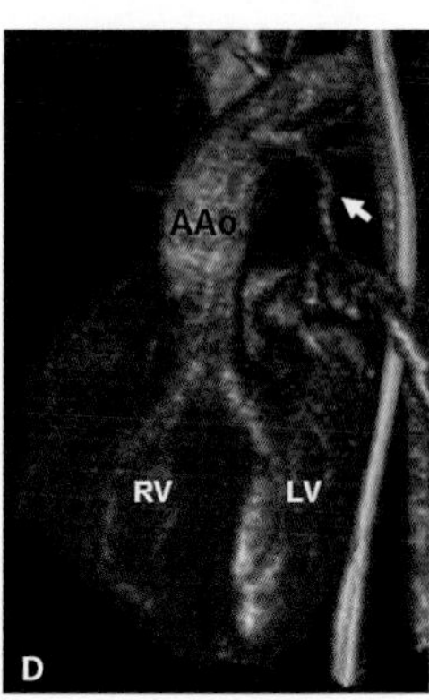

(A) A posteroanterior view of an aortogram shows opacification of the ascending aorta (*A*) and a patent ductus arteriosus (PDA) (*white arrow*) and left pulmonary artery (*black arrow*). **(B)** A left posterior oblique view of the heart in a reconstructed computed tomography (CT) image shows the PDA (*white arrow*) and ascending aorta (*AAo*). **(C)** An anteroposterior view of the heart from the CT image also shows the ascending aorta (*AAo*), PDA (*white arrow*), and left pulmonary artery (*black arrow*). **(D)** An angled superior view of the heart with altered window and level settings reveals the overriding position of the ascending aorta (AAo) (PDA, *white arrow*), which receives outflow from the right (*RV*) and left (*LV*) ventricles.

Differential Diagnosis

- ***Pulmonary artery atresia, tetralogy of Fallot:*** The main and right pulmonary arteries are absent. The left pulmonary artery arises from the PDA, which fills from the aorta.
- *PDA:* Although the ductus arteriosus is patent, the other abnormalities indicate more serious congenital heart disease. The pulmonary circulation is "ductus-dependent."
- *Vascular ring:* A vascular ring occurs when vascular structures surround the trachea and the esophagus. Although this patient has a right-sided aortic arch and PDA, a vascular ring is not complete because there is discontinuity of the left and main pulmonary arteries.

Essential Facts

- Four cardiac malformations are found in patients with tetralogy of Fallot:
  - Pulmonary valve atresia; main, branch, or peripheral pulmonary artery atresia and/or stenoses
  - Hypertrophy of the right ventricular myocardium due to increased work by the ventricle pumping blood through the pulmonary valve and arteries
  - A ventricular septal defect (VSD), typically with malalignment of the atrial and ventricular septa, allowing decompression of the right ventricle
  - Malalignment of the VSD allowing the aortic valve to override the defect, so that blood from both ventricles is ejected into the ascending aorta
- The aortic arch is right-sided in 25% of patients with tetralogy of Fallot.
- Tetralogy of Fallot is the most common type of cyanotic congenital heart disease (5–7% of cases).
- Infants are most often cyanotic because of decreased pulmonary blood flow.

Other Imaging Findings

- Although not seen in this patient, the cardiac apex may be displaced upward by hypertrophy of the right ventricle.
- This finding is the "boot-shaped" cardiac silhouette seen on chest radiographs.
- Chest radiographs and CT also show decreased pulmonary vascularity.

✔ Pearls & ✘ Pitfalls

✔ If the distance between the right ventricular outflow tract (RVOT) and confluent pulmonary arteries is minimal, it may be possible to surgically repair the RVOT to physiologic status.

✘ The origin of the pulmonary arteries may be from the right ventricle, aorta, or ductus arteriosus in patients with tetralogy of Fallot.

Case 87

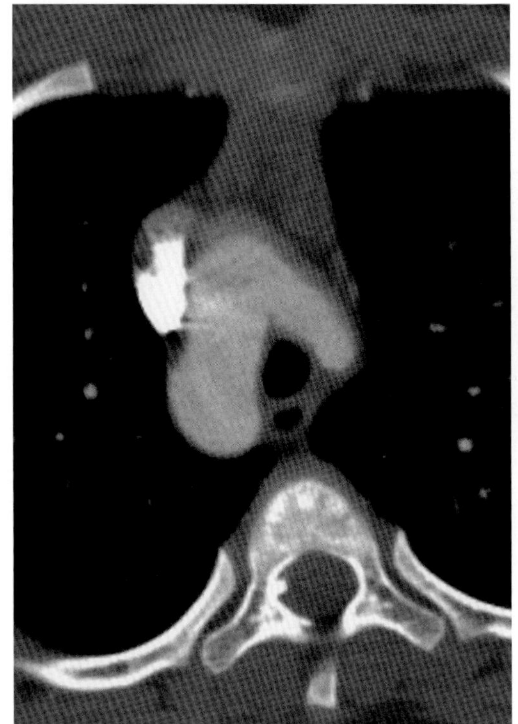

A

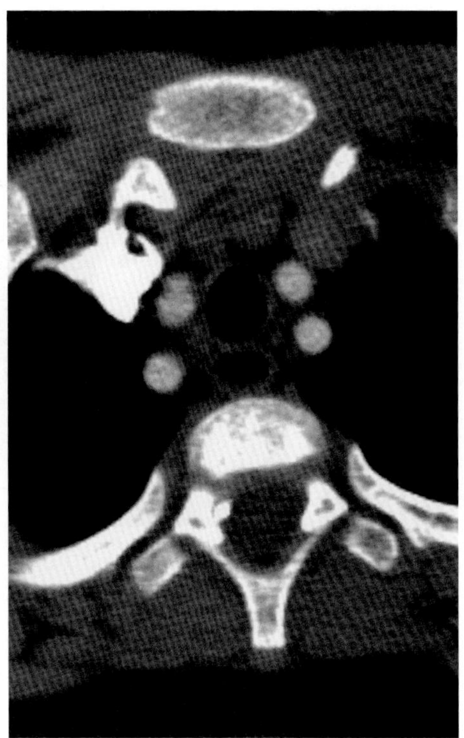

B

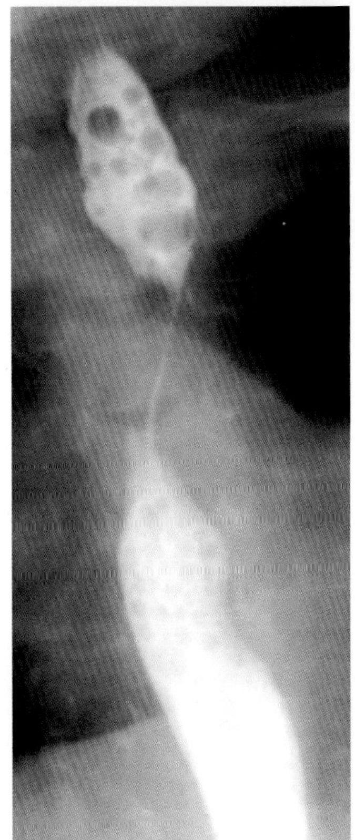

C

■ Clinical Presentation

A 6-year-old boy presents with lifelong difficulty swallowing and a history of “asthma.”

Imaging Findings

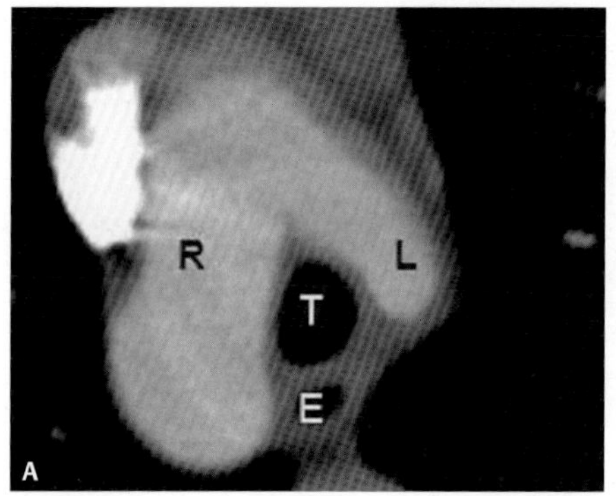

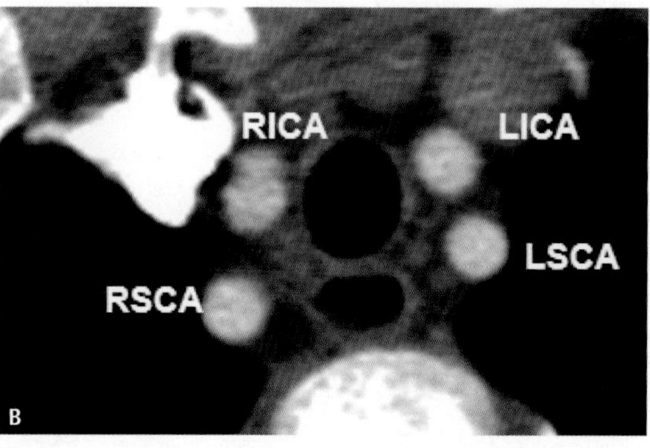

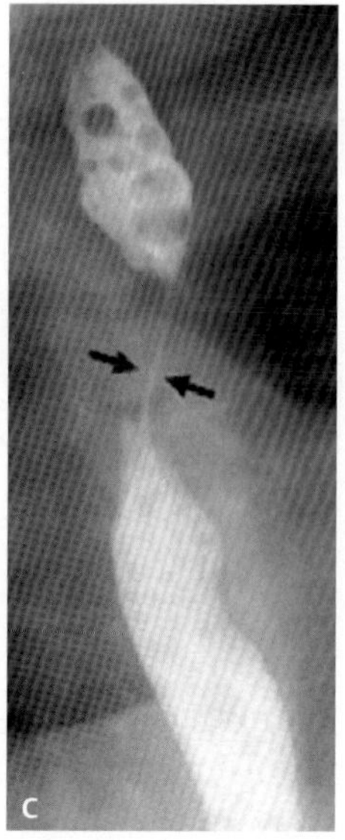

(A) The right (*R*) and left (*L*) aortic arches are patent, encircling the trachea (*T*) and esophagus (*E*). **(B)** The right (*RICA*) and left (*LICA*) internal carotid arteries and the right (*RSCA*) and left (*LSCA*) subclavian arteries arise individually from each arch. **(C)** An esophagogram in this patient shows marked right- and left-sided extrinsic narrowing of the lumen (*arrows*) and slight displacement of the esophagus to the right, indicating a left-sided descending thoracic aorta.

Differential Diagnosis

- ***Double aortic arch:*** The proximal ascending aorta is divided into two major branches because of persistence of the fourth aortic arch. The right and left brachiocephalic arteries arise from their respective arches. The arches then converge to form the descending aorta, which may be on the right or left, or in the midline.
- *Right aortic arch:* A right-sided arch is present and is the dominant vessel as its caliber is larger; however, the smaller left-sided arch remains patent.
- *Right-sided aortic arch and large-caliber left brachiocephalic artery:* Dilatation of the left ventricular chamber can be seen in patients with ischemic cardiomyopathy, but the myocardial signal should remain normal on nonenhanced images.

Essential Facts

- Double aortic arch occurs when the fourth through sixth right-sided pharyngeal arch arteries do not regress.
- The right-sided arch is the dominant arch in up to 70% of patients.
- The left arch may be atretic, persisting only as a ligamentous or fibrous structure that completes the vascular ring.
- Double aortic arch is one of the most common types of vascular ring, accounting for up to 65% of treated patients.
- There are usually no other associated cardiac lesions.
- Chromosome 22q11 is abnormal in ~20% of patients with double aortic arch, manifesting as CATCH-22 (chromosome 22q11 deletion), DiGeorge and velocardiofacial syndromes, and conotruncal facial anomalies.
- These syndromes include abnormalities of the palate, larynx, and trachea; speech and developmental delay; characteristic facial features; T-cell immune dysfunction; hypercalcemia; and neurologic defects.
- When these defects are not present, surgical release of the vascular ring is curative.

Other Imaging Findings

- Tracheal compression may not be completely relieved following surgery.

✔ Pearls & ✘ Pitfalls

✔ Review craniofacial and neurologic imaging studies when asked to image patients with possible double aortic arch.

✘ The left arch may be atretic and therefore not fill with contrast on computed tomography (CT) or produce a flow void on magnetic resonance imaging. Look for a fibrous structure on CT.

✘ Differentiate an atretic left arch from the ligament of the ductus arteriosus.

Case 88

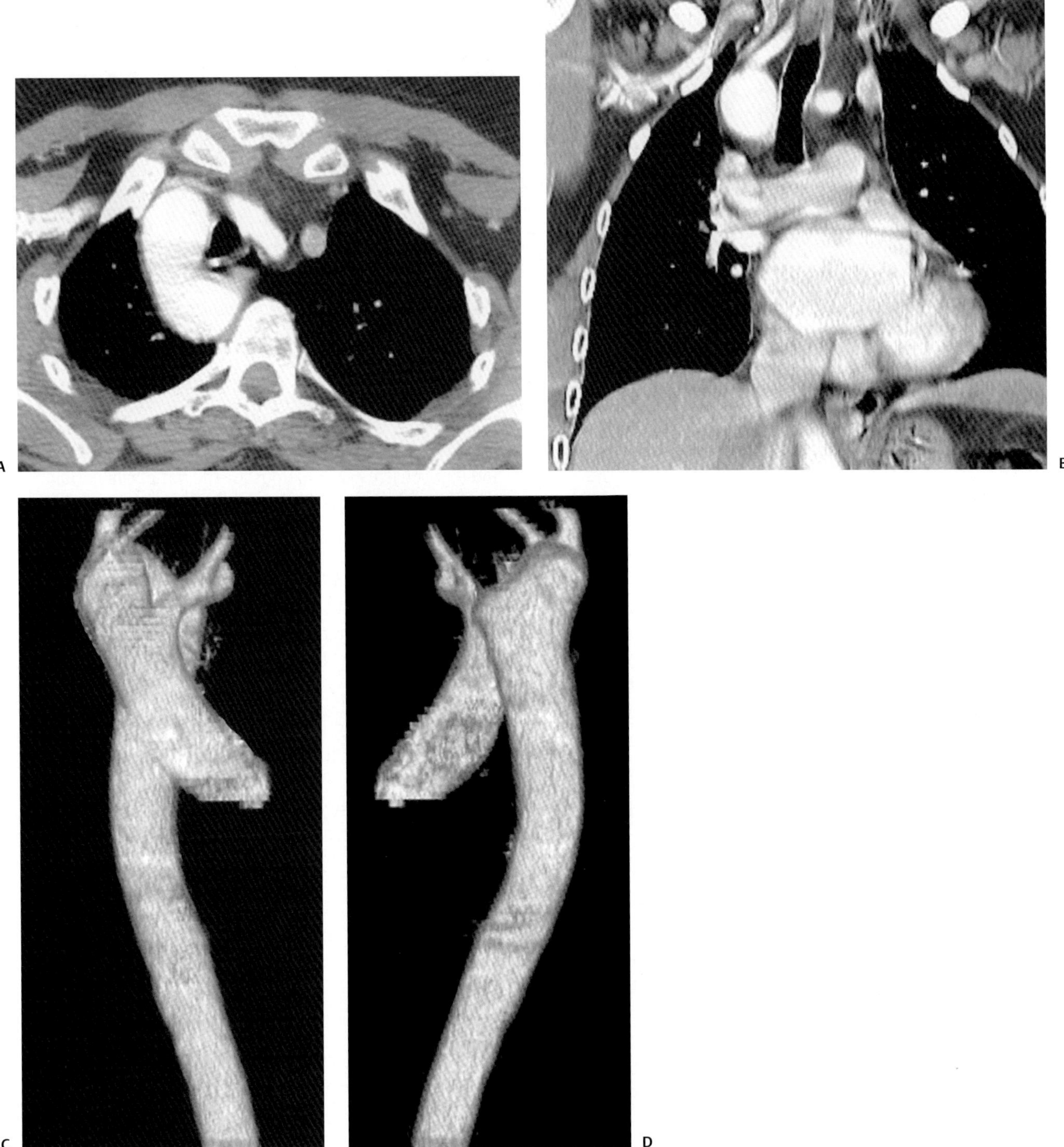

Clinical Presentation

A 58-year-old woman presents with a long history of dysphagia.

Imaging Findings

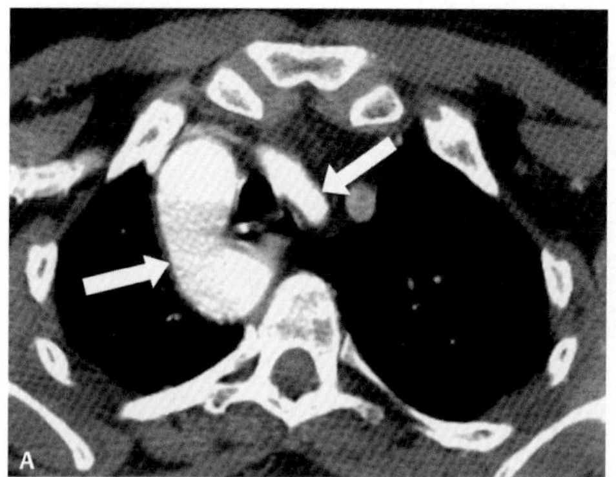

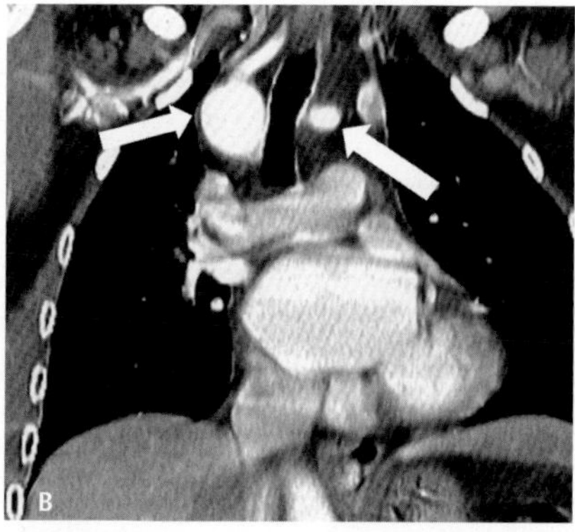

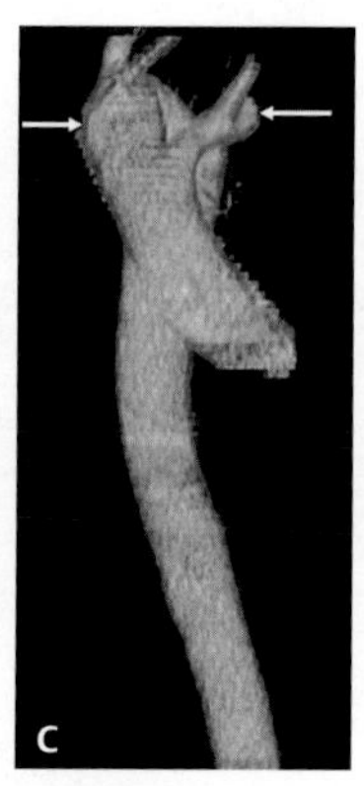

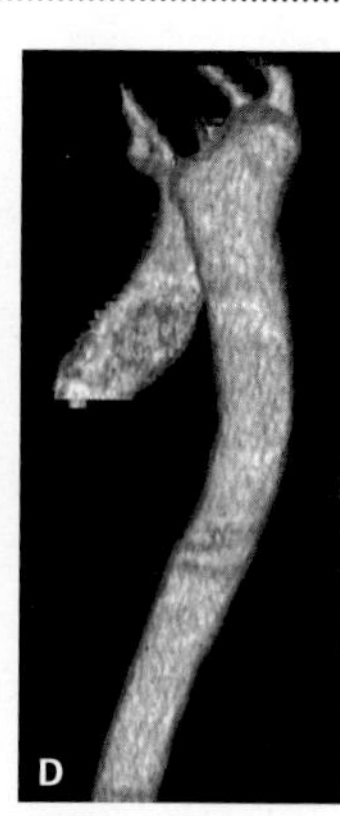

(A) Axial, **(B)** coronal, and **(C,D)** volume-rendered contrast-enhanced computed tomography (CT) images demonstrate vascular structures to the right and left of the trachea (*arrows*), consistent with a duplication of the aortic arch, with a dilated and dominant right-sided arch.

Differential Diagnosis

- ***Double aortic arch:*** In a duplication of the aortic arch, one arch is usually larger and dominant compared with the contralateral.
- *Incomplete double aortic arch with atresia of the distal left arch:* This is a form of incomplete double aortic arch in which atresia of the left arch results in a nonpatent fibrous cord, which can be a potentially symptomatic vascular ring.
- *Right-sided aortic arch:* A right-sided aortic arch that traverses the mediastinum to the right of the trachea and esophagus is seen in 0.1% of adults. Several variations of this anomaly have been described, but the three typical forms are a right aortic arch with an aberrant left subclavian artery, a right aortic arch with mirror image branching, and a right aortic arch with an isolated left subclavian artery.

Essential Facts

- A double aortic arch results from persistence of the embryologic double aortic arch. Left and right aortic arches arise from the ascending aorta and join posteriorly, forming a single descending aorta, after each one has given off its respective carotid and subclavian arteries.
- A double aortic arch is the most common symptomatic vascular ring.
- One arch is usually larger than the other; the right limb is generally higher and dominant and passes posterior to the trachea and esophagus to merge with the contralateral arch and from the descending aorta.
- Respiratory symptoms are more common (e.g., stridor) than gastrointestinal symptoms (e.g., choking with feeding).
- Associated congenital heart diseases are uncommon (18%), including ventricular septal defect, atrial septal defect, patent ductus arteriosus, and tetralogy of Fallot.
- Postoperative respiratory symptoms persist in 50% of patients.

Other Imaging Findings

- Chest radiographs and barium esophagograms are simple and inexpensive examinations for the initial evaluation. The frontal radiograph shows a soft-tissue density to the right and left of the trachea, and the lateral radiograph shows an abnormal retrotracheal opacity. In the barium esophagogram, bilateral persistent compression of the esophagus (anteroposterior view) and posterior esophageal indentation (lateral view) are typically seen.

✔ Pearls & ✘ Pitfalls

✔ A double aortic arch is the most common symptomatic vascular ring.

✘ Differentiation between a right aortic arch and a double aortic arch with an atretic distal left segment may be difficult.

Case 89

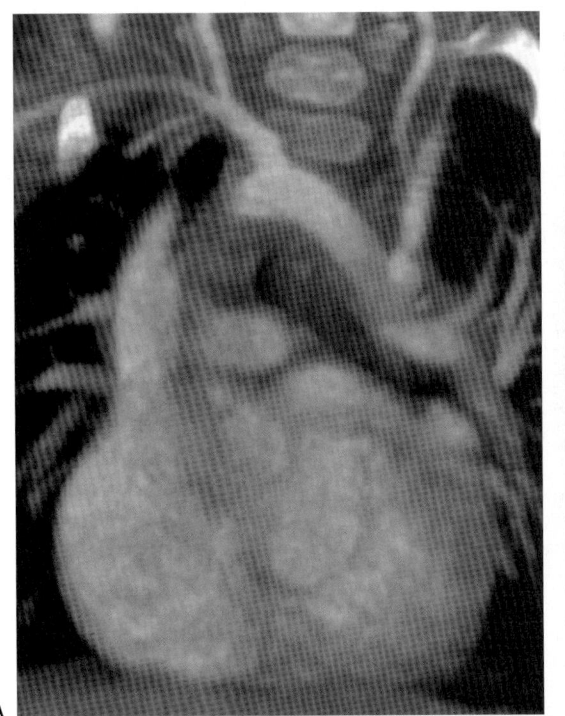
A

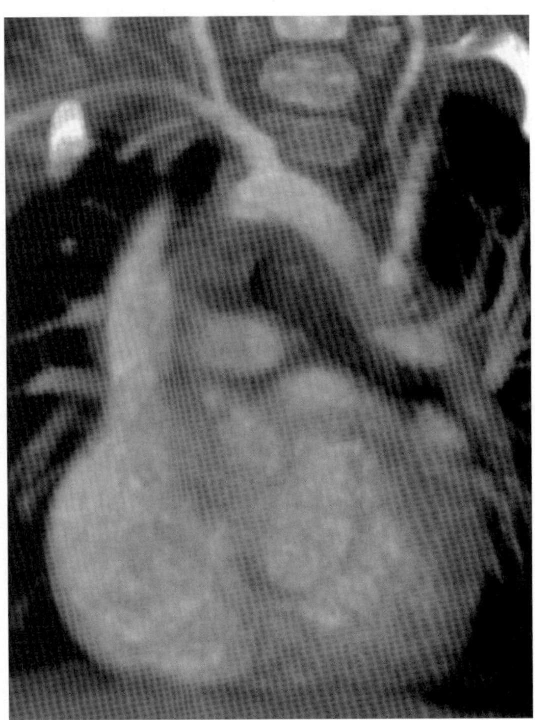
B

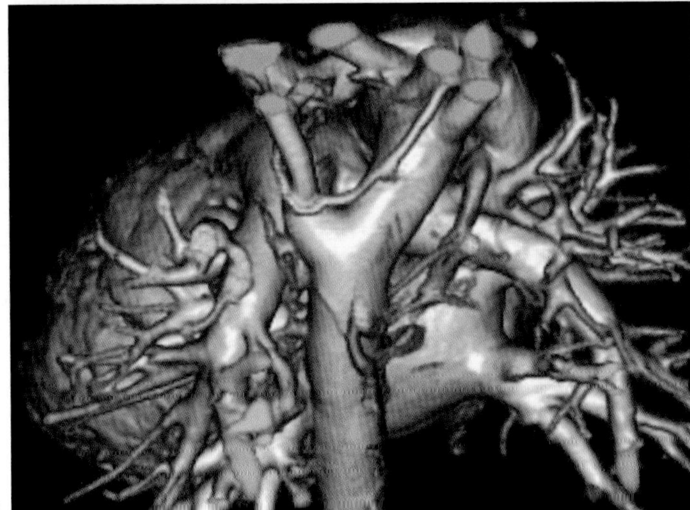
C

Clinical Presentation

A 10-month-old boy presents with a history of stridor.

Imaging Findings

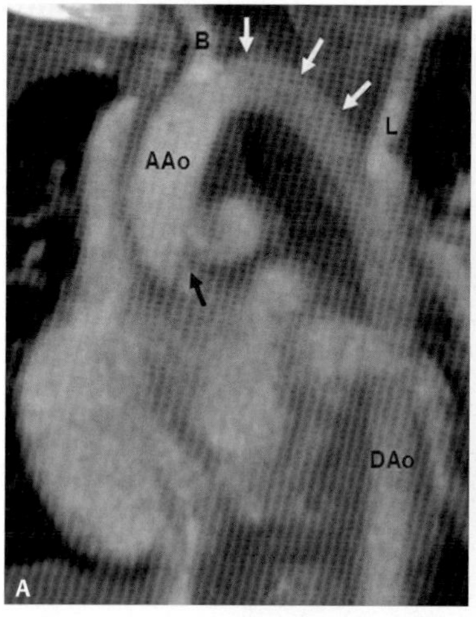

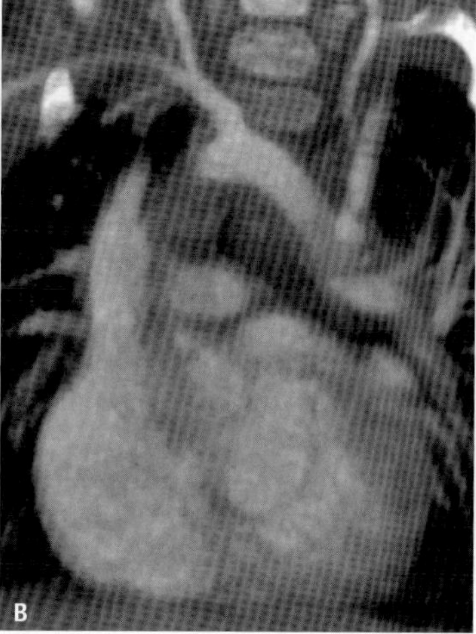

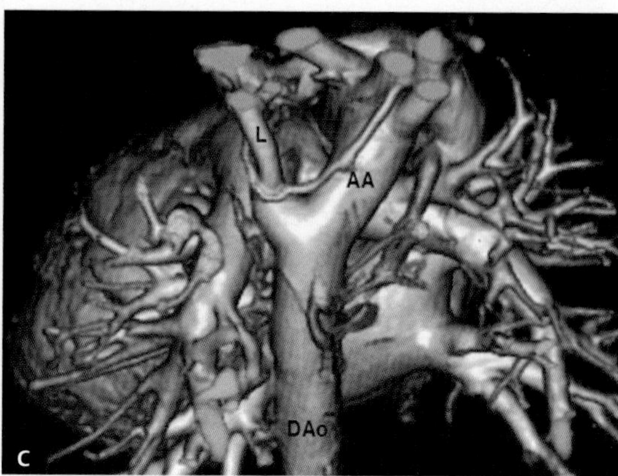

(A) A coronal oblique view of the ascending aorta (*AAo*), aortic arch (*white arrows*), and descending thoracic aorta (*DAo*) shows the aortic valve (*black arrow*) and the origins of the brachiocephalic (*B*) and the left subclavian (*L*) arteries. **(B)** The retroesophageal segment of the aortic arch seen in a direct coronal view shows the origins of the brachiocephalic and subclavian arteries and the proximal vertebral arteries as the arch courses from right to left ventral to the vertebral bodies. **(C)** A three-dimensional surface-rendered view of the heart shows the aortic ach (*AA*), descending thoracic aorta (*DAo*), and origin of the left subclavian artery (*L*).

Differential Diagnosis

- ***Circumflex right aortic arch:*** The ascending aorta is on the right, and the descending aorta is on the left. The transverse arch courses behind the esophagus (retroesophageal), partially encircling the trachea and esophagus; hence the descriptive name.
- *Right aortic arch with aberrant left subclavian artery:* This is found when a right aortic arch is associated with a right-sided or midline descending aorta and the last vessel branching from the arch is the left subclavian artery. The retroesophageal vessel is the left subclavian artery rather than the aortic arch. This is the most common type of right aortic arch and is usually not associated with other forms of congenital heart disease.
- *Double aortic arch:* With a double aortic arch, the right arch is most often larger than the left. The left arch may be atretic (i.e., does not fill with contrast). When atretic, the ligamentous structure does not have a connection with the left pulmonary artery as a ductus ligament would.

Essential Facts

- The retroesophageal segment of the aortic arch usually causes only a mild and extrinsic impression on the lumen of the esophagus, which can be seen on an esophagogram.
- A vascular ring can be present, completely encircling the aorta and esophagus, if there is a left-sided ductus arteriosus or ductus ligament.
- The trachea is displaced to the left by the right-sided aortic arch.
- A circumflex left aortic arch is rarer, occurring when a left-sided aortic arch and a right-sided descending aorta are present.

Other Imaging Findings

- Chest radiographs may indicate the presence of a double aortic arch because the left-sided descending aorta and the larger right-sided arch can be seen.

✔ Pearls & ✘ Pitfalls

✔ The ductus arteriosus is almost always left-sided.

✔ With a left-sided aortic arch, the first brachiocephalic branch is to the right.

✔ With a right-sided aortic arch, the first brachiocephalic branch is to the left.

✘ It is often difficult to distinguish a circumflex right aortic arch from a double aortic arch with an atretic left-sided arch.

Case 90

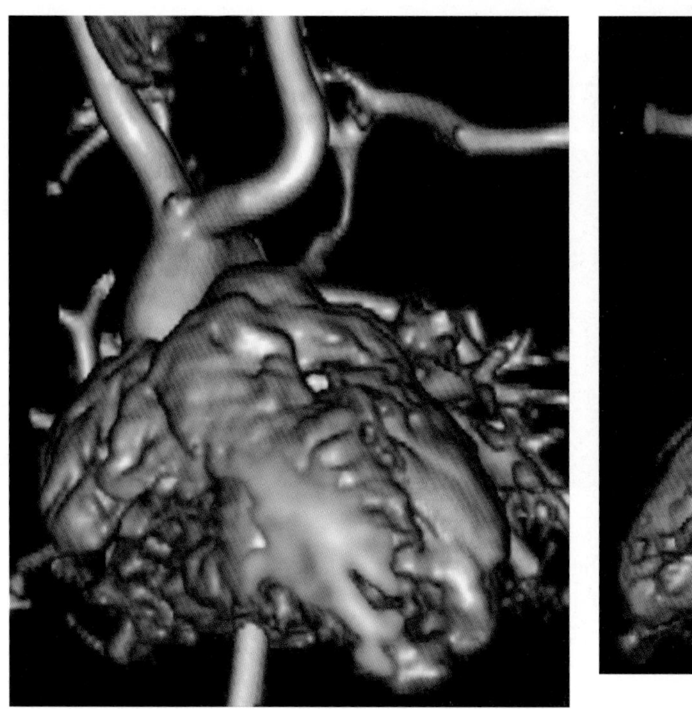
A

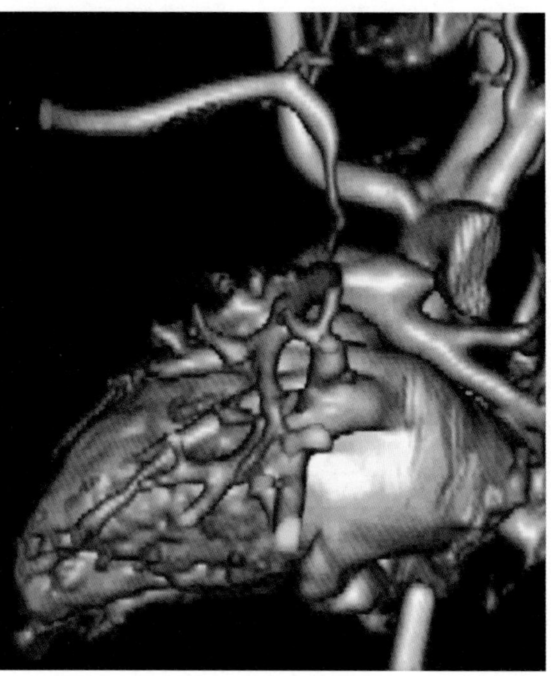
B

Clinical Presentation

A 3-day-old (34-week gestation) male infant presents with diminished left upper extremity pulse and hypotension. Although the aortic arch was clearly visualized on echocardiogram, the left subclavian artery origin was not seen.

Imaging Findings

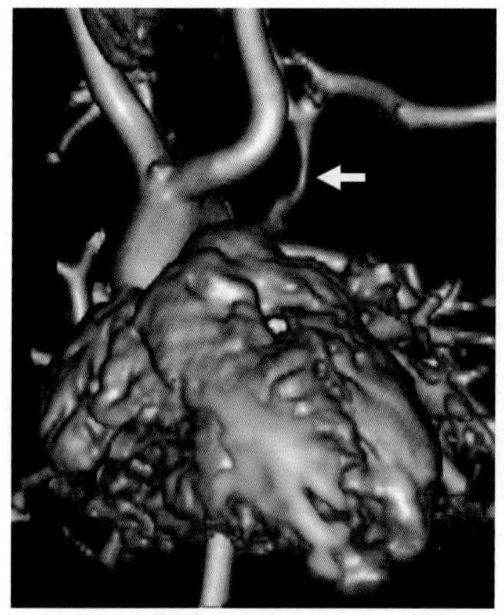

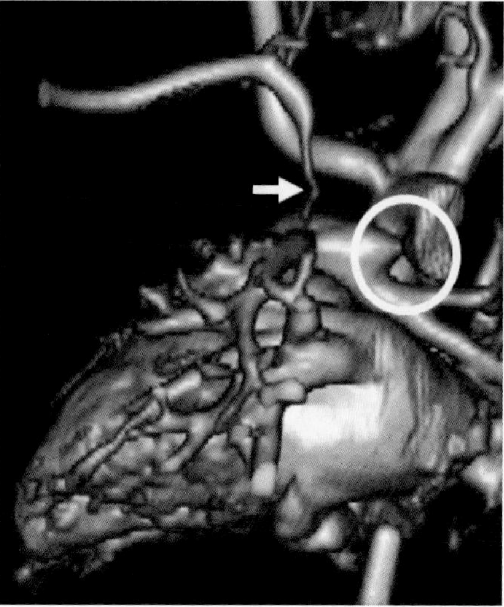

(A) In this anterior oblique view, the left subclavian artery arises from the left pulmonary artery (*white arrow*). Although its origin is narrowed, the distal vessel is of normal caliber because there is a vertebral artery steal supplying the distal vessel. **(B)** In a posterior oblique view, the origin of the left subclavian artery from the left pulmonary artery (*white arrow*) and a patent right sided ductus arteriosus (*white circle*) are seen.

Differential Diagnosis

- ***Isolated left subclavian artery:*** The left subclavian artery does not arise from the aortic arch as it should, but from the left pulmonary artery.
- *Patent ductus arteriosus:* The narrow segment of the left subclavian artery is actually the patent ductus arteriosus, but the normal left subclavian artery origin from the aortic arch is not present, so the primary problem is of the origin of the left subclavian artery.
- *Dissection of the left subclavian artery:* Although possible, dissection would most likely be the result of traumatic injury, which was not present in this patient.

Essential Facts

- Isolated left subclavian artery was initially reported in 1970. The original paper documented three types:
  - Left subclavian with patent ductus: no vascular ring
  - Atretic left subclavian origin from a retroesophageal aortic diverticulum: with vascular ring
  - Brachiocephalic vessels in mirror image configuration and an atretic innominate artery
- A right-sided aortic arch may have a varied order of brachiocephalic artery branching:
  - Mirror image branching: the arteries branch in the following order—left brachiocephalic, right common carotid, and right subclavian arteries.
  - Aberrant left subclavian artery: this branching pattern may or may not be associated with a vascular ring. When present, the vascular ring is completed by a patent ductus arteriosus or ductus ligament.
  - Isolated left subclavian artery: the left subclavian artery does not originate from the aortic arch, but rather is isolated from the arch, arising from the left pulmonary artery.
- There is a reported association with tetralogy of Fallot.
- There may also be an association with 22q11 chromosomal deletion.
- Left upper extremity pulses and blood pressure should be diminished compared with the right.

Other Imaging Findings

- The ductus arteriosus is patent in this patient and has a separate origin from the left pulmonary artery.
- There may be ductal tissue in the isolated subclavian artery origin, which may lead to stenosis or complete closure of the origin of the vessel.
- Collateral blood flow to the left upper extremity occurs via the chest wall, thyrocervical trunk, and/or vertebral system (steal phenomenon).

✔ Pearls & ✘ Pitfalls

✔ There is no connection between the aortic arch and the left subclavian artery.

✔ If a vascular connection with the left subclavian artery is not found, the vessel most likely arises from the pulmonary artery and is narrowed because of closure of ductal tissue.

✔ The origin of the left subclavian artery is from the left pulmonary artery, but there may be a separate lumen from the ductus arteriosus.

✔ Prostaglandin maintains patency of the ductus arteriosus.

✔ Indomethacin speeds closure of the ductus arteriosus.

✔ In a vertebral steal phenomenon, antegrade blood flow from one vertebral artery is "stolen" as it flows in a retrograde manner through the contralateral vertebral artery to the upper extremity.

✔ With a right aortic arch, there may be a right-sided ductus arteriosus.

✘ Look for an aberrant origin of a subclavian artery.

Case 91

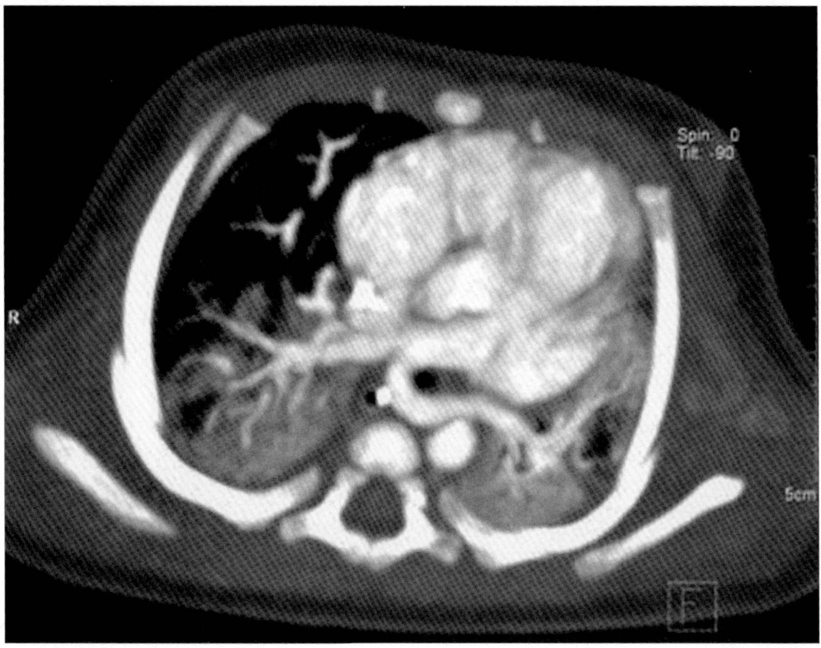

Clinical Presentation

A 7-week-old female infant presents with shortness of breath and wheezing.

Imaging Findings

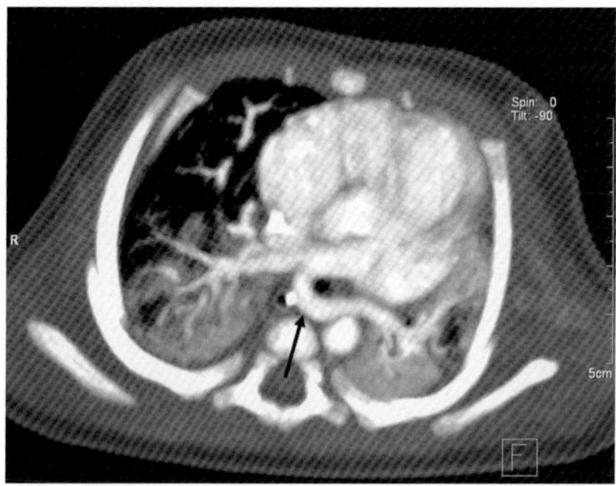

Contrast-enhanced computed tomography (CT) image of the chest shows an abnormal origin of the left pulmonary artery from the right pulmonary artery. The aberrant left pulmonary artery passes above the right main bronchus and courses between a narrow distal trachea and the esophagus (nasogastric tube) to the left pulmonary hilum. Bibasilar parenchymal opacities are also appreciated.

Differential Diagnosis

- ***Pulmonary artery sling:*** Pulmonary artery sling or aberrant origin of the left pulmonary artery is characterized by an abnormal origin of the left pulmonary artery from the right pulmonary artery.
- *Pulmonary sequestration:* An aberrant origin of a feeding vessel to the pulmonary vasculature can be seen in the case of pulmonary sequestration, with systemic circulation from the aorta providing vascular supply to the lung.

Essential Facts

- Associated anomalies of the tracheobronchial tree are common (48–54%). The most common are hypoplasia of the distal trachea or right main bronchus, usually associated with complete cartilaginous ring ("napkin ring" cartilage), tracheomalacia, and bronchus suis.
- Cardiovascular anomalies are also common (> 50%), including persistent left superior vena cava draining into the coronary sinus, atrial septal defect, ventricular septal defect, patent ductus arteriosus, aortic arch anomalies, and tetralogy of Fallot.
- Ninety percent of patients present with respiratory symptoms during the first year of life, the majority either at the time of birth or before 6 months.

Other Imaging Findings

- Chest radiographs may show hyperlucent right lung and deviation of the trachea to the left, with narrowing of the distal tracheal air column.
- A barium esophagogram is often diagnostic, showing an anterior indentation of the esophagus, a finding that is seen only in this type of vascular ring.

✔ Pearls & ✘ Pitfalls

✔ Patients often present with aberrant origin of the left pulmonary artery (pulmonary artery sling) with associated tracheobronchial or cardiovascular malformations. Despite significant improvement with early surgical correction, the mortality rate remains high.

✘ Vascular rings may present with extrinsic compression of the esophagus and trachea. However, both plain radiographs and esophagograms are limited in the evaluation of these conditions and in delineating the complex anatomy of these cases. Further evaluation with cross-sectional imaging (CT or magnetic resonance imaging) is required.

Case 92

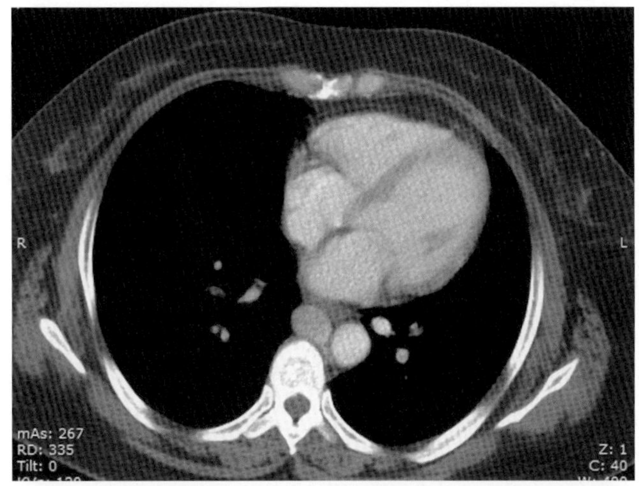

A

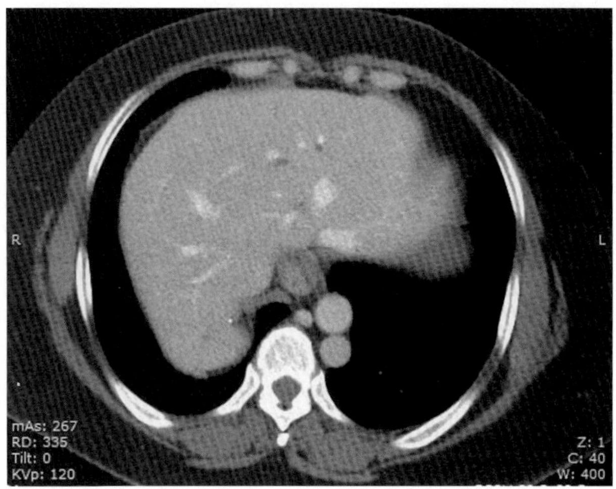

B

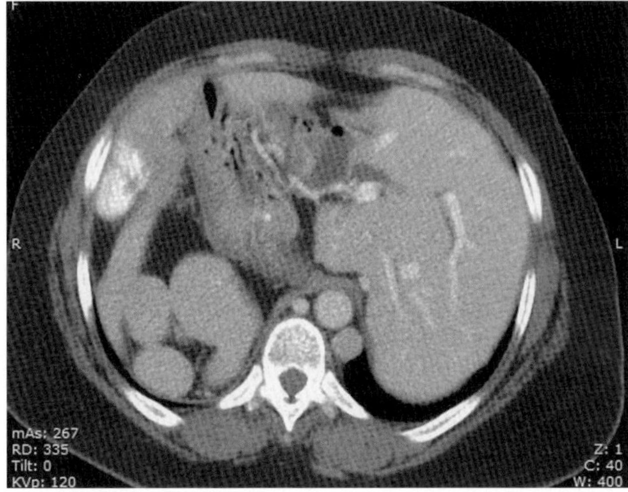

C

Clinical Presentation

Young male patient with abnormal findings in a routine clinical examination

Imaging Findings

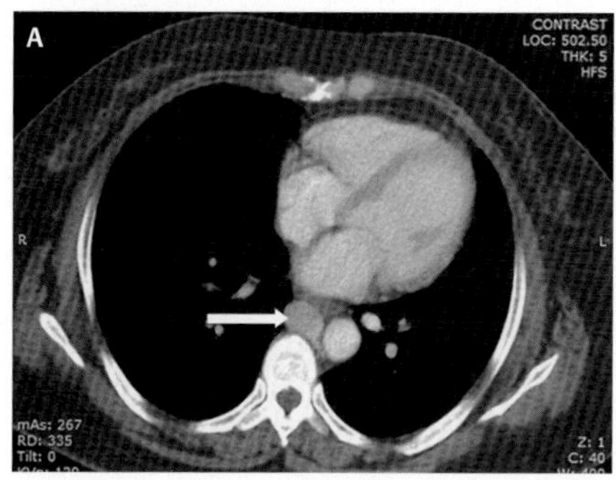
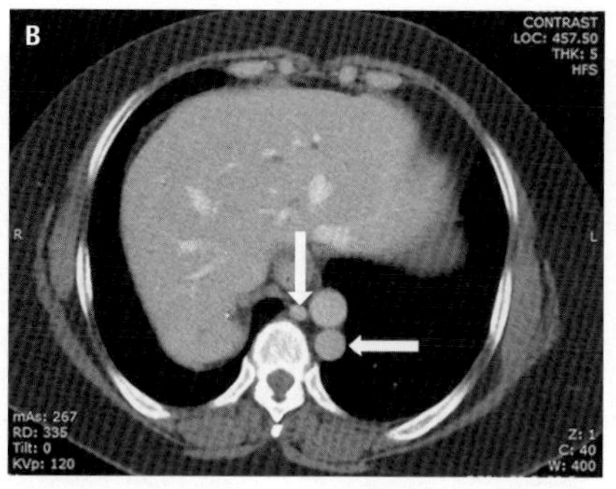
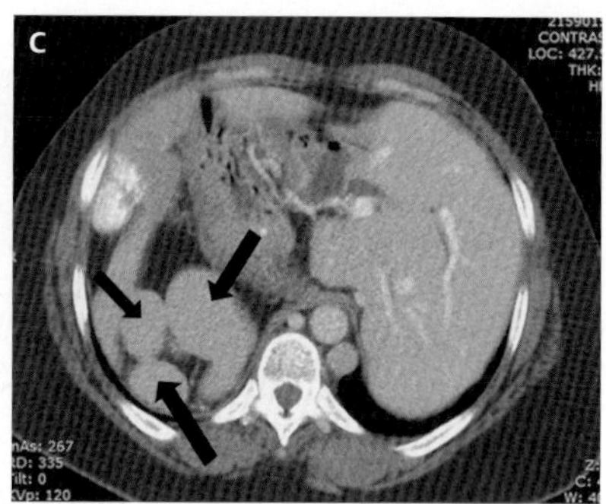

(A–C) Contrast-enhanced computed tomography (CT) axial images at two different levels show the absence of the intrahepatic segment of the inferior vena cava (IVC) and prominent azygos and hemiazygos veins. Note that the liver is in the left upper quadrant, the stomach is to the right of the midline, and multiple spleens are present under the right hemidiaphragm.

Differential Diagnosis

- ***Azygos continuation of intrahepatic interruption of the IVC:*** CT shows dilated azygos and hemiazygos veins in the retrocrural space, absence of the intrahepatic portion of the IVC, and situs inversus and polysplenia in the right lower quadrant of the abdomen.
- *Enlarged lymph nodes:* Dilated azygos and/or hemiazygos veins can be tracked as vascular structures in contiguous levels, different from enlarged lymph nodes. The presence of situs inversus and multiple soft-tissue-density structures in the expected position of the spleen also allows differentiation from lymph nodes.

Essential Facts

- Azygos continuation of the IVC can be seen as an isolated finding, or it can be associated with complex congenital anomalies.
- This is a common finding in patients with heterotaxia syndrome with polysplenia.
- In those with heterotaxia syndrome with polysplenia, complex congenital heart disease (e.g., atrioventricular canal) and situs anomalies (situs ambiguus) are common.
- An association among heterotaxia, congenital heart disease, and primary ciliary dyskinesia, such as in Kartagener syndrome, has been reported.

Other Imaging Findings

- The increased flow to the azygos system and azygos vein arch also produces prominence of the superior vena cava. The hepatic vein can be seen normally draining through a small suprahepatic segment of the IVC into the right atrium.

✔ Pearls & ✘ Pitfalls

✔ In patients with azygos continuation of intrahepatic interruption of the IVC, polysplenia, and situs ambiguus (heterotaxia syndrome, left-sided isomerism), the association with congenital heart disease is less common than in patients with heterotaxia syndrome and asplenia (right-sided isomerism).

✘ In patients with deep vein thrombosis and an IVC filter, an abnormal venous return may provide alternative routes for emboli to reach the pulmonary circulation.

Case 93

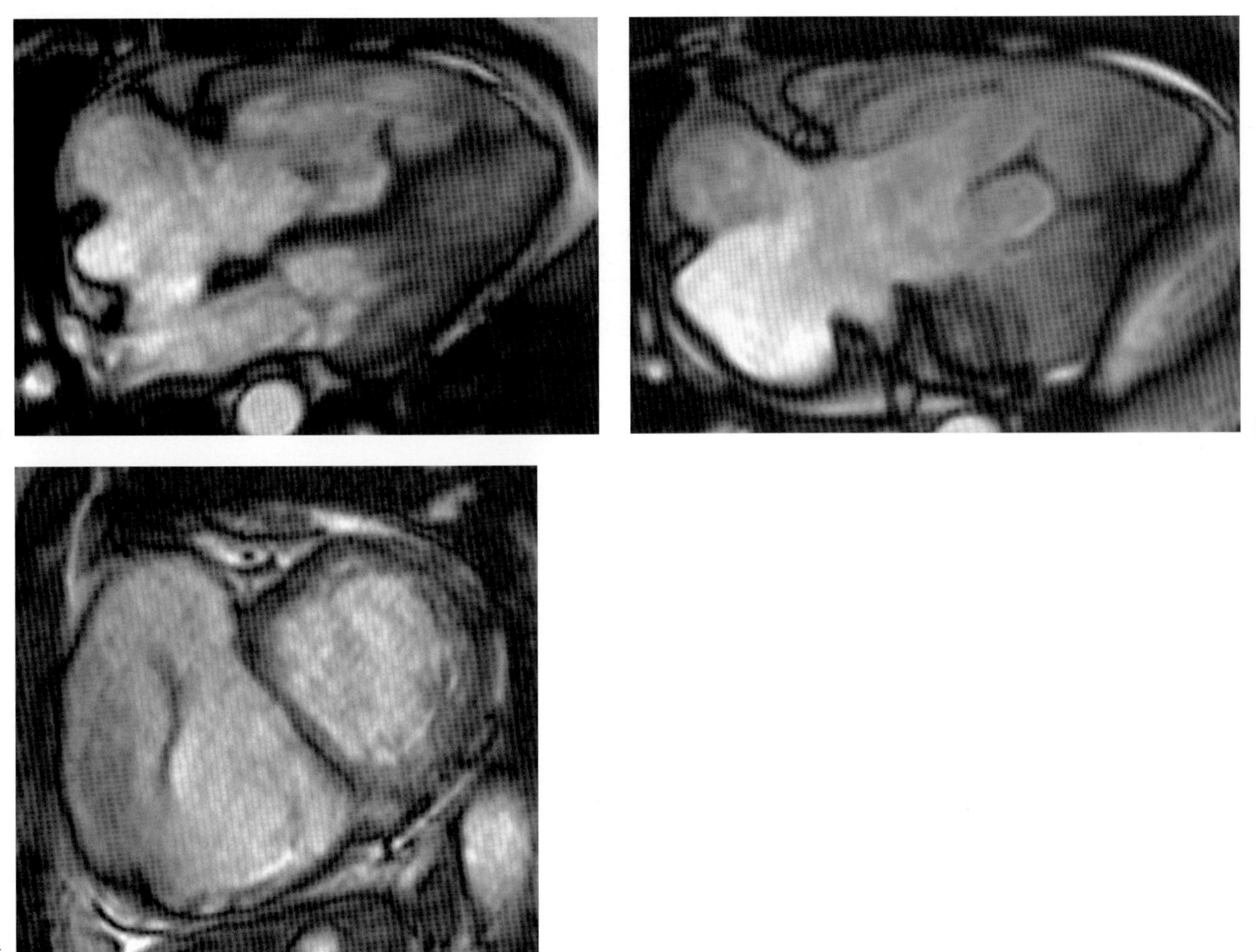

Clinical Presentation

A 28-year-old woman presents with a history of congenital heart disease.

Imaging Findings

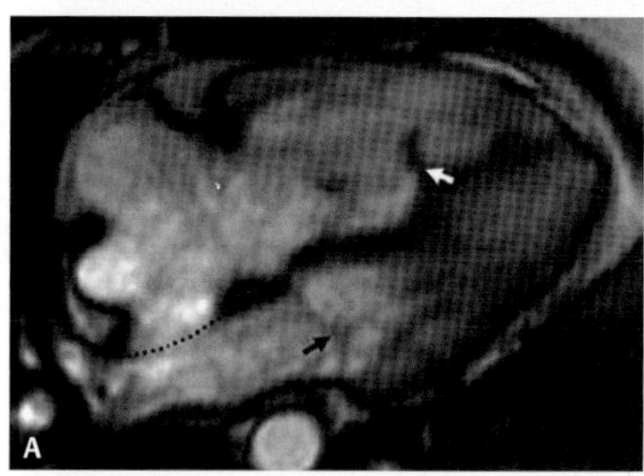

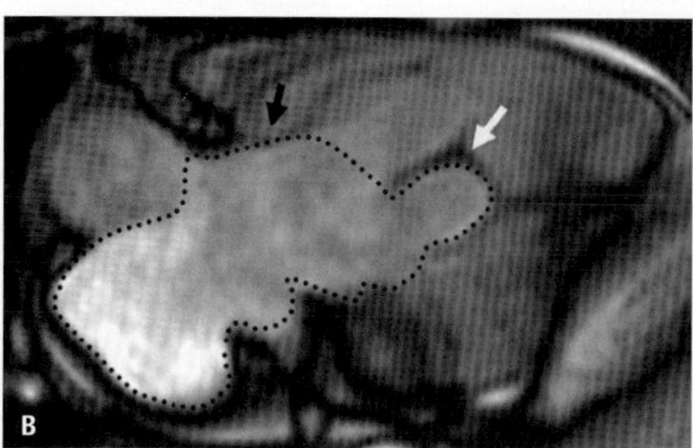

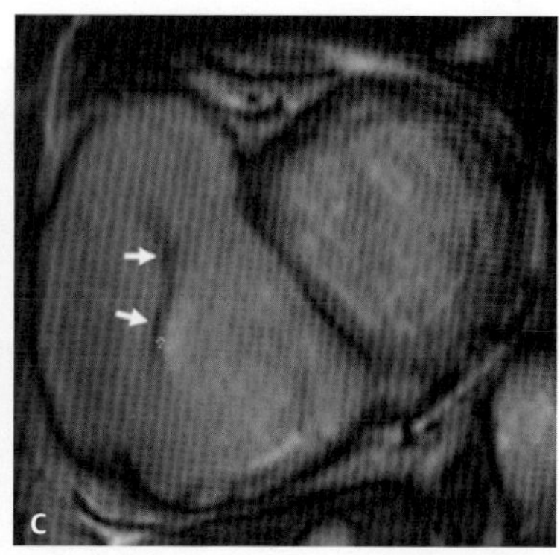

(A) The septal leaflet of the tricuspid valve is displaced toward the right ventricular (RV) apex (*white arrow*). The upper portion of the RV is therefore functionally part of the atrium. The mitral valve is in the normal position (*black arrow*). Although the atrial septum is thin, it is intact (*dotted line*). **(B)** The posterior leaflet of the tricuspid valve (*white arrow*) is also displaced inferiorly. The right atrium is large because part of the RV is "atrialized" (*dotted black line*). **(C)** In a short-axis view of the heart, in a plane just below the mitral annulus, only the anterior leaflet of the tricuspid valve is seen (*white arrows*).

Differential Diagnosis

- ***Ebstein anomaly:*** The tricuspid valve is malformed; the septal and posterior leaflets are displaced toward the RV apex. The portion of the RV above the displaced valve is "atrialized."
- *Tricuspid atresia:* Incomplete formation of the tricuspid valve and RV inflow are seen. An atrial septal defect (ASD) is always present to decompress the right side of the heart.
- *Tricuspid regurgitation:* Given malalignment of the tricuspid valve leaflets in this case, regurgitation is certainly present but is not the primary disease.

Essential Facts

- Congenital abnormalities of the tricuspid valve include atresia, regurgitation, and Ebstein anomaly.
- Ebstein anomaly is a form of structural congenital heart disease in which the septal and posterior tricuspid valve leaflets (and sometimes the anterior leaflet) are displaced toward the RV apex.
- Tricuspid regurgitation is mild if there is minimal displacement of the tricuspid leaflets.
- If the hemodynamic effects are mild, the patient may be asymptomatic in adolescence or adulthood.
- When severe, tricuspid regurgitation may lead to severe dilatation of the right atrium.
- Supraventricular tachycardia, an arrhythmia that can be due to accessory electrical pathways, may be found in patients with Ebstein anomaly.
- If tricuspid regurgitation is severe, the RV is unable to pump blood forward, resulting in functional pulmonic valve atresia and dependence on the ductus arteriosus.
- If a right-to-left shunt is present, or when the patent ductus arteriosus closes, the patient may become cyanotic.
- Indications for surgical repair include heart failure, cyanosis, and acidosis associated with tricuspid regurgitation, depressed RV function, and severe cardiomegaly.

Other Imaging Findings

- Tricuspid regurgitation
- ASD
- Ventricular septal defect
- Right atrial enlargement
- Moderate to massive cardiomegaly
- Pulmonary stenosis
- Four-chamber views on magnetic resonance (MR) and computed tomography images clearly show the displaced septal leaflet of the tricuspid valve.

✔ Pearls & ✘ Pitfalls

✔ When calculating the volume of the RV, use short-axis and axial images of the heart. This makes it easier to see the displaced valve, so the volume calculation is more accurate.

✘ Tricuspid regurgitation is difficult or impossible to quantify with MR flow studies.

Case 94

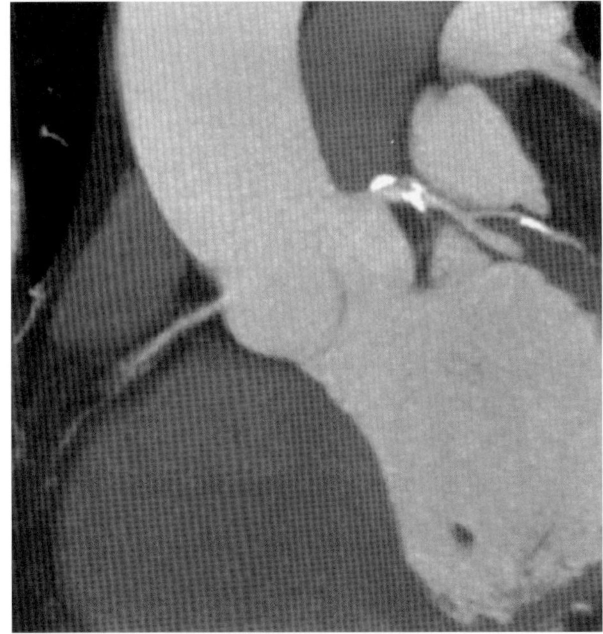
A

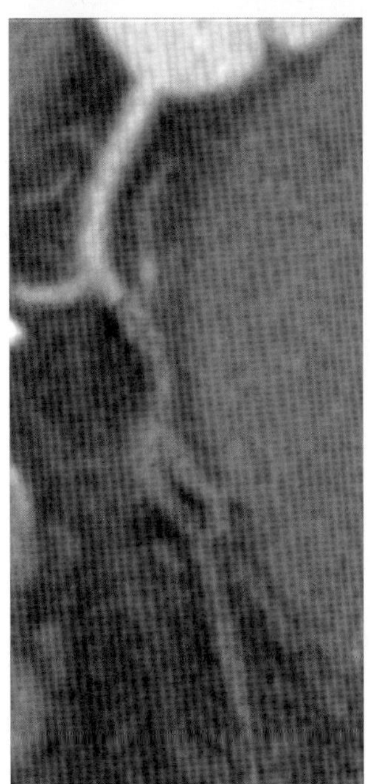
B

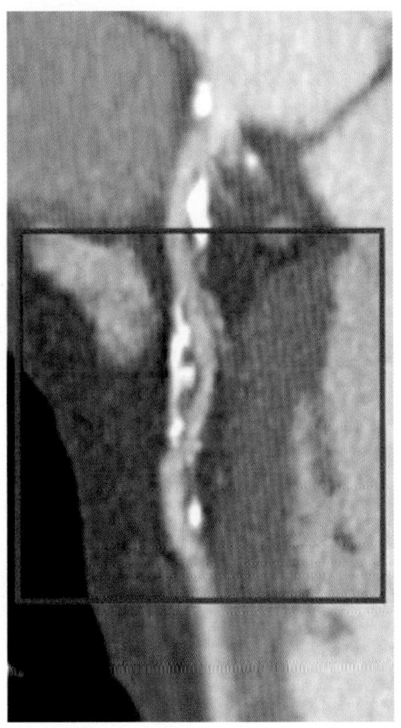
C

Clinical Presentation

A 56-year-old woman presents with a 1-day history of mild chest pain and a long history of tobacco use, although she has not smoked for 5 years. She has a normal electrocardiogram and no troponin leak for 6 hours.

Imaging Findings

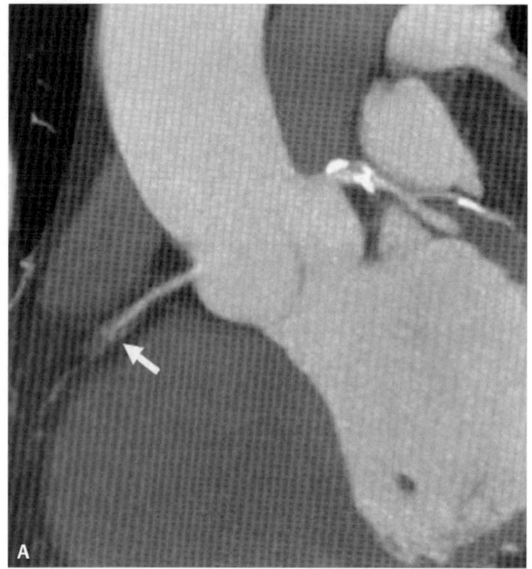

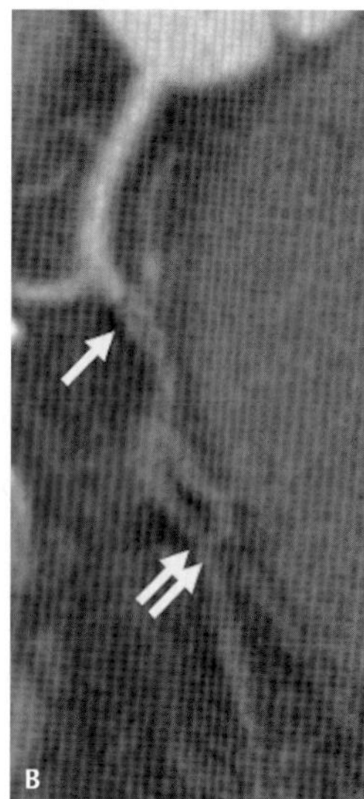

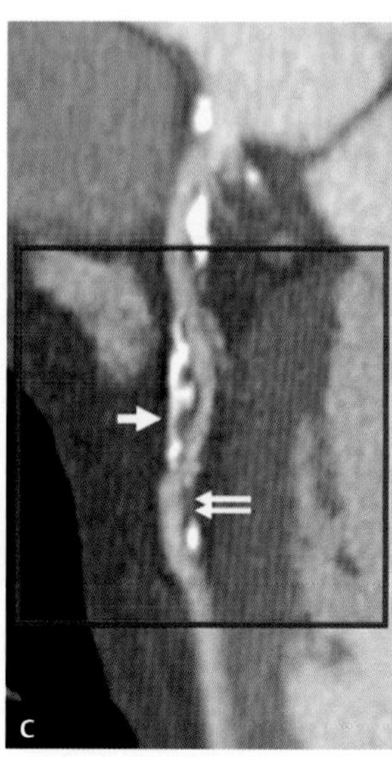

(A) The coronal plane shows the origins of the coronary arteries. The right coronary artery (RCA) is small caliber, and its enhancing lumen ends abruptly (*white arrow*). **(B)** A curved planar reconstruction of the RCA shows the abrupt cutoff of the patent lumen (*white arrow*) and the nonenhancing but still normal-caliber of the distal RCA and branch vessel (*double white arrows*).

(C) A curved planar reconstruction of the left main and proximal left anterior descending (LAD) coronary arteries shows severe mixed atherosclerotic disease; calcified (*white arrow*) and noncalcified plaque (*double white arrows*) cause only mild narrowing of the LAD artery.

Differential Diagnosis

- ***Acute coronary syndrome due to RCA thrombosis, LAD atherosclerosis:*** The proximal RCA lumen is occluded. Calcified and noncalcified atherosclerotic disease in the LAD artery causes luminal irregularity, although the vessel lumen remains patent.
- *Severe LAD and RCA stenosis:* The LAD lumen is clearly visualized adjacent to the calcified plaque, indicating that the narrowing of the lumen is mild to moderate (i.e., not hemodynamically significant, which is defined as > 70% based on angiographic visual measurements).
- *"Widow maker" lesion:* A "widow maker" lesion is a severe stenosis of the left main coronary artery that is likely to lead to a catastrophic myocardial infarction, thereby creating a widow or widower. Although the degree of left main and LAD disease is important, the reason for acute chest pain in this patient is the acute thrombosis of the RCA.

Essential Facts

- This is the most common cause of sudden cardiac death in middle-aged men and women.
- Because of endothelial injury on the surface of an atheromatous plaque, thrombus formation is induced.
- Thrombosis sometimes occurs on superficial plaque erosion without discrete plaque rupture.
- Nonocclusive coronary artery thrombosis is associated with distal embolization and extensive myocardial damage.

Other Imaging Findings

- The distal RCA is visualized because the tissue of the wall of the vessel is more radiodense than the fat in the atrioventricular groove.
- This patient has a calcium score of 1700.
- Even with a very high calcium score, the coronary artery computed tomography angiogram (CTA) is diagnostic of the acute occlusion because there is no calcium in the RCA.

✔ Pearls & ✘ Pitfalls

✔ The high negative predictive value of coronary artery CTA is valuable; if coronary artery disease is not seen on CTA, the patient does not have coronary artery disease.

✘ A high calcium score does not necessarily preclude a diagnostic coronary artery CTA.

Case 95

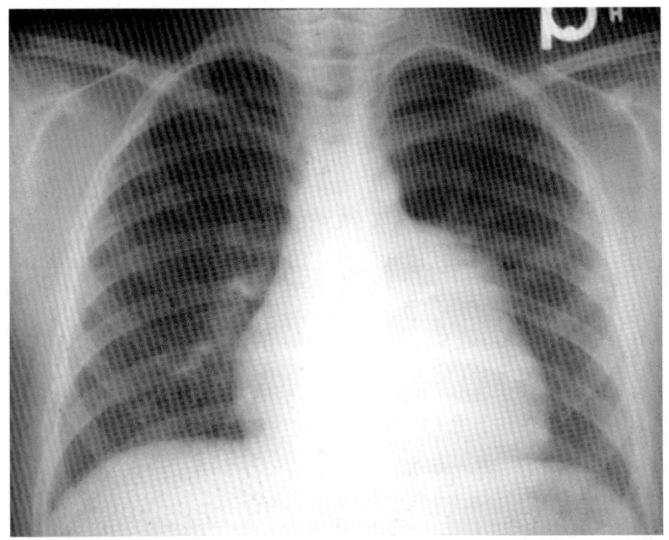
A

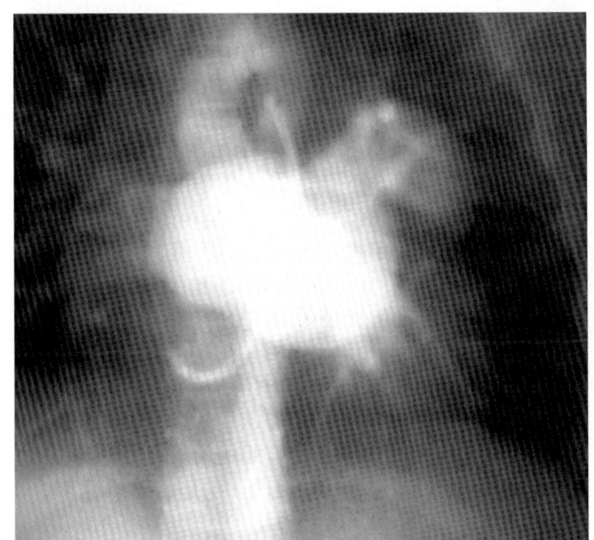
B

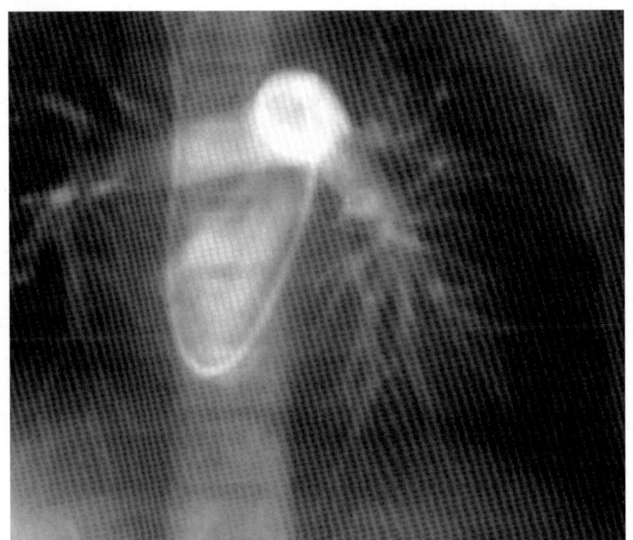
C

Clinical Presentation

A 16-year-old boy presents with chest pain.

Imaging Findings

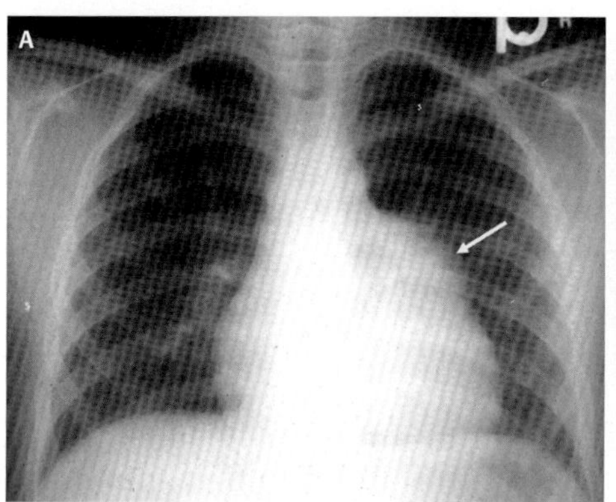
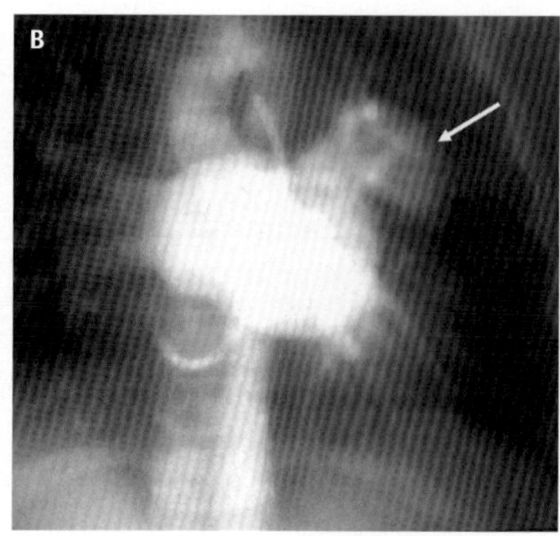
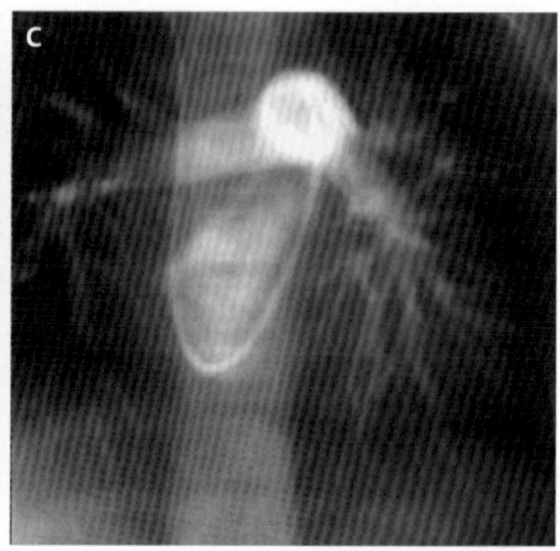

(A) Plain film of the chest shows an abnormal prominence on the left atrial appendage (*arrow*), which is confirmed with **(B)** contrast filling (*arrow*) of the enlarged appendage during the venous phase of a catheter angiography. **(C)** Arterial phase after contrast injection shows normal pulmonary arteries.

Differential Diagnosis

- ***Partial congenital absence of the pericardium (PCAP):*** PCAP may manifest clinically with chest pain and abnormal prominence of the left atrial appendage, secondary to herniation.
- *Mitral stenosis:* The increased pressure in the left atrium is associated with prominence of the left atrial appendage and other signs of left atrial enlargement, not present in this patient.
- *Pulmonary hypertension:* Abnormal prominence of the main trunk of the pulmonary artery can produce a prominence in the left side of the cardiac silhouette. Anatomical location and appearance differ from that of left atrial enlargement, and differentiation should not be difficult. Cross-sectional imaging with computed tomography or magnetic resonance (MR) can easily differentiate between vascular and nonvascular prominence (e.g., mass or lymph nodes) in this anatomical region.

Essential Facts

- Congenital pericardial defects are rare.
- Whereas a complete left-sided pericardial defect has little clinical relevance, a partial left-sided pericardial defect is more serious and can be a life-threatening condition.
- Patients with left-sided PCAP are at risk for herniation of the left atrial appendage or left ventricle with secondary fatal myocardial strangulation.
- In patients with complete left-sided congenital absence of the pericardium, the cardiac silhouette is significantly displaced posteriorly and to the left. On MR and CT lung tissue is appreciated interposed between the main pulmonary artery and the aorta occupying and replacing the preaortic recess of the pericardium.

Other Imaging Findings

- Elevation of the apex of the heart and interposition of lung parenchyma between the heart and the diaphragm are additional imaging findings that have been reported in congenital pericardial defects.

✔ Pearls & ✘ Pitfalls

✔ The bulging of the left atrial appendage without gross leftward cardiac displacement and without evidence of mitral valve disease is consistent with atrial herniation through a PCAP.

✘ Affected patients typically present with paroxysmal stabbing chest pain. Symptomatic apical defects need to be detected as soon as possible, as patients with ventricular herniation and strangulation can die in hours.

Case 96

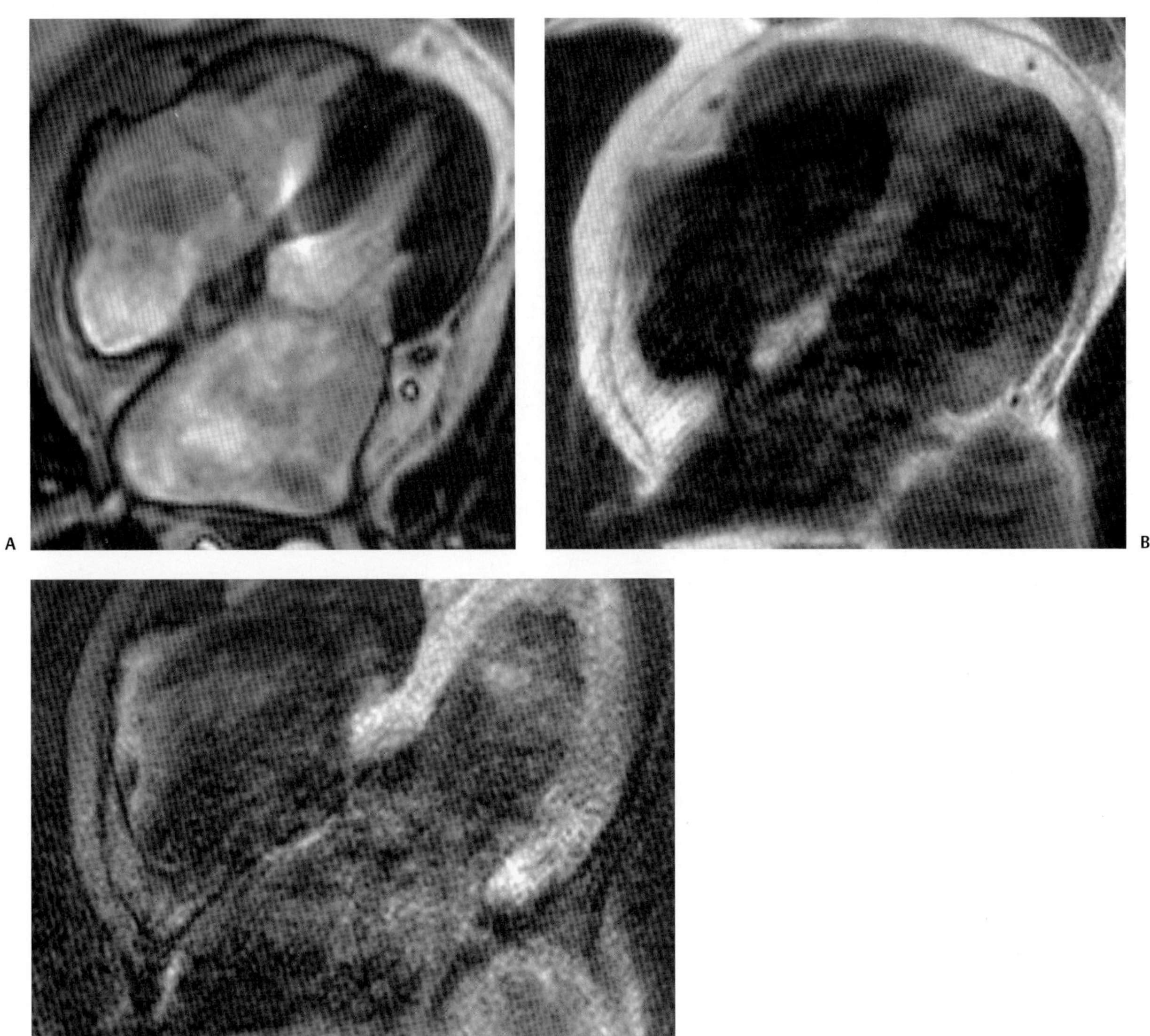

Clinical Presentation

A 65-year-old man presents with a hyperechoic mass in the interatrial septum on echocardiography.

Imaging Findings

All three images are four-chamber views of the heart.

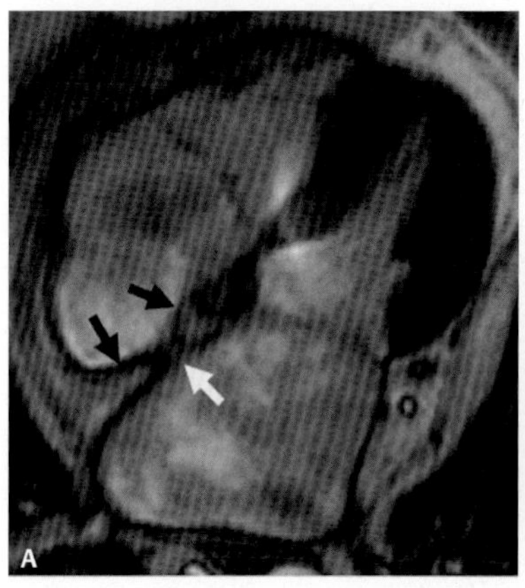

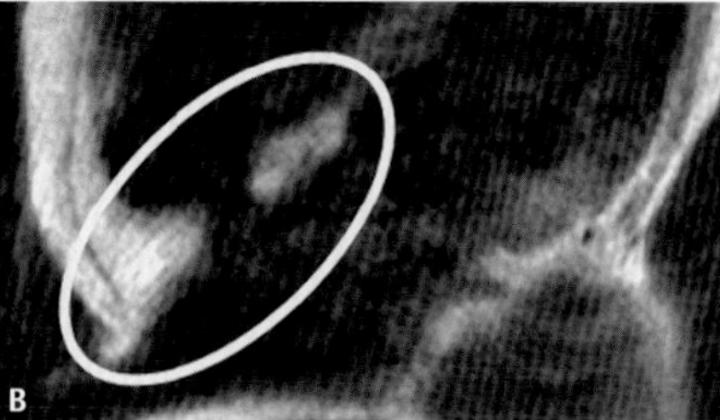

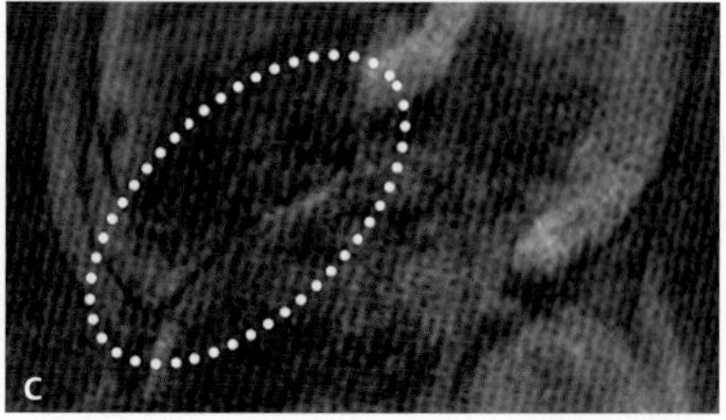

(A) This balanced fast-field echo image shows heterogeneous signal in the thickened interatrial septum (*black arrows*) and a waist in the mass centrally (*white arrow*). **(B)** With a spin echo sequence, the interatrial septum is homogeneously high-signal, as is the pericardial fat (*white oval*). **(C)** After addition of a fat saturation pulse to a spin echo sequence, the signal of the interatrial mass is completely saturated (*dotted white oval*).

Differential Diagnosis

- ***Interatrial lipoma or lipomatous hypertrophy of the atrial septum:*** Fetal and adult types of adipose tissue accumulate in the interatrial septum and can result in massive enlargement of the septum. This thickening of the septum typically spares the foramen ovale.
- *Atrial myxoma:* This entity is a not uncommonly diagnosed benign cardiac mass in adults. The mass is most often in the left atrium (50%) and has mixed signal on magnetic resonance imaging (MRI). Myxomas are most often exophytic in the left atrium.
- *Atrial fibroma:* Fibrous tissue is of low to intermediate attenuation on computed tomography (CT) but is usually lower-signal than fat on T1- and T2-weighted MRI sequences and does not change signal with a fat saturation pulse.

Essential Facts

- Lipomatous hypertrophy is not a true neoplasm.
- Lipomatous hypertrophy is more common in elderly obese women.
- The patient may experience supraventricular arrhythmias.
- Interatrial lipomas usually contain Kupffer (reticuloendothelial) cells that take up sulfur colloid.

Other Imaging Findings

- Although most often diagnosed with echocardiography, the finding is not uncommonly seen on chest CT and coronary artery CT angiography.

✔ Pearls & ✘ Pitfalls

✔ Low attenuation in a thickened interatrial septum is characteristic of the presence of fat on CT.

✔ Fat saturation sequences in cardiac MRI are essential to confirm the diagnosis.

✔ Lipomas of the interatrial septum almost never cause obstruction of the atrioventricular valves, but they may partially obstruct the inferior or superior vena cava.

✔ Lipomas typically spare the foramen ovale, resulting in a characteristic “dumbbell” shape.

✘ Other benign and malignant cardiac tumors rarely imitate lipomatous hypertrophy of the interatrial septum.

Case 97

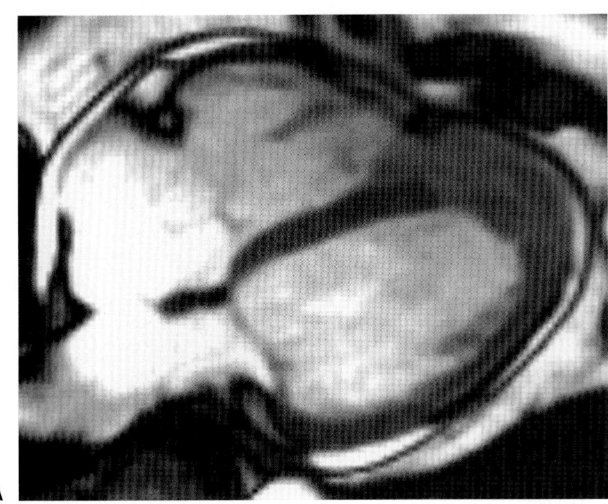

A

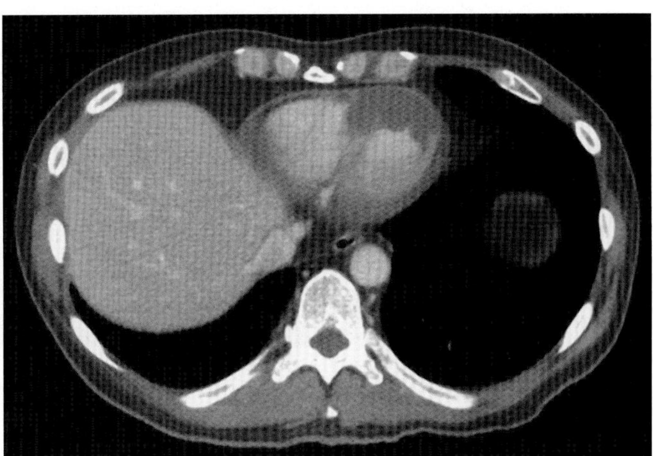

B

Clinical Presentation

A 61-year-old man with a history of lung cancer presents with new stress-induced ST elevation on electrocardiogram (ECG). The apex was not seen well on echocardiography but was not moving normally.

Imaging Findings

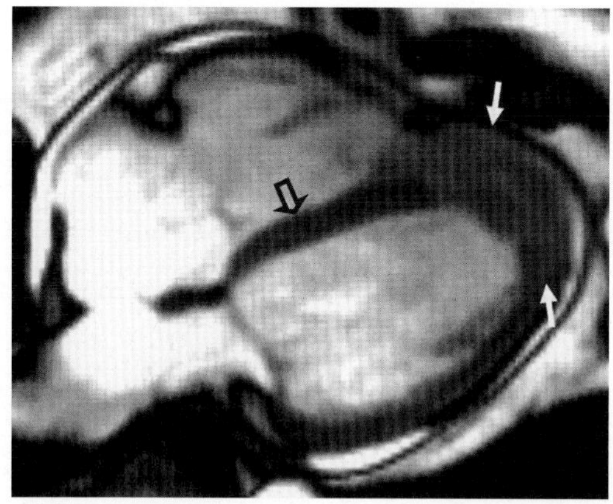

A

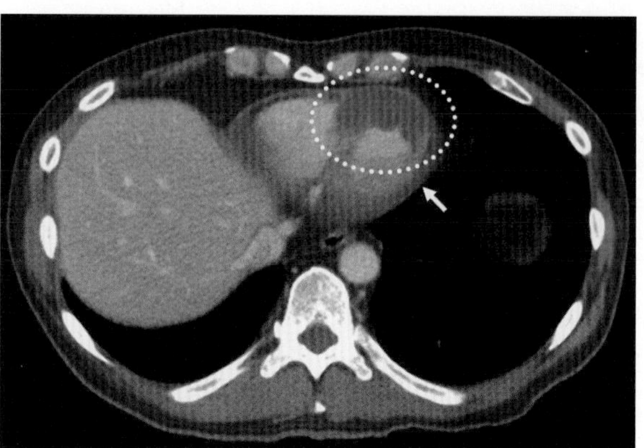

B

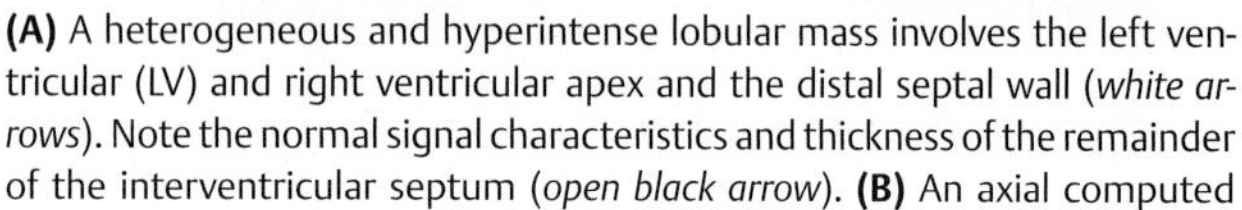

(A) A heterogeneous and hyperintense lobular mass involves the left ventricular (LV) and right ventricular apex and the distal septal wall (*white arrows*). Note the normal signal characteristics and thickness of the remainder of the interventricular septum (*open black arrow*). **(B)** An axial computed tomography (CT) image performed to monitor the status of the patient's lung cancer also shows the mass of the cardiac apex (*dotted white oval*). The mass shows low attenuation compared with the normal LV myocardium (*white arrow*).

Differential Diagnosis

- ***Lung cancer metastases to the LV apex:*** In a patient with a known malignancy and a mass in the myocardium, metastasis is a leading consideration. Benign cardiac masses are usually within a cardiac chamber.
- *Myocarditis:* The apical myocardium is thickened and nodular, and the right ventricular apex is also involved. Myocarditis is more typically seen in the lateral wall of the LV.
- *Myocardial infarction:* Although the ECG findings suggest infarction, they are nonspecific, and the appearance of the myocardium does not suggest infarction.

Essential Facts

- Primary cardiac tumors are rare; 75% of cardiac tumors of all types are benign, most commonly myxomas.
- Primary cardiac neoplasms are usually located within a cardiac chamber.
- Metastatic cardiac tumors are ~100 times more frequent than primary cardiac neoplasms.
- Cardiac metastases are found during autopsy in up to 25% of cancer patients and are more frequent in those with disseminated disease.
- Metastatic cardiac masses are usually in the myocardium or pericardium rather than in a cardiac chamber.
- The tumors most commonly found to be metastatic to the heart are carcinomas of the lung and breast, melanoma, esophageal and renal cancer, lymphoma, and leukemia.

Other Imaging Findings

- Cardiac metastases may be multifocal.
- Diffuse pericardial thickening is seen.
- Pericardial effusion is present.
- New valve insufficiency is noted.
- The right and left sides of the heart may be affected.

✔ Pearls & ✘ Pitfalls

✔ Tumor spread to the heart may be hematogenous, via direct invasion, or intravascular (usually via the inferior vena cava).

✘ Pericardial effusion in a patient with cancer is more likely to be secondary to chemotherapy or radiation therapy.

✘ The blood of patients with malignancy is also hypercoagulable. Consider intracavitary thrombus when a mass is seen within a cardiac chamber.

Case 98

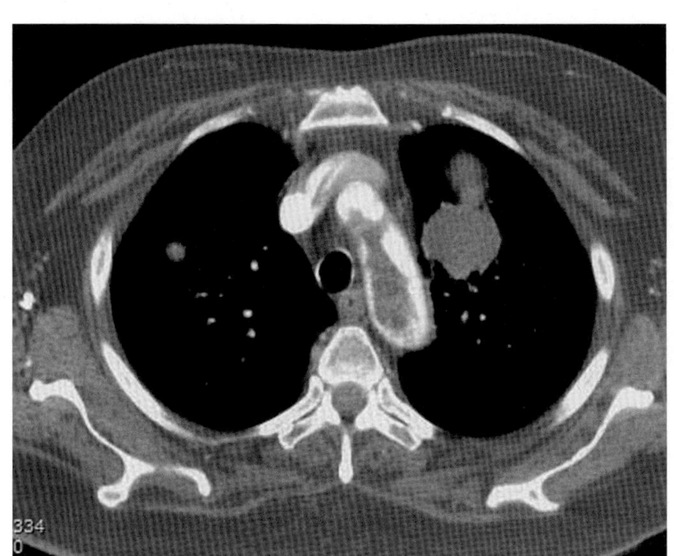

A

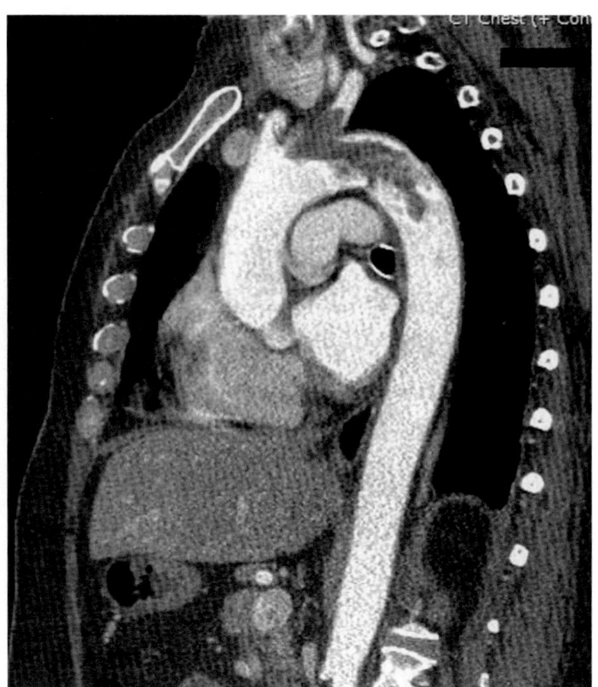

B

Clinical Presentation

A 65-year-old woman presents with a history of syncope.

Imaging Findings

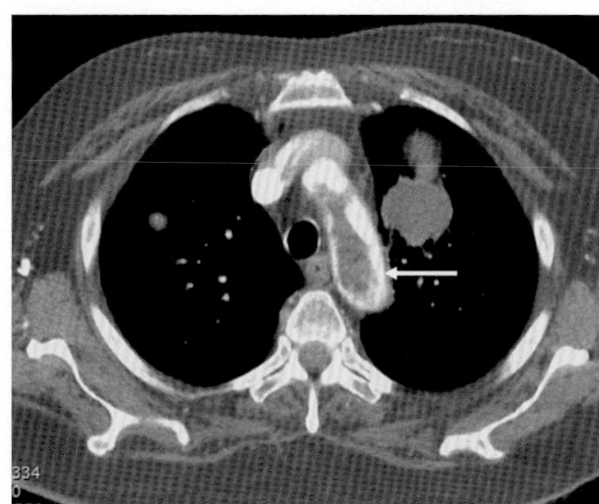

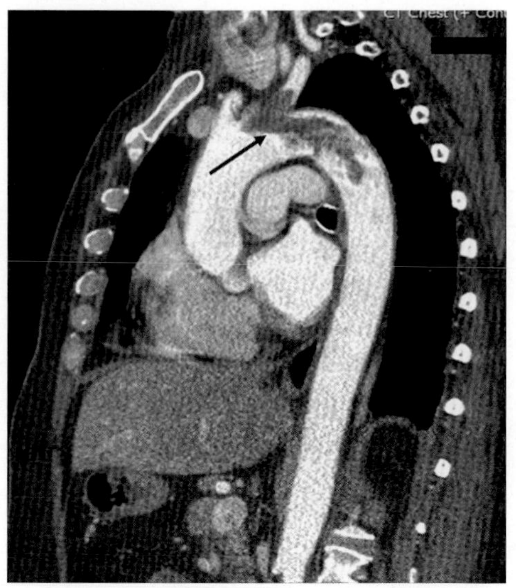

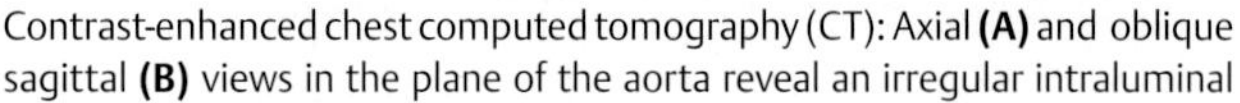

Contrast-enhanced chest computed tomography (CT): Axial **(A)** and oblique sagittal **(B)** views in the plane of the aorta reveal an irregular intraluminal mass in the aortic lumen with extension into the left subclavian artery, as well as a pulmonary mass and nodules.

Differential Diagnosis

- ***Aortic sarcoma:*** Aortic sarcomas are rare primary malignant tumors that more often affect the aortic arch. On CT, they present as an irregular soft-tissue mass with a broad-based attachment to the endothelial surface.
- *Aortic metastasis:* Different tumors may secondarily involve the aorta, but in general aortic metastases are uncommon. The most common presentation is extrinsic invasion by proximity (e.g., lung cancer, esophageal cancer, and lymphomas).
- *Aortic thrombus:* Aortic thrombi are commonly seen as concentric, low-density tissue in aortic aneurysms or as occluding tissue density in smaller vessels. They are by far more common than primary or secondary tumors, presenting as an endovascular filling defect in the aorta.
- *Atherosclerotic disease:* Aortic wall and luminal changes from atherosclerotic disease are the most common cause of abnormal thickening of the aortic wall. This can significantly produce wall thickening with soft-tissue and calcium density and compromise of the vascular lumen.

Essential Facts

- Most common aortic tumors are secondary to local invasion by lung or esophageal cancer in the chest, or by retroperitoneal tumors in the abdomen (e.g., lymphomas and seminomas).
- Primary aortic tumors are rare. The most common tumors are sarcomas (poorly differentiated sarcomas, angiosarcomas, or leiomyosarcomas), followed by malignant fibrous histiocytomas, and malignant hemangioendotheliomas.
- Clinical presentation relates to peripheral embolization, claudication, or ischemia from aortic occlusion.
- Some patients may present with symptoms suggestive of vasculitis or arteritis (fatigue, weight loss, and high blood sedimentation rate).
- The mean age at diagnosis is ~60 years.
- Men are affected more often than women.
- In general, the prognosis is poor. Distant metastases, including of the bones, liver, and lungs, are common.

Other Imaging Findings

- The appearance of aortic tumors on imaging depends on whether the tumor is intimal or mural in origin. Intimal tumors tend to develop in the vascular lumen and are more likely to metastasize downstream and cause embolic events. Mural types present as an abnormal thickening of the aortic wall, are less emboligenic, and manifest few symptoms.

✔ Pearls & ✘ Pitfalls

✔ Benign primary tumors of the aorta are also rare and include papillary fibroelastoma (aortic valve and ascending aorta), myxoma, leiomyoma, and lipoma.

✘ Aortic tumors and intramural or endoluminal thrombi can have a similar appearance. Contrast-enhanced magnetic resonance imaging can help in their differentiation, as sarcomas exhibit contrast enhancement.

Case 99

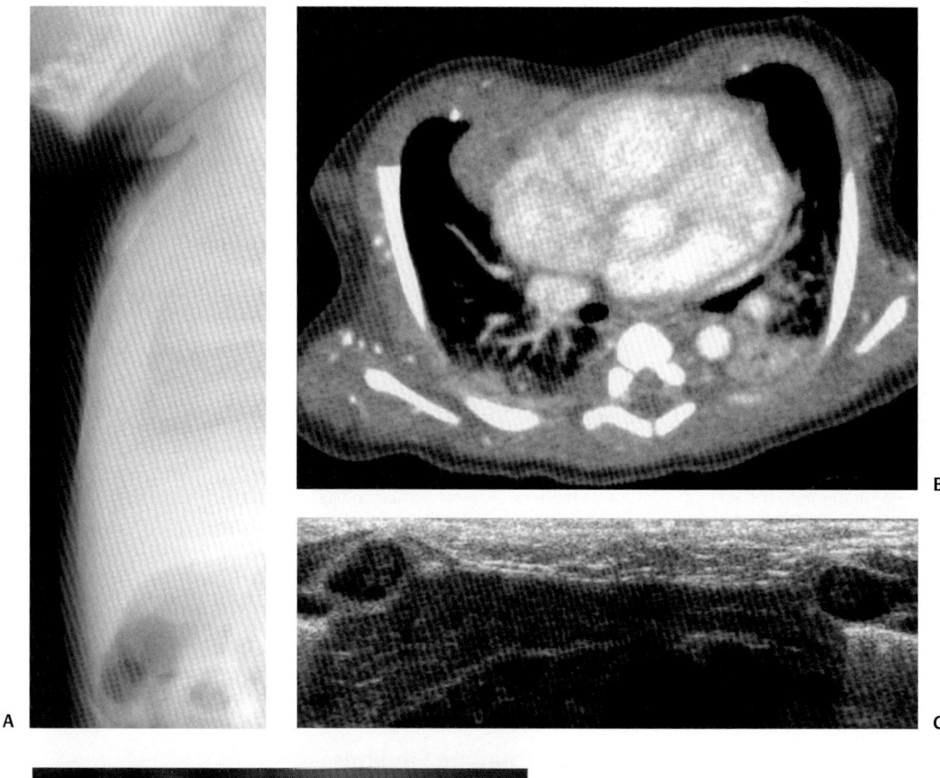

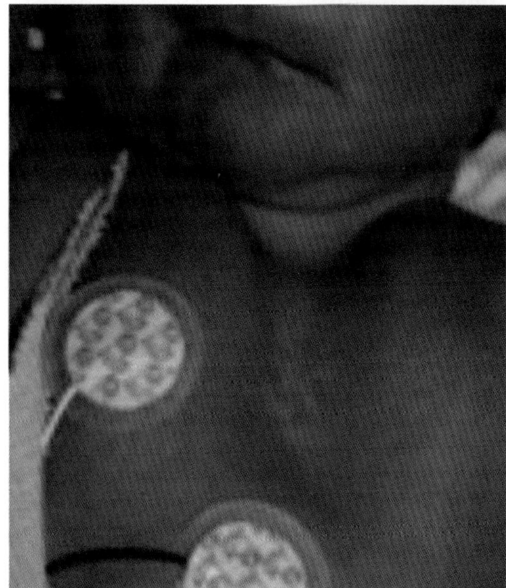

Clinical Presentation

A newborn girl presents with an anterior chest wall deformity. The diagnosis was anticipated by antenatal sonography and was confirmed in the neonatal period with a variety of imaging modalities.

Imaging Findings

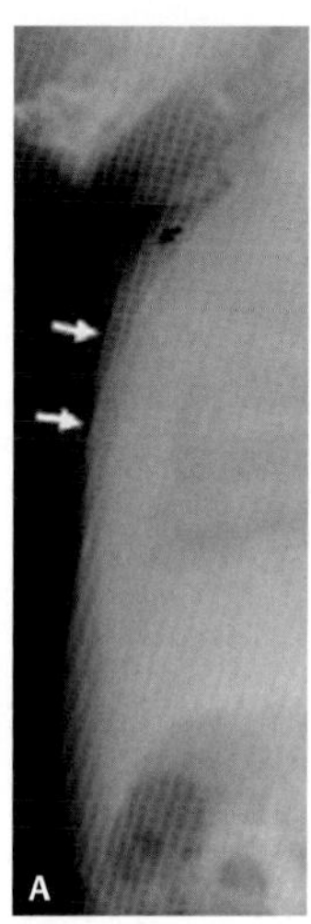

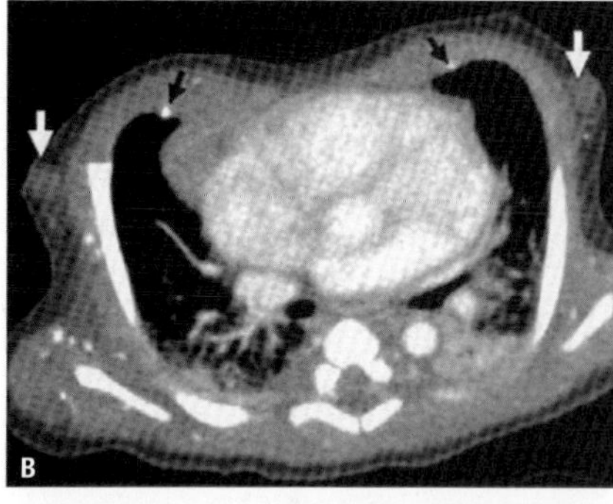

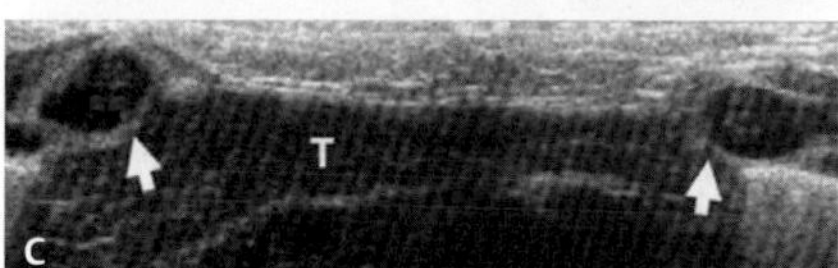

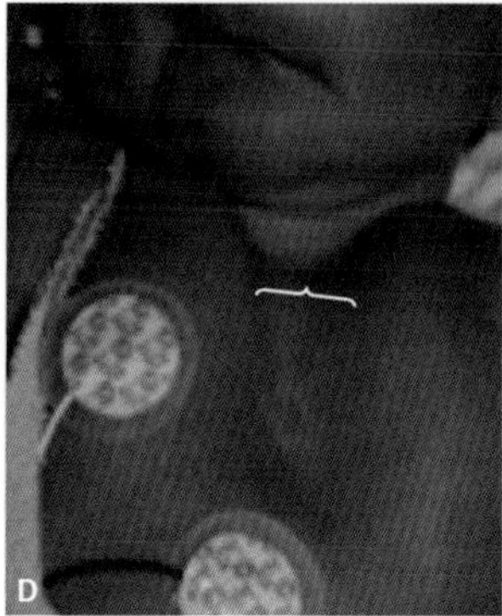

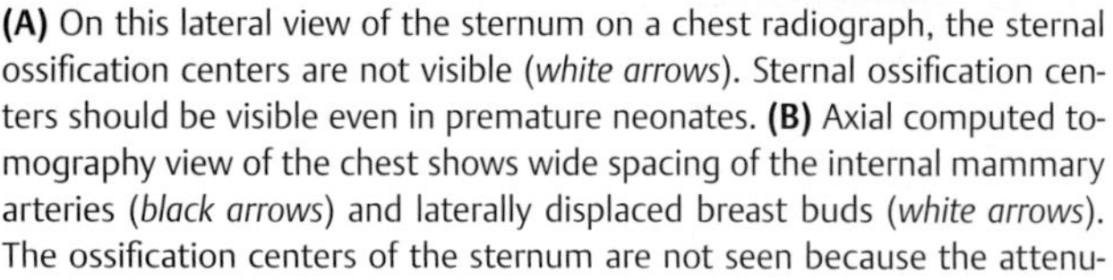

(A) On this lateral view of the sternum on a chest radiograph, the sternal ossification centers are not visible (*white arrows*). Sternal ossification centers should be visible even in premature neonates. **(B)** Axial computed tomography view of the chest shows wide spacing of the internal mammary arteries (*black arrows*) and laterally displaced breast buds (*white arrows*). The ossification centers of the sternum are not seen because the attenuation of their cartilage is similar to that of muscle in the chest wall. The anterior chest wall is indented slightly. **(C)** Wide spacing of the sternal ossification centers is seen in this sonographic image (*arrows*). The thymus (*T*) lies directly under the subcutaneous fat. **(D)** In this image, the superior anterior chest wall is depressed in the midline (*bracket*) because the sternum is deficient.

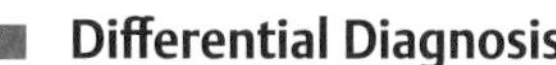

Differential Diagnosis

- ***Ectopia cordis:*** This entity includes a range of congenital abnormalities of the anterior chest wall that result in various defects of the anterior chest wall. These may in turn result in placement of the heart completely outside the thorax.
- *Pectus excavatum:* The slight depression of the anterior chest wall in this patient is not due to a deformity of the sternum, but rather to the wide separation of the sternal ossification centers, which failed to fuse normally in the midline. Pectus excavatum is a posterior depression of the inferior aspect of the sternum caused by idiopathic overgrowth of the costal cartilages.
- *Poland syndrome:* Asymmetric hypoplasia of the pectoralis major muscles, along with breast or nipple and upper extremity anomalies extending from the scapula to the digits, characterizes Poland syndrome. The chest wall musculature and breast buds are symmetric in this patient.

Essential Facts

- Sternal ossification centers are usually visible (sonographically) by 6 months' gestation.
- The ossification centers initially comprise two centers at each level that fuse during infancy or childhood.
- Separate superior and inferior manubrial ossification centers are common in patients with Down syndrome, but they are much less likely to be seen other patients.
- Pentalogy of Cantrell consists of lower sternal defect, high omphalocele, pericardial and diaphragmatic defect, and ventral diverticulum of the left ventricle.
- The heart may be completely covered with skin and subcutaneous tissue and the thymus intact in the anterior mediastinum, as in this patient.
- The heart may be completely exposed, lying outside the thorax and not covered by skin.

Other Imaging Findings

- The medial ends of the clavicles are laterally displaced.
- Sternal ossification centers are difficult to visualize on frontal chest radiographs. Lateral and oblique views of the chest easily show normal sternal ossification centers.
- Ectopia cordis is divided into five types: cervical, cervicothoracic, thoracic, thoracoabdominal, and abdominal.
- In the thoracic type, there is a cleft sternum.
- Other cardiac malformations associated with ectopia cordis are ventricular septal defect, common atrium, atrioventricular septal defect, tricuspid atresia, pulmonary stenosis, pulmonary atresia, and transposition of the great arteries.

✔ Pearls & ✘ Pitfalls

✔ The sternal ossification centers are normally visible radiographically at birth.

✔ Midline upper abdominal and lower chest wall abnormalities accompany one another, as the lateral folds of the thorax and abdominal wall do not fuse normally during the 4th week of gestation.

✔ Omphalocele is differentiated from gastroschisis by the presence of a peritoneal covering over the exposed bowel.

✔ Omphalocele has a much greater association with other congenital anomalies, such as other forms of congenital heart disease.

✘ Given the rarity of ectopia cordis, one may fail to recognize the subtle findings of an incomplete sternal cleft.

✘ Defects in the pericardium may be visualized only with magnetic resonance.

Case 100

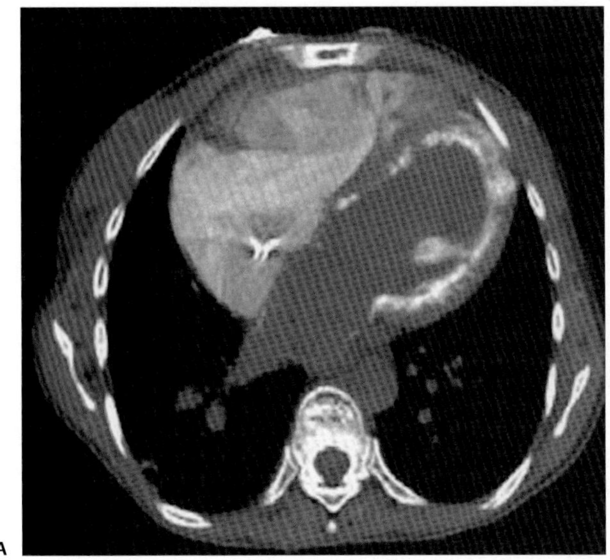

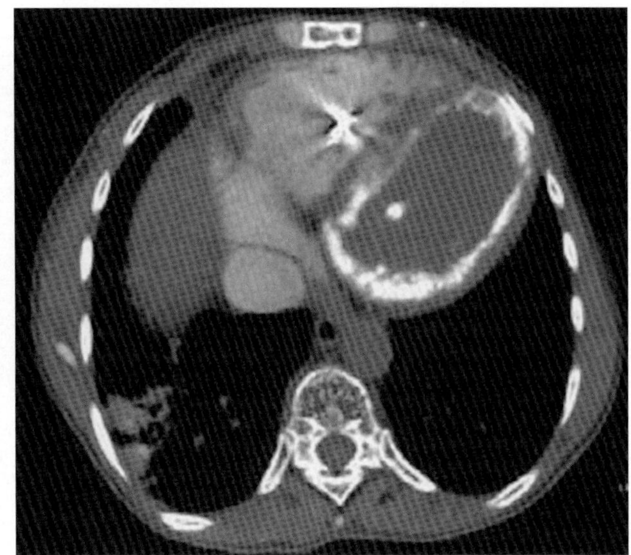

A B

Clinical Presentation

Congestive heart failure in a 56-year-old woman on long-term dialysis

Imaging Findings

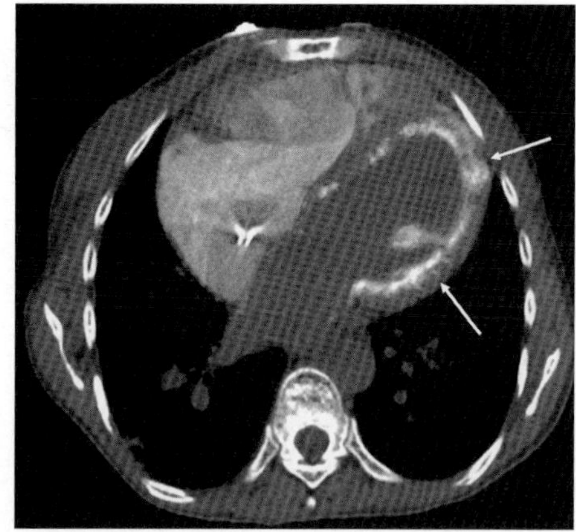

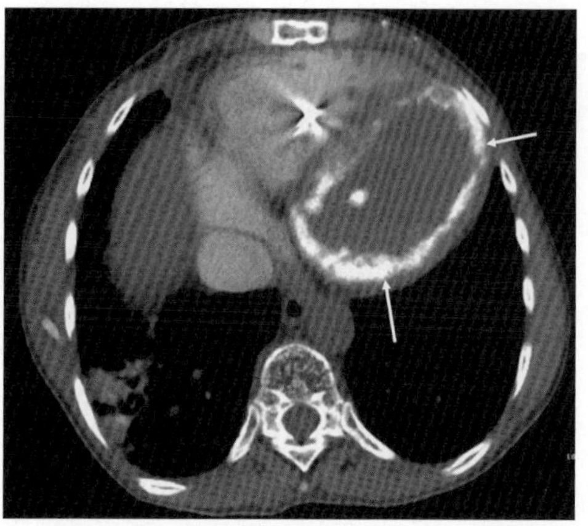

(A,B) Contrast-enhanced cardiac computed tomography images show diffuse extensive calcification of the myocardium, involving mainly the left ventricle and to a lesser extent the left atrium. Global cardiomegaly is also noted, as well as parenchymal pulmonary opacity in the right lower lobe. Electrodes from an automatic implantable cardioverter-defibrillator are seen.

Differential Diagnosis

- ***Metastatic cardiac calcification secondary to chronic renal failure:*** The deposit of calcium in previously normal tissue, seen in patients with chronic renal failure, is the result of abnormal serum levels of calcium and phosphorus. It can present involving the myocardium and is known as metastatic calcification.
- *Dystrophic calcification secondary to ischemia or inflammation:* A late consequence of myocardial infarction or extensive inflammatory changes is abnormal calcification of the affected tissue.

Essential Facts

- Metastatic calcification is a very common finding at autopsy of patients who have been on long-term dialysis.
- Clinical manifestations include refractory cardiac failure and conduction abnormalities (atrioventricular block).
- Pathophysiology is closely related to the serum imbalance of calcium and phosphorus, as well as elevated levels of parathyroid hormone (secondary or tertiary parathyroidism) that result in abnormal calcium deposits in previously healthy tissue.
- Affected tissues and organs include skin, joints, vessels, cornea, conjunctiva, heart, lungs, bowel, and kidneys.
- In the heart, the left ventricle wall, including the interventricular septum, is the more extensively affected.
- Chronic renal insufficiency and long-term dialysis are also associated with calcification of cardiac valves and coronary arteries.

Other Imaging Findings

- Radionuclide imaging with technetium Tc 99m pyrophosphate may show increased myocardial uptake in the presence of metastatic cardiac calcification.

✔ Pearls & ✘ Pitfalls

✔ Increased myocardial calcification is strongly associated with myocardial dysfunction in patients with chronic renal failure undergoing dialysis.

✘ Chronic inflammation resulting from prior surgery, infection, radiation therapy, or lupus may produce extensive pericardial calcification. The location, distribution, and clinical significance of pericardial calcification should be differentiated from that of myocardial calcification.

Further Readings

Case 1 Normal cardiac conduction system

Cardiac conduction system. Available at: http://www.americanheart.org/presenter.jhtml?identifier=68 Accessed November 4, 2008.

Case 2 Atrial myxoma

Araoz PA, Mulvag hSL, Tazelaar HD, Julsrud PR, Breen JF. CT and MR imaging of benign primary cardiac neoplasms with echocardiographic correlation. Radiographics 2000;20(5):1303–1319

Grebenc ML, Rosado de Christenson ML, Green CE, Burke AP, Galvin JR. Cardiac myxoma: imaging features in 83 patients. Radiographics 2002;22(3):673–689

Restrepo CS, Largoza A, Lemos DF, et al. CT and MR imaging findings of benign cardiac tumors. Curr Probl Diagn Radiol 2005;34(1):12–21

Tsuchiya F, Kohno A, Saitoh R, Shigeta A. CT findings of atrial myxoma. Radiology 1984;151(1):139–143

Case 3 Papillary fibroelastoma

Basso C, Bottio T, Valente M, Bonato R, Casarotto D, Thiene G. Primary cardiac valve tumours. Heart 2003;89(10):1259–1260

Bootsveld A, Puetz J, Grube E. Incidental finding of a papillary fibroelastoma on the aortic valve in 16 slice multi-detector row computed tomography. Heart 2004;90(6):e35

Lembcke A, Meyer R, Kivelitz D, et al. Images in cardiovascular medicine: papillary fibroelastoma of the aortic valve—appearance in 64-slice spiral computed tomography, magnetic resonance imaging, and echocardiography. Circulation 2007;115(1):e3–e6

Sun JP, Asher CR, Yang XS, et al. Clinical and echocardiographic characteristics of papillary fibroelastomas: a retrospective and prospective study in 162 patients. Circulation 2001;103(22):2687–2693

Case 4 Left ventricular (LV) apical infarction

Anzai T, Yoshikawa T, Kaneko H, et al. Association between serum C-reactive protein elevation and left ventricular thrombus formation after first anterior myocardial infarction. Chest 2004;125(2):384-389

Hunold P, Schlosser T, Vogt FM, et al. Myocardial late enhancement in contrast-enhanced cardiac MRI: distinction between infarction scar and non-infarction-related disease. AJR Am J Roentgenol 2005;184(5):1420-1426

Tóth C, Ujhelyi E, Fülöp T, Istvan E. Clinical predictors of early left ventricular thrombus formation in acute myocardial infarction. Acta Cardiol 2002;57(3):205-211

Case 5 Membranous ventricular septal defect (VSD)

Braunwald E. Ventricular Septal Defect in Adult Congenital Heart Disease: A Practical Guide. Malden, MA: Blackwell; 2005:82–91

Miller SM. Congenital Heart Disease in Cardiac Imaging: The Requisites. Philadelphia: Elsevier Mosby; 2005:331–334

Case 6 Patent left interior mammary artery to left anterior descending artery (LIMA–LAD) coronary artery bypass graft (CABG)

Dikkers R, Willems TP, Tio RA, Anthonio RL, Zijlstra F, Oudkerk M. The benefit of 64-MDCT prior to invasive coronary angiography in symptomatic post-CABG patients. Int J Cardiovasc Imaging 2007;23(3):369–377

Doi H, Koshima R, Suzuki M, Takahashi K, Yokoyama H, Yoshida N. Can 64-row computed tomography replace angiography after coronary bypass? Asian Cardiovasc Thorac Ann 2008;16(6):444–449

Le Breton H, Pavin D, Langanay T, et al. Aneurysms and pseudoaneurysms of saphenous vein coronary artery bypass grafts. Heart 1998;79(5):505–508

Case 7 Anomalous origin of the left coronary artery from the pulmonary artery (ALCAPA)

Brotherton H, Philip RK. Anomalous left coronary artery from pulmonary artery (ALCAPA) in infants: a 5-year review in a defined birth cohort. Eur J Pediatr 2008;167:43–46

Fierens C, Budts W, Denef B, Van de Werf F. A 72 year old woman with ALCAPA. Heart 2000;83:e2

Kang WC, Chung W-J, Choi CH, et al. A rare case of anomalous left coronary artery from the pulmonary artery (ALCAPA) presenting congestive heart failure in an adult. Int J Cardiol 2007;115:e63–e67

Khanna A, Torigian DA, Ferrari VA, Bross RJ, Rosen MA. Anomalous origin of the left coronary artery from the pulmonary artery in adulthood on CT and MRI. AJR Am J Roentgenol 2005;185:326–329

Case 8 Anomalous right coronary artery from the pulmonary artery (ARCAPA)

Glanz S, Gordon DH, Mesko Z, Griepp R. Anomalous origin of the right coronary artery from the pulmonary artery. Cardiovasc Intervent Radiol 1981;4(4):256–258

Luciani GB, Vendrametto F, Barozzi L, Oberhollenzer R, Pitscheider W, Mazzucco A. Repair of anomalous right and circumflex coronary arteries arising from the pulmonary artery. J Thorac Cardiovasc Surg 2006;132(4):970–972

Case 9 Constrictive pericarditis

Kim JS, Kim HH, Yoon Y. Imaging of pericardial diseases. Clin Radiol 2007;62(7):626–631

Maisch B, Seferović PM, Ristić AD, et al; Task Force on the Diagnosis and Management of Pricardial Diseases of the European Society of Cardiology. Guidelines on the diagnosis and management of pericardial diseases executive summary. Eur Heart J 2004;25(7):587–610

Wang ZJ, Reddy GP, Gotway MB, Yeh BM, Hetts SW, Higgins CB. CT and MR imaging of pericardial disease. Radiographics 2003;23(Spec No):S167–S180

Case 10 LV apical aneurysm and early thrombus formation secondary to infarction

Francone M, Carbone I, Napoli A, et al. Imaging of myocardial infarction using a 64-slice MDCT scanner: correlation between infarcted region and status of territory-dependent coronary artery. Radiol Med (Torino) 2007;112(8):1100–1116

Hoffmann U, Pena AJ, Moselewski F, et al. MDCT in early triage of patients with acute chest pain. AJR Am J Roentgenol 2006;187(5):1240–1247

Lardo AC, Cordeiro MAS, Silva C, et al. Contrast-enhanced multidetector computed tomography viability imaging after myocardial infarction: characterization of myocyte death, microvascular obstruction, and chronic scar. Circulation 2006;113(3):394–404

Case 11 Discrete subaortic stenosis (SAS)

Aboulhosn J, Child JS. Left ventricular outflow obstruction: subaortic stenosis, bicuspid aortic valve, supravalvar aortic stenosis, and coarctation of the aorta. Circulation 2006;114(22):2412–2422

Oliver JM, González A, Gallego P, Sánchez-Recalde A, Benito F, Mesa JM. Discrete subaortic stenosis in adults: increased prevalence and slow rate of progression of the obstruction and aortic regurgitation. J Am Coll Cardiol 2001;38(3):835–842

Tentolouris K, Kontozoglou T, Trikas A, et al. Fixed subaortic stenosis revisited. congenital abnormalities in 72 new cases and review of the literature. Cardiology 1999;92(1):4–1010640790

Van Arsdell G, Tsoi K. Subaortic stenosis: at risk substrates and treatment strategies. Cardiol Clin 2002;20(3):421–429

Case 12 Myocardial bridge

Bonvini RF, Alibegovic J, Perret X, et al. Coronary myocardial bridge: an innocent bystander? Heart Vessels 2008;23(1):67–7018273549

WanL, WuQ. Myocardial bridge, surgery or stenting? Interact Cardiovasc Thorac Surg 2005;4(6):517–520

Zeina A-R, Odeh M, Blinder J, Rosenschein U, Barmeir E. Myocardial bridge: evaluation on MDCT. AJR Am J Roentgenol 2007;188(4):1069–1073

Case 13 Coronary artery fistula (CAF)

Kim SY, Seo JB, Do K-H, et al. Coronary artery anomalies: classification and ECG-gated multi-detector row CT findings with angiographic correlation. Radiographics 2006;26(2):317–333, discussion 333–334

McMahon CJ, Nihill MR, Kovalchin JP, Mullins CE, Grifka RG. Coronary artery fistula: management and intermediate-term outcome after transcatheter coil occlusion. Tex Heart Inst J 2001;28(1):21–25

Case 14 Noncalcified atherosclerotic plaques

Budoff MJ. Prevalence of soft plaque detection with computed tomography. J Am Coll Cardiol 2006;48(2):319–321

Glagov S, Weisenberg E, Zarins CK, Stankunavicius R, Kolettis GJ. Compensatory enlargement of human atherosclerotic coronary arteries. N Engl J Med 1987;316(22):1371–1375

Hausleiter J, Meyer T, Hadamitzky M, Kastrati A, Martinoff S, Schömig A. Prevalence of noncalcified coronary plaques by 64-slice computed tomography in patients with an intermediate risk for significant coronary artery disease. J Am Coll Cardiol 2006;48(2):312–318

Kelly JL, Thickman D, Abramson SD, et al. Coronary CT angiography findings in patients without coronary calcification. AJR Am J Roentgenol 2008;191(1):50–55

Leber AW, Knez A, White CW, et al. Composition of coronary atherosclerotic plaques in patients with acute myocardial infarction and stable angina pectoris determined by contrast-enhanced multislice computed tomography. Am J Cardiol 2003;91(6):714–718

Case 15 Pulmonary vein extension and left atrial invasion by lung cancer

Ibrahim NBN, Burnley H, Gaber KA, et al. Segmental pulmonary veno-occlusive disease secondary to lung cancer. J Clin Pathol 2005;58(4):434–436

Ratto GB, Costa R, Vassallo G, Alloisio A, Maineri P, Bruzzi P. Twelve-year experience with left atrial resection in the treatment of non-small cell lung cancer. Ann Thorac Surg 2004;78(1):234–237

Spaggiari L, D' Aiuto M, Veronesi G, et al. Extended pneumonectomy with partial resection of the left atrium, without cardiopulmonary bypass, for lung cancer. Ann Thorac Surg 2005;79(1):234–240

Takahashi K, Furuse M, Hanaoka H, et al. Pulmonary vein and left atrial invasion by lung cancer: assessment by breath-hold gadolinium-enhanced three-dimensional MR angiography. J Comput Assist Tomogr 2000;24(4):557–561

Case 16 Bronchopulmonary sequestration

Deguchi E, Furukawa T, Ono S, Aoi S, Kimura O, Iwai N. Intralobar pulmonary sequestration diagnosed by MR angiography. Pediatr Surg Int 2005;21(7):576-577

Lee EY, Dillon JE, Callahan MJ, Voss SD. 3D multidetector CT angiographic evaluation of extralobar pulmonary sequestration with anomalous venous drainage into the left internal mammary vein in a paediatric patient. Br J Radiol 2006;79(945):e99-e102

Case 17 Effusive constrictive pericarditis (ECP)

Rienmüller R, Gröll R, Lipton MJ. CT and MR imaging of pericardial disease. Radiol Clin North Am 2004;42(3):587–601

Sagristà-Sauleda J, Angel J, Sánchez A, Permanyer-Miralda G, Soler-Soler J. Effusive-constrictive pericarditis. N Engl J Med 2004;350(5):469–475

Zagol B, Minderman D, Munir A, D'Cruz I. Effusive constrictive pericarditis: 2D, 3D echocardiography and MRI imaging. Echocardiography 2007;24(10):1110–1114

Case 18 Coronary artery calcification (CAC)

Budoff MJ, Achenbach S, Blumenthal RS, et al; American Heart Association Committee on Cardiovascular Imaging and Intervention; American Heart Association Council on Cardiovascular Radiology and Intervention; American Heart Association Committee on Cardiac Imaging, Council on Clinical Cardiology. Assessment of coronary artery disease by cardiac computed tomography: a scientific statement from the American Heart Association Committee on Cardiovascular Imaging and Intervention, Council on Cardiovascular Radiology and Intervention, and Committee on Cardiac Imaging, Council on Clinical Cardiology. Circulation 2006;114(16):1761–1791

Greenland P, Bonow RO, Brundage BH, et al; American College of Cardiology Foundation Clinical Expert Consensus Task Force (ACCF/AHA Writing Committee to Update the 2000 Expert Consensus Document on Electron Beam Computed Tomography); Society of Atherosclerosis Imaging and Prevention; Society of Cardiovascular Computed Tomography. ACCF/AHA 2007 clinical expert consensus document on coronary artery calcium scoring by computed tomography in global cardiovascular risk assessment and in evaluation of patients with chest pain: a report of the American College of Cardiology Foundation Clinical Expert Consensus Task Force (ACCF/AHA Writing Committee to Update the 2000 Expert Consensus Document on Electron Beam Computed Tomography). Circulation 2007;115(3):402–426

Pletcher MJ, Tice JA, Pignone M, Browner WS. Using the coronary artery calcium score to predict coronary heart disease events: a systematic review and meta-analysis. Arch Intern Med 2004;164(12):1285–1292

Case 19 Secundum atrial septal defect (ASD)

Boxt LM, Rozenshtein A. MR imaging of congenital heart disease. Magn Reson Imag Clin N Am 2003;11:27-48

Craig RJ, Selzer A. Natural history and prognosis of atrial septal defect. Circulation 1968;37(5):805-815

Swan L, Gatzoulis MA. Closure of atrial septal defects: is the debate over? Eur Heart J 2003;24(2):130-132

Case 20 Takayasu arteritis

Gotway MB, Araoz PA, Macedo TA, et al. Imaging findings in Takayasu's arteritis. AJR Am J Roentgenol 2005;184(6):1945–1950 PubMed

Matsunaga N, Hayashi K, Sakamoto I, Ogawa Y, Matsumoto T. Takayasu arteritis: protean radiologic manifestations and diagnosis. Radiographics 1997;17(3):579–594 PubMed

Sueyoshi E, Sakamoto I, Hayashi K. Aortic aneurysms in patients with Takayasu's arteritis: CT evaluation. AJR Am J Roentgenol 2000;175(6):1727–1733 PubMed

Sueyoshi E, Sakamoto I, Uetani M. MRI of Takayasu's arteritis: typical appearance and complications. AJR 2006;186(7):W569–W575

Yamada I, Nakagawa T, Himeno Y, Numano F, Shibuya H. Takayasu arteritis: evaluation of the thoracic aorta with CT angiography. Radiology 1998;209(1):103–109 PubMed

Case 21 Multifocal acute and chronic myocardial infarction

Gerber BL, Garot J, Bluemke DA, Wu KC, Lima JAC. Accuracy of contrast-enhanced magnetic resonance imaging in predicting improvement of regional myocardial function in patients after acute myocardial infarction. Circulation 2002;106(9):1083–1089

Hunold P, Schlosser T, Vogt FM, et al. Myocardial late enhancement in contrast-enhanced cardiac MRI: distinction between infarction scar and non-infarction-related disease. AJR Am J Roentgenol 2005;184(5):1420–1426

Jackson E, Bellenger N, Seddon M, Harden S, Peebles C. Ischaemic and non-ischaemic cardiomyopathies—cardiac MRI appearances with delayed enhancement. Clin Radiol 2007;62(5):395–403

Case 22 Pericardial cyst (mesothelial)

Jeung M-Y, Gasser B, Gangi A, et al. Imaging of cystic masses of the mediastinum. Radiographics 2002;22(Spec No):S79–S93

Kim JS, Kim HH, Yoon Y. Imaging of pericardial diseases. Clin Radiol 2007;62(7):626–631

Stoller JK, Shaw C, Matthay RA. Enlarging, atypically located pericardial cyst: recent experience and literature review. Chest 1986;89(3):402–406

Wang ZJ, Reddy GP, Gotway MB, Yeh BM, Hetts SW, Higgins CB. CT and MR imaging of pericardial disease. Radiographics 2003;23(Spec No):S167–S180

Case 23 Acute right ventricular dysfunction secondary to pulmonary embolism

Ghaye B, Ghuysen A, Bruyere P-J, D'Orio V, Dondelinger RF. Can CT pulmonary angiography allow assessment of severity and prognosis in patients presenting with pulmonary embolism? What the radiologist needs to know. Radiographics 2006;26(1):23–39, discussion 39–40

He H, Stein MW, Zalta B, Haramati LB. Computed tomography evaluation of right heart dysfunction in patients with acute pulmonary embolism. J Comput Assist Tomogr 2006;30(2):262–266

Schoepf UJ, Kucher N, Kipfmueller F, Quiroz R, Costello P, Goldhaber SZ. Right ventricular enlargement on chest computed tomography: a predictor of early death in acute pulmonary embolism. Circulation 2004;110(20):3276–3280

van der Meer RW, Pattynama PM, van Strijen MJL, et al. Right ventricular dysfunction and pulmonary obstruction index at helical CT: prediction of clinical outcome during 3-month follow-up in patients with acute pulmonary embolism. Radiology 2005;235(3):798–803

Case 24 Giant thrombosed aneurysm of right coronary artery (RCA)

Konen E, Feinberg MS, Morag B, et al. Giant right coronary aneurysm: CT angiographic and echocardiographic findings. AJR Am J Roentgenol 2001;177(3):689–691

Madsen EH, Villadsen AB, Frøbert O. Acute coronary artery thrombosis and a giant coronary artery aneurysm: an atypical combination and an unconventional catheter-based intervention. Catheter Cardiovasc Interv 2006;68(3):399–402

Case 25 Bicuspid aortic valve

Baron MG. Abnormalities of the mitral valve in endocardial cushion defects. Circulation 1972;45(3):672–680

Piccoli GP, Gerlis LM, Wilkinson JL, Lozsadi K, Macartney FJ, Anderson RH. Morphology and classification of atrioventricular defects. Br Heart J 1979;42(6):621–632

Case 26 Supravalvular aortic stenosis (SVAS)

Aboulhosn J, Child JS. Left ventricular outflow obstruction: subaortic stenosis, bicuspid aortic valve, supravalvular aortic stenosis, and coarctation of the aorta. Circulation 2006;114(22):2412–2422

Sharma BK, Fujiwara H, Hallman GL, Ott DA, Reul GJ, Cooley DA. Supravalvular aortic stenosis: a 29-year review of surgical experience. Ann Thorac Surg 1991;51(6):1031–1039

Vaideeswar P, Shankar V, Deshpande JR, et al. Pathology of the diffuse variant of supravalvular aortic stenosis. Cardiovasc Pathol 2001;10:33–37

Case 27 RCA to coronary sinus fistula

Armsby LR, Keane JF, Sherwood MC, Forbess JM, Perry SB, Lock JE. Management of coronary artery fistulae: patient selection and results of transcatheter closure. J Am Coll Cardiol 2002;39(6):1026–1032

McMahon CJ, Nihill MR, Kovalchin JP, Mullins CE, Grifka RG. Coronary artery fistula: management and intermediate-term outcome after transcatheter coil occlusion. Tex Heart Inst J 2001;28(1):21–25

Parga JR, Ikari NM, Bustamante LNP, Rochitte CE, de Avila LFR, Oliveira SA. Case report: MRI evaluation of congenital coronary artery fistulae. Br J Radiol 2004;77(918):508–511

Case 28 Saphenous vein graft aneurysm (SVGA)

Lupetin AR, Gabriele FJ, Kramer CM, Reichek N. Magnetic resonance imaging diagnosis of an aortocoronary saphenous vein graft aneurysm. Cardiovasc Intervent Radiol 1995;18(5):330–332

Nölke L, McGovern E, Wood AE. Saphenous vein graft aneurysms; the true, false and ugly! Interact Cardiovasc Thorac Surg 2004;3(4):631–633

Trop I, Samson L, Cordeau M-P, Leblanc P, Thérasse E. Anterior mediastinal mass in a patient with prior saphenous vein coronary artery bypass grafting. Chest 1999;115(2):572–576

Case 29 Cardiac amyloidosis

Garg P, Gupta R, Hsi DH, Sheils LA, DiSalle MR, Woodlock TJ. Hypertrophic cardiomyopathy and symptomatic conduction system disease in cardiac amyloidosis. South Med J 2006;99(12):1390–1392

vanden Driesen RI, Slaughter RE, Strugnell WE. MR findings in cardiac amyloidosis. AJR Am J Roentgenol 2006;186(6):1682–1685

White JA, Patel MR. The role of cardiovascular MRI in heart failure and the cardiomyopathies. Magn Reson Imaging Clin N Am 2007;15(4):541–564, vi

Case 30 Anomalous origin of the left coronary artery (LCA) from the right aortic sinus

Budoff MJ, Ahmed V, Gul KM, Mao SS, Gopal A. Coronary anomalies by cardiac computed tomographic angiography. Clin Cardiol 2006;29(11):489–493

Datta J, White CS, Gilkeson RC, et al. Anomalous coronary arteries in adults: depiction at multi-detector row CT angiography. Radiology 2005;235(3):812–818

Kim SY, Seo JB, Do KH, et al. Coronary artery anomalies: classification and ECG-gated multi-detector row CT findings with angiographic correlation. Radiographics 2006;26(2):317–333, discussion 333–334

Case 31 Cardiac sarcoidosis

Nemeth MA, Muthupillai R, Wilson JM, Awasthi M, Flamm SD. Cardiac sarcoidosis detected by delayed-hyperenhancement magnetic resonance imaging. Tex Heart Inst J 2004;31(1):99–102

Swanson N, Goddard M, McCann G, Ng GA. Sarcoidosis presenting with tachy- and brady-arrhythmias. Europace 2007;9(2):134–136

Vignaux O. Cardiac sarcoidosis: spectrum of MRI features. AJR Am J Roentgenol 2005;184(1):249–254

Vogel-Claussen J, Rochitte CE, Wu KC, et al. Delayed enhancement MR imaging: utility in myocardial assessment. Radiographics 2006;26(3):795–810

Case 32 Endoleak after endovascular aneurysm repair (EVAR)

Corriere MA, Feurer ID, Becker SY, et al. Endoleak following endovascular abdominal aortic aneurysm repair: implications for duration of screening. Ann Surg 2004;239(6):800–805, discussion 805–807

Stavropoulos SW, Charagundla SR. Imaging techniques for detection and management of endoleaks after endovascular aortic aneurysm repair. Radiology 2007;243(3):641–655

Therasse E, Soulez G, Giroux MF, et al. Stent-graft placement for the treatment of thoracic aortic diseases. Radiographics 2005;25(1):157–173

Case 33 Dextro-transposition of the great arteries (d-TGA)

Brickner ME, Hillis LD, Lange RA. Congenital heart disease in adults: second of two parts. N Engl J Med 2000;342(5):334–342

Sommer RJ, Hijazi ZM, Rhodes JF. Pathophysiology of congenital heart disease in the adult: 3. Complex congenital heart disease. Circulation 2008;117(10):1340–1350

Warnes CA. Transposition of the great arteries. Circulation 2006;114(24):2699–2709

Case 34 Arrhythmogenic right ventricular cardiomyopathy (ARVC)

Abbara S, Migrino RQ, Sosnovik DE, Leichter JA, Brady TJ, Holmvang G. Value of fat suppression in the MRI evaluation of suspected arrhythmogenic right ventricular dysplasia. AJR Am J Roentgenol 2004;182(3):587–591

Kayser HW, van der Wall EE, Sivananthan MU, Plein S, Bloomer TN, de Roos A. Diagnosis of arrhythmogenic right ventricular dysplasia: a review. Radiographics 2002;22(3):639–648, discussion 649–650

Case 35 Hypertrophic obstructive cardiomyopathy (HOCM) with middle chamber obstruction

Hansen MW, Merchant N. MRI of hypertrophic cardiomyopathy: 1. MRI appearances. AJR Am J Roentgenol 2007;189(6):1335–1343

Hansen MW, Merchant N. MRI of hypertrophic cardiomyopathy: 2. Differential diagnosis, risk stratification, and posttreatment MRI appearances. AJR Am J Roentgenol 2007;189(6):1344–1352

Moon JCC, McKenna WJ, McCrohon JA, Elliott PM, Smith GC, Pennell DJ. Toward clinical risk assessment in hypertrophic cardiomyopathy with gadolinium cardiovascular magnetic resonance. J Am Coll Cardiol 2003;41(9):1561–1567

Case 36 Cardiac tamponade

Asher CR, Klein AL. Diastolic heart failure: restrictive cardiomyopathy, constrictive pericarditis, and cardiac tamponade: clinical and echocardiographic evaluation. Cardiol Rev 2002;10(4):218–229

Restrepo CS, Lemos DF, Lemos JA, et al. Imaging findings in cardiac tamponade with emphasis on CT. Radiographics 2007;27(6):1595–1610

Rienmüller R, Gröll R, Lipton MJ. CT and MR imaging of pericardial disease. Radiol Clin North Am 2004;42(3):587–601, vi

Spodick DH. Acute cardiac tamponade. N Engl J Med 2003;349(7):684–690

Case 37 Hypoplastic left heart syndrome (HLHS)

Bardo DME, Frankel DG, Applegate KE, Murphy DJ, Saneto RP. Hypoplastic left heart syndrome. Radiographics 2001;21(3):705–717

Tweddell JS, Hoffmann GM, Mussatto KA, et al. Improved survival of patients undergoing palliation of hypoplastic left heart syndrome: lessons learned from 115 consecutive patients. Circulation 2002;106:182–189

Case 38 False aneurysm of the LV (FALV)

Brown SL, Gropler RJ, Harris KM. Distinguishing left ventricular aneurysm from pseudoaneurysm: a review of the literature. Chest 1997;111(5):1403–1409

Frances C, Romero A, Grady D. Left ventricular pseudoaneurysm. J Am Coll Cardiol 1998;32(3):557–561

Ghersin E, Kerner A, Gruberg L, Bar-El Y, Abadi S, Engel A. Left ventricular pseudoaneurysm or diverticulum: differential diagnosis and dynamic evaluation by catheter left ventriculography and ECG-gated multidetector CT. Br J Radiol 2007;80(957):e209–e211

Moreno R, Gordillo E, Zamorano J, et al. Long-term outcome of patients with postinfarction left ventricular pseudoaneurysm. Heart 2003;89(10):1144–1146

Case 39 Pulmonary arterial hypertension

Chin KM, Rubin LJ. Pulmonary arterial hypertension. J Am Coll Cardiol 2008;51(16):1527–1538

Frazier AA, Galvin JR, Franks TJ, Rosado-De-Christenson ML. From the archives of the AFIP: pulmonary vasculature: hypertension and infarction. Radiographics 2000;20(2):491–524, quiz 530–531, 532

Nguyen ET, Silva CIS, Seely JM, Chong S, Lee KS, Müller NL. Pulmonary artery aneurysms and pseudoaneurysms in adults: findings at CT and radiography. AJR Am J Roentgenol 2007;188(2):W126–W34

Remy-Jardin M, Remy J. Spiral CT angiography of the pulmonary circulation. Radiology 1999;212(3):615–636

Tan RT, Kuzo R, Goodman LR, Siegel R, Haasler GB, Presberg KW; Medical College of Wisconsin Lung Transplant Group. Utility of CT scan evaluation for predicting pulmonary hypertension in patients with parenchymal lung disease. Chest 1998;113(5):1250–1256

Case 40 Ruptured thoracic aortic aneurysm

Castañer E, Andreu M, Gallardo X, Mata JM, Cabezuelo MA, Pallardó Y. CT in nontraumatic acute thoracic aortic disease: typical and atypical features and complications. Radiographics 2003;23(Spec No):S93–S110

Gotway MB. Helical CT evaluation of the thoracic aorta. Appl Radiol 2000;29:7–28

Halliday KE, al-Kutoubi A. Draped aorta: CT sign of contained leak of aortic aneurysms. Radiology 1996;199(1):41–43

Macura KJ, Szarf G, Fishman EK, Bluemke DA. Role of computed tomography and magnetic resonance imaging in assessment of acute aortic syndromes. Semin Ultrasound CT MR 2003;24(4):232–254

Case 41 Dilated cardiomyopathy (DCM)

Andreini D, Pontone G, Pepi M, et al. Diagnostic accuracy of multidetector computed tomography coronary angiography in patients with dilated cardiomyopathy. J Am Coll Cardiol 2007;49(20):2044–2050

LimaJ AC, Hare J. Visualizing the coronaries in patients presenting with heart failure of unknown etiology. J Am Coll Cardiol 2007;49(20):2051–2052

Mohan SB, Parker M, Wehbi M, Douglass P. Idiopathic dilated cardiomyopathy: a common but mystifying cause of heart failure. Cleve Clin J Med 2002;69(6):481–487

Case 42 Chronic infarct of the anterior wall of the LV and acute infarct versus ischemia

Francone M, Carbone I, Napoli A, et al. Imaging of myocardial infarction using a 64-slice MDCT scanner: correlation between infarcted region and status of territory-dependent coronary artery. Radiol Med (Torino) 2007;112(8):1100–1116

Hoffmann U, Pena AJ, Moselewski F, et al. MDCT in early triage of patients with acute chest pain. AJR Am J Roentgenol 2006;187(5):1240–1247

Lardo AC, Cordeiro MAS, Silva C, et al. Contrast-enhanced multidetector computed tomography viability imaging after myocardial infarction: characterization of myocyte death, microvascular obstruction, and chronic scar. Circulation 2006;113(3):394–404

Case 43 Chronic anterolateral LV wall infarction and LIMA CABG

Francone M, Carbone I, Napoli A, et al. Imaging of myocardial infarction using a 64-slice MDCT scanner: correlation between infarcted region and status of territory-dependent coronary artery. Radiol Med (Torino) 2007;112(8):1100–1116

Hoffmann U, Pena AJ, Moselewski F, et al. MDCT in early triage of patients with acute chest pain. AJR Am J Roentgenol 2006;187(5):1240–1247

Lardo AC, Cordeiro MAS, Silva C, et al. Contrast-enhanced multidetector computed tomography viability imaging after myocardial infarction: characterization of myocyte death, microvascular obstruction, and chronic scar. Circulation 2006;113(3):394–404

Case 44 Eisenmenger syndrome secondary to a large atrial septal defect (ASD)

Broberg C, Ujita M, Babu-Narayan S, et al. Massive pulmonary artery thrombosis with haemoptysis in adults with Eisenmenger's syndrome: a clinical dilemma. Heart 2004;90(11):e63

Diller G-P, Gatzoulis MA. Pulmonary vascular disease in adults with congenital heart disease. Circulation 2007;115(8):1039–1050

Griffin N, Allen D, Wort J, Rubens M, Padley S. Eisenmenger syndrome and idiopathic pulmonary arterial hypertension: do parenchymal lung changes reflect aetiology? Clin Radiol 2007;62(6):587–595

Vongpatanasin W, Brickner ME, Hillis LD, Lange RA. The Eisenmenger syndrome in adults. Ann Intern Med 1998;128(9):745–755

Case 45 Caseous calcification of the mitral annulus

Alkadhi H, Leschka S, Prêtre R, Perren A, Marincek B, Wildermuth S. Caseous calcification of the mitral annulus. J Thorac Cardiovasc Surg 2005;129(6):1438–1440

Harpaz D, Auerbach I, Vered Z, Motro M, Tobar A, Rosenblatt S. Caseous calcification of the mitral annulus: a neglected, unrecognized diagnosis. J Am Soc Echocardiogr 2001;14(8):825–831

Lubarsky L, Jelnin VJ, Marino N, Hecht HS. Images in cardiovascular medicine: caseous calcification of the mitral annulus by 64-detector-row computed tomographic coronary angiography—a rare intracardiac mass. Circulation 2007;116(5):e114–e115

Vanovermeire OM, Duerinckx AJ, Duncan DA, Russell WG. Caseous calcification of the mitral annulus imaged with 64-slice multidetector CT and magnetic resonance imaging. Int J Cardiovasc Imaging 2006;22(3-4):553–559

Case 46 Hypertrophic cardiomyopathy (HCM)

Ghersin E, Lessick J, Litmanovich D, Engel A, Reisner S. Comprehensive multidetector CT assessment of apical hypertrophic cardiomyopathy. Br J Radiol 2006;79(948):e200–e204

Maron BJ. Hypertrophic cardiomyopathy: a systematic review. JAMA 2002;287(10):1308–1320

Park JH, Kim YM. MR imaging of cardiomyopathy. Magn Reson Imaging Clin N Am 1996;4(2):269–286

Case 47 Avulsion of a cusp of the aortic valve

Hirata K, Kakazu M, Wake M, et al. Acute aortic valvular regurgitation secondary to avulsion of aortic valve commissure in a patient with pseudoxanthoma elasticum. Intern Med 2000;39(11):940–942

Kan CD, Yang YJ. Traumatic aortic and mitral valve injury following blunt chest injury with a variable clinical course. Heart 2005;91(5):568–570

Case 48 Mitral valve stenosis

Bonow RO, Carabello BA, Chatterjee K, et al; American College of Cardiology; American Heart Association Task Force on Practice Guidelines (Writing Committee to Revise the 1998 Guidelines for the Management of Patients with Valvular Heart Disease); Society of Cardiovascular Anesthesiologists. ACC/AHA 2006 guidelines for the management of patients with valvular heart disease: a report of the American College of Cardiology/American Heart Association Task Force on Practice Guidelines (Writing Committee to Revise the 1998 Guidelines for the Management of Patients with Valvular Heart Disease) developed in collaboration with the Society of Cardiovascular Anesthesiologists, endorsed by the Society for Cardiovascular Angiography and Interventions and the Society of Thoracic Surgeons. J Am Coll Cardiol 2006;48(3):e1–e148

Mahnken AH, Mühlenbruch G, Das M, et al. MDCT detection of mitral valve calcification: prevalence and clinical relevance compared with echocardiography. AJR Am J Roentgenol 2007;188(5):1264–1269

Messika-Zeitoun D, Serfaty JM, Laissy JP, et al. Assessment of the mitral valve area in patients with mitral stenosis by multislice computed tomography. J Am Coll Cardiol 2006;48(2):411–413

Case 49 Thrombus of the LV apex with subsequent emboli to the kidneys and brain

Stratton JR. Common causes of cardiac emboli—left ventricular thrombi and atrial fibrillation. West J Med 1989;151(2):172–179

Visser CA, Kan G, Meltzer RS, Dunning AJ, Roelandt J. Embolic potential of left ventricular thrombus after myocardial infarction: a two-dimensional echocardiographic study of 119 patients. J Am Coll Cardiol 1985;5(6):1276–1280

Case 50 Constrictive pericarditis

Kim JS, Kim HH, Yoon Y. Imaging of pericardial diseases. Clin Radiol 2007;62(7):626–631

Maisch B, Seferović PM, Ristić AD, et al; Task Force on the Diagnosis and Management of Pericardial Diseases of the European

Society of Cardiology. Guidelines on the diagnosis and management of pericardial diseases executive summary: the Task Force on the Diagnosis and Management of Pericardial Diseases of the European Society of Cardiology. Eur Heart J 2004;25(7):587–610

Wang ZJ, Reddy GP, Gotway MB, Yeh BM, Hetts SW, Higgins CB. CT and MR imaging of pericardial disease. Radiographics 2003;23(Spec No):S167–S180

Case 51 Noncompaction of the left ventricular myocardium

Chin TK, Perloff JK, Williams RG, Jue K, Mohrmann R. Isolated noncompaction of left ventricular myocardium: a study of eight cases. Circulation 1990;82(2):507–513

Moreira FC, Miglioransa MH, Mautone MP, Müller KR, Lucchese F. Noncompaction of the left ventricle: a new cardiomyopathy is presented to the clinician. Sao Paulo Med J 2006;124(1):31–35

Pignatelli RH, McMahon CJ, Dreyer WJ, et al. Clinical characterization of left ventricular noncompaction in children: a relatively common form of cardiomyopathy. Circulation 2003;108(21):2672–2678

Case 52 Apical infarction, thrombus, hypokinesis, and poor wall thickening

Anzai T, Yoshikawa T, Kaneko H, et al. Association between serum C-reactive protein elevation and left ventricular thrombus formation after first anterior myocardial infarction. Chest 2004;125(2):384–389

Hunold P, Schlosser T, Vogt FM, et al. Myocardial late enhancement in contrast-enhanced cardiac MRI: distinction between infarction scar and non-infarction-related disease. AJR Am J Roentgenol 2005;184(5):1420–1426

Tóth C, Ujhelyi E, Fülöp T, Istvan E. Clinical predictors of early left ventricular thrombus formation in acute myocardial infarction. Acta Cardiol 2002;57(3):205–211

Case 53 Myocardial fatty replacement in old infracted myocardium

Baroldi G, Silver MD, De Maria R, Parodi O, Pellegrini A. Lipomatous metaplasia in left ventricular scar. Can J Cardiol 1997;13(1):65–719039067

Goldfarb JW, Arnold S, Roth M, Han J. T1-weighted magnetic resonance imaging shows fatty deposition after myocardial infarction. Magn Reson Med 2007;57(5):828–834

Su L, Siegel JE, Fishbein MC. Adipose tissue in myocardial infarction. Cardiovasc Pathol 2004;13(2):98–102

Zafar HM, Litt HI, Torigian DA. CT imaging features and frequency of left ventricular myocardial fat in patients with CT findings of chronic left ventricular myocardial infarction. Clin Radiol 2008;63(3):256–262

Case 54 Degenerative aortic valve stenosis with secondary dilatation of the ascending aorta and LV hypertrophy

Miller SW. Cardiac Imaging of the Requisites. 2nd ed. Philadelphia: Mosby; 2005:159–168

Case 55 True left ventricular aneurysm (LVA)

Brown SL, Gropler RJ, Harris KM. Distinguishing left ventricular aneurysm from pseidoaneurysm: a review of the literature. Chest 1997;111:1403–1409

Konen E, Merchant N, Gutierrez C, et al. True versus false left ventricular aneurysm: differentiation with MR imaging—initial experience. Radiology 2005;236:65–70

Kumbasar B, Wu K, Kamel IR, et al. Left ventricular aneurysm: diagnosis of myocardial viability shown on MR imaging. AJR Am J Roentgenol 2002;179:472–474

Paul M, Schafers M, Grude M, et al. Idiopathic left ventricular aneurysms and sudden cardiac death in young adults. Europace 2006;8:607–612

Case 56 False tendons (cords) of the myocardium

Sutton MG, Dubrey S, Oldershaw PJ. Muscular false tendons, aberrant left ventricular papillary musculature, and severe electrocardiographic repolarisation abnormalities: a new syndrome. Br Heart J 1994;71(2):187–190

Suwa M, Hirota Y, Nagao H, Kino M, Kawamura K. Incidence of the coexistence of left ventricular false tendons and premature ventricular contractions in apparently healthy subjects. Circulation 1984;70(5):793–798

Case 57 Calcified left myocardial infarction and ventricular thrombus

Cameron CS, Roberts WC. Clinical and necropsy findings in patients with calcified myocardial infarcts. Baylor U Med Center Proc 2004;17:420–424

Gowda RM, Box tLM. Calcifications of the heart. Radiol Clin North Am 2004;42(3):603–617

Mousseaux E, Hernigou A, Azencot M, et al. Endomyocardial fibrosis: electron-beam CT features. Radiology 1996;198(3):755–760

Robles P, Sonlleva A. Myocardial calcification and subendocardial fatty replacement of the left ventricle following myocardial infarction. Int J Cardiovasc Imaging 2007;23(5):667–670

Case 58 Penetrating atherosclerotic aortic ulcer

Castañer E, Andreu M, Gallardo X, Mata JM, Cabezuelo MA, Pallardó Y. CT in nontraumatic acute thoracic aortic disease: typical and atypical features and complications. Radiographics 2003;23(Spec No):S93–S110

Macura KJ, Corl FM, Fishman EK, Bluemke DA. Pathogenesis in acute aortic syndromes: aortic dissection, intramural hematoma, and penetrating atherosclerotic aortic ulcer. AJR Am J Roentgenol 2003;181(2):309–316

Quint LE, Williams DM, Francis IR, et al. Ulcerlike lesions of the aorta: imaging features and natural history. Radiology 2001;218(3):719–723

Sueyoshi E, Matsuoka Y, Imada T, Okimoto T, Sakamoto I, Hayashi K. New development of an ulcerlike projection in aortic intramural hematoma: CT evaluation. Radiology 2002;224(2):536–541

Case 59 Ventricular diverticulum

Ghersin E, Kerner A, Gruberg L, Bar-El Y, Abadi S, Engel A. Left ventricular pseudoaneurysm or diverticulum: differential diagnosis and dynamic evaluation by catheter left ventriculography and ECG-gated multidetector CT. Br J Radiol 2007;80(957):e209–e211

Parthenakis FI, Kochiadakis GE, Patrianakos AP, et al. Peripheral arterial embolism due to a left ventricular diverticulum in a young adult. Chest 2005;127(4):1452–1454

Srichai MB, Hecht EM, Kim DC, Jacobs JE. Ventricular diverticula on cardiac CT: more common than previously thought. AJR Am J Roentgenol 2007;189(1):204–208

Case 60 LV myocarditis

Laissy JP, Hyafil F, Feldman LJ, et al. Differentiating acute myocardial infarction from myocarditis: diagnostic value of early- and delayed-perfusion cardiac MR imaging. Radiology 2005;237(1):75–82

Laissy JP, Messin B, Varenne O, et al. MRI of acute myocarditis: a comprehensive approach based on various imaging sequences. Chest 2002;122(5):1638–1648

Mahrholdt H, Goedecke C, Wagner A, et al. Cardiovascular magnetic resonance assessment of human myocarditis: a comparison to histology and molecular pathology. Circulation 2004;109(10):1250–1258

Case 61 Interatrial septal aneurysm (IASA)

Dodd JD, Aquino SL, Holmvang G, et al. Cardiac septal aneurysm mimicking pseudomass: appearance on ECG-gated cardiac MRI and MDCT. AJR Am J Roentgenol 2007;188(6):W550–553

Duerinckx AJ, Vanovermeire O. Accessory appendages of the left atrium as seen during 64-slice coronary CT angiography. Int J Cardiovasc Imaging 2008;24(2):215–221

Marazanof M, Roudaut R, Cohen A, et al. Atrial septal aneurysm: morphological characteristics in a large population—pathological associations. Int J Cardiol 1995;52(1):59–65

Mügge A, Daniel WG, Angermann C, et al. Atrial septal aneurysm in adult patients: a multicenter study using transthoracic and transesophageal echocardiography. Circulation 1995;91(11):2785–2792

Case 62 Coarctation of the aorta, aberrant right subclavian artery, and moyamoya disease

Lutterman J, Scott M, Nass R, Geva T. Moyamoya syndrome associated with congenital heart disease. Pediatrics 1998;101(1 Pt 1):57–60

Manceau E, Giroud M, Dumas R. Moyamoya disease in children: a review of the clinical and radiological features and current treatment. Childs Nerv Syst 1997;13(11-12):595–600

Nowak-Göttl U, Günther G, Kurnik K, Sträter R, Kirkham F. Arterial ischemic stroke in neonates, infants, and children: an overview of underlying conditions, imaging methods, and treatment modalities. Semin Thromb Hemost 2003;29(4):405–41414517752

Case 63 Restrictive cardiomyopathy (RCM)

Hancock EW. Differential diagnosis of restrictive cardiomyopathy and constrictive pericarditis. Heart 2001;86(3):343–349

Kushwaha SS, Fallon JT, Fuster V. Restrictive cardiomyopathy. N Engl J Med 1997;336(4):267–276

Masui T, Finck S, Higgins CB. Constrictive pericarditis and restrictive cardiomyopathy: evaluation with MR imaging. Radiology 1992;182(2):369–373

vanden Driesen RI, Slaughter RE, Strugnell WE. MR findings in cardiac amyloidosis. AJR Am J Roentgenol 2006;186(6):1682–1685

Case 64 LAA thrombus

Alam G, Addo F, Malik M, Levinsky R, Lieb D. Detection of left atrial appendage thrombus by spiral CT scan. Echocardiography 2003;20(1):99–100

Al-Saady NM, Obel OA, Camm AJ. Left atrial appendage: structure, function, and role in thromboembolism. Heart 1999;82(5):547–554

Nakanishi T, Hamada S, Takamiya M, et al. A pitfall in ultrafast CT scanning for the detection of left atrial thrombi. J Comput Assist Tomogr 1993;17(1):42–45

Ostermayer SH, Reisman M, Kramer PH, et al. Percutaneous left atrial appendage transcatheter occlusion (PLAATO system) to prevent stroke in high-risk patients with non-rheumatic atrial fibrillation: results from the international multi-center feasibility trials. J Am Coll Cardiol 2005;46(1):9–14

Case 65 Anomalous coronary artery origin

Angelini P, Velasco JA, Flamm S. Coronary anomalies: incidence, pathophysiology, and clinical relevance. Circulation 2002;105(20):2449–2454

Davis JA, Cecchin F, Jones TK, Portman MA. Major coronary artery anomalies in a pediatric population: incidence and clinical importance. J Am Coll Cardiol 2001;37(2):593–597

Jahnke C, Nagel E, Ostendorf PC, Tangcharoen T, Fleck E, Paetsch I. Images in cardiovascular medicine: diagnosis of a "single" coronary artery and determination of functional significance of concomitant coronary artery disease. Circulation 2006;113(9):e386–e387

Case 66 Coarctation of the aorta, hypoplastic aortic arch, and aorta-aortic bypass

Oliver JM, Gallego P, Gonzalez A, Aroca A, Bret M, Mesa JM. Risk factors for aortic complications in adults with coarctation of the aorta. J Am Coll Cardiol 2004;44(8):1641–1647

Russell GA, Berry PJ, Watterson K, Dhasmana JP, Wisheart JD. Patterns of ductal tissue in coarctation of the aorta in the first three months of life. J Thorac Cardiovasc Surg 1991;102(4):596–601

Case 67 Angiosarcoma of the right atrium

Ananthasubramaniam K, Farha A. Primary right atrial angiosarcoma mimicking acute pericarditis, pulmonary embolism, and tricuspid stenosis. Heart 1999;81(5):556–558

Grebenc ML, Rosado de Christenson ML, Burke AP, Green CE, Galvin JR. Primary cardiac and pericardial neoplasms: radiologic-pathologic correlation. Radiographics 2000;20(4):1073–1103, quiz 1110–1112

Restrepo CS, Largoza A, Lemos DF, et al. CT and MR imaging findings of malignant cardiac tumors. Curr Probl Diagn Radiol 2005;34(1):1–11

Case 68 Loculated postoperative pericardial effusion

Meurin P, Weber H, Renaud N, et al. Evolution of the postoperative pericardial effusion after day 15: the problem of the late tamponade. Chest 2004;125(6):2182–2187

Wang ZJ, Reddy GP, Gotway MB, Yeh BM, Hetts SW, Higgins CB. CT and MR imaging of pericardial disease. Radiographics 2003;23(Spec No):S167–S180

Yousem D, Traill TT, Wheeler PS, Fishman EK. Illustrative cases in pericardial effusion misdetection: correlation of echocardiography and CT. Cardiovasc Intervent Radiol 1987;10(3):162–167

Case 69 Mycotic pseudoaneurysms of the aortic root, complicating an aortic valve endocarditis

Akins EW, Slone RM, Wiechmann BN, Browning M, Martin TD, Mayfield WR. Perivalvular pseudoaneurysm complicating bacterial endocarditis: MR detection in five cases. AJR Am J Roentgenol 1991;156(6):1155–1158

Anguera I, Miro JM, Vilacostal, et al; Aorto-cavitary Fistula in Endocarditis Working Group. Aorto-cavitary fistulous tract formation in infective endocarditis: clinical and echocardiographic features of 76 cases and risk factors for mortality. Eur Heart J 2005;26(3):288–297

Feigl D, Feigl A, Edwards JE. Mycotic aneurysms of the aortic root: a pathologic study of 20 cases. Chest 1986;90(4):553–557

Salanitri GC, Huo E, Miller FH, Gupta A, Pereles FS. MRI of mycotic sinus of valsalva pseudoaneurysm secondary to Aspergillus pericarditis. AJR Am J Roentgenol 2005;184(3, Suppl):S25–S27

Case 70 Traumatic aortic injury (TAI)

Creasy JD, Chiles C, Routh WD, Dyer RB. Overview of traumatic injury of the thoracic aorta. Radiographics 1997;17(1):27–45

Dyer DS, Moore EE, Mestek MF, et al. Can chest CT be used to exclude aortic injury? Radiology 1999;213(1):195–202

Gavant ML, Menke PG, Fabian T, Flick PA, Graney MJ, Gold RE. Blunt traumatic aortic rupture: detection with helical CT of the chest. Radiology 1995;197(1):125–133

Mirvis SE, Shanmuganathan K, Miller BH, White CS, Turney SZ. Traumatic aortic injury: diagnosis with contrast-enhanced thoracic CT—five-year experience at a major trauma center. Radiology 1996;200(2):413–422

Case 71 Interruption of the aortic arch (IAA)

Everett AD, Lim DS. The Illustrated Field Guide to Congenital Heart Disease and Repair. 2nd ed. Charlottesville, VA: Scientific Software Solutions 2005:74, 75, 248

Case 72 Aortic dissection

Castañer E, Andreu M, Gallardo X, Mata JM, Cabezuelo MA, Pallardó Y. CT in nontraumatic acute thoracic aortic disease: typical and atypical features and complications. Radiographics 2003;23(Spec No):S93–S110

Hayter RG, Rhea JT, Small A, Tafazoli FS, Novelline RA. Suspected aortic dissection and other aortic disorders: multi-detector row CT in 373 cases in the emergency setting. Radiology 2006;238(3):841–852

Macura KJ, Szarf G, Fishman EK, Bluemke DA. Role of computed tomography and magnetic resonance imaging in assessment of acute aortic syndromes. Semin Ultrasound CT MR 2003;24(4):232–254

Case 73 Complete atrioventricular septal defect (AVSD)

Everett AD, Lim DS. Illustrated Field Guide to Congenital Heart Disease and Repair. 2nd ed. Charlottesville, VA: Scientific Software Solutions; 2005:52, 53

Gatzoulis MA, Swan L, Therrien J, Pantley GA. Adult Congenital Heart Disease: A Practical Guide. Oxford: Blackwell; 2005:87–91

Case 74 Intramural hematoma of the aorta

Evangelista A, Mukherjee D, Mehta RH, et al; International Registry of Aortic Dissection (IRAD) Investigators. Acute intramural hematoma of the aorta: a mystery in evolution. Circulation 2005;111(8):1063–1070

Macura KJ, Szarf G, Fishman EK, Bluemke DA. Role of computed tomography and magnetic resonance imaging in assessment of acute aortic syndromes. Semin Ultrasound CT MR 2003;24(4):232–254

Murray JG, Manisali M, Flamm SD, et al. Intramural hematoma of the thoracic aorta: MR image findings and their prognostic implications. Radiology 1997;204(2):349–355

von Kodolitsch Y, Csösz SK, Koschyk DH, et al. Intramural hematoma of the aorta: predictors of progression to dissection and rupture. Circulation 2003;107(8):1158–1163

Case 75 Aberrant origin of the RCA from the left aortic sinus

Budoff MJ, Ahmed V, Gul KM, Mao SS, Gopal A. Coronary anomalies by cardiac computed tomographic angiography. Clin Cardiol 2006;29(11):489–493

Datta J, White CS, Gilkeson RC, et al. Anomalous coronary arteries in adults: depiction at multi-detector row CT angiography. Radiology 2005;235(3):812–818

Ghersin E, Litmanovich D, Ofer A, et al. Anomalous origin of right coronary artery: diagnosis and dynamic evaluation with multidetector computed tomography. J Comput Assist Tomogr 2004;28(2):293–294

Kim SY, Seo JB, Do KH, et al. Coronary artery anomalies: classification and ECG-gated multi-detector row CT findings with angiographic correlation. Radiographics 2006;26(2):317–333, discussion 333–334

Case 76 Aortic assist device

Gregoric ID, Kosir R, Smart FW, et al. Left ventricular assist device implantation in a patient with congenitally corrected transposition of the great arteries. Tex Heart Inst J 2005;32(4):567–569

Medical assist device. Available at: http://www.heartandstroke.com/site/c.ikIQLcMWJtE/b.3831923/k.4C25/Mechanical_assist_device.htm. Accessed November 4, 2008

Case 77 Pulmonary and cardiac sarcoidosis

Nemeth MA, Muthupillai R, Wilson JM, Awasthi M, Flamm SD. Cardiac sarcoidosis detected by delayed-hyperenhancement magnetic resonance imaging. Tex Heart Inst J 2004;31(1):99–102

Vignaux O. Cardiac sarcoidosis: spectrum of MRI features. AJR Am J Roentgenol 2005;184(1):249–254

Vogel-Claussen J, Rochitte CE, Wu KC, et al. Delayed enhancement MR imaging: utility in myocardial assessment. Radiographics 2006;26(3):795–810

Case 78 Pseudoaneurysm of the thoracic aorta

Takach TJ, Cervera RD, Gregoric ID. Aortic pseudoaneurysm. Tex Heart Inst J 2005;32(2):235–237

Case 79 Pulmonary artery stenosis (PAS)

Clark SC, Levine AJ, Hasan A, Hilton CJ, Forty J, Dark JH. Vascular complications of lung transplantation. Ann Thorac Surg 1996;61(4):1079–1082

Kreutzer J, Landzberg MJ, Preminger TJ, et al. Isolated peripheral pulmonary artery stenoses in the adult. Circulation 1996;93(7):1417–1423

Mahnken AH, Breuer C, Haage P. Silicosis-induced pulmonary artery stenosis: demonstration by MR angiography and perfusion MRI. Br J Radiol 2001;74(885):859–861

Sachweh J, Däbritz S, Didilis V, Vazquez-Jimenez JF, v Bernuth G, Messmer BJ. Pulmonary artery stenosis after systemic-to-pulmonary shunt operations. Eur J Cardiothorac Surg 1998;14(3):229–234

Shaj R, Cestone P, Muller C. Congenital multiple peripheral pulmonary artery stenosis (pulmonary branch stenosis or supravalvular pulmonary stenosis). AJR Am J Roentgenol 2000;175:856–857

Case 80 Bicuspid aortic valve (BAV)

Bonow RO, Carabello BA, ChaterjeeK, et al. ACC/AHA 2006 guidelines for the management of patients with valvular heart disease: a report of the American College of Cardiology/American Heart Association Task Force on Practice Guidelines (Writing Committee to Revise the 1998 Guidelines for the Management of Patients with Valvular Heart Disease) developed in collaboration with the Society of Cardiovascular Anesthesiologists, endorsed by the Society of Cardiovascular Angiography and Intervention and the Society of Thoracic Surgeons. J Am Coll Cardiol 2006;48:1–148

De Mozzi P, Longo UG, Galanti G, Maffulli N. Bicuspid aortic valve: a literature review and its impact on sport activity. Br Med Bull 2008;85:63–85

Vogel-Claussen J, Pannu H, Spevak PJ, Fishman EK, Bluemke DA. Cardiac valve assessment with MR imaging and 64-section multi-detector row CT. Radiographics 2006;26(6):1769–1784

Case 81 Isolation of the left coronary artery ostia and SVAS

Amrani M, Rubay J, Pirenne B, Col J, Dion R. Isolation of the left coronary artery ostium by an aortic cusp attachment: a rare cause of myocardial ischemia. Eur J Cardiothorac Surg 1994;8(12):663–664

Gilon D, Cape EG, Handschumacher MD, et al. Effect of three-dimensional valve shape on the hemodynamics of aortic stenosis: three-dimensional echocardiographic stereolithography and patient studies. J Am Coll Cardiol 2002;40(8):1479–1486

Line DE, Babb JD, Pierce WS. Congenital aortic valve anomaly: aortic regurgitation with left coronary artery isolation. J Thorac Cardiovasc Surg 1979;77(4):533–535

Case 82 Mitral valve prolapse

Avierinos JF, Brown RD, Foley DA, et al. Cerebral ischemic events after diagnosis of mitral valve prolapse: a community-based study of incidence and predictive factors. Stroke 2003;34(6):1339–1344

Klues HG, Maron BJ, Dollar AL, Roberts WC. Diversity of structural mitral valve alterations in hypertrophic cardiomyopathy. Circulation 1992;85(5):1651–1660

Case 83 Mitral annulus calcification

Atar S, Jeon DS, Luo H, Siegel RJ. Mitral annular calcification: a marker of severe coronary artery disease in patients under 65 years old. Heart 2003;89(2):161–164

Choe YH, Kim EA, Yoon Y-C, et al. Cardiac calcifications found at CT: spectrum of diseases. Radiologist 2002;9:147–154

Fox CS, Vasan RS, Parise H, et al. Framingham Heart Study. Mitral annular calcification predicts cardiovascular morbidity and mortality: the Framingham Heart Study. Circulation 2003;107(11):1492–1496

Gowda RM, Boxt LM. Calcifications of the heart. Radiol Clin North Am 2004;42(3):603–617

Kizer JR, Wiebers DO, Whisnant JP, et al. Mitral annular calcification, aortic valve sclerosis, and incident stroke in adults free of clinical cardiovascular disease: the Strong Heart Study. Stroke 2005;36(12):2533–2537

Case 84 Sinus venosus atrial septal defect (ASD) with partial anomalous pulmonary venous return (PAPVR)

Agrawal SK, Khanna SK, Tampe D. Sinus venosus atrial septal defects: surgical follow-up. Eur J Cardiothorac Surg 1997;11(3):455–457

Lembcke A, Razek V, Kivelitz D, Rogalla N, Rogalla P. Sinus venosus atrial septal defect with partial anomalous pulmonary venous return: diagnosis with 64-slice spiral computed tomography at low radiation dose. J Pediatr Surg 2008;43(2):410–411

Webb G, Gatzoulis MA. Atrial septal defects in the adult: recent progress and overview. Circulation 2006;114(15):1645–1653

Case 85 Patent ductus arteriosus (PDA)

Goitein O, Fuhrman CR, Lacomis JM. Incidental finding on MDCT of patent ductus arteriosus: use of CT and MRI to assess clinical importance. AJR Am J Roentgenol 2005;184(6):1924–1931

Morgan-Hughes GJ, Marshall AJ, Roobottom C. Morphologic assessment of patent ductus arteriosus in adults using retrospectively ECG-gated multidetector CT. AJR Am J Roentgenol 2003;181(3):749–754

Schneider DJ, Moore JW. Patent ductus arteriosus. Circulation 2006;114(17):1873–1882

Case 86 Pulmonary artery atresia, tetralogy of Fallot

Salaymeh KJ, Kimball TR, Manning PB. Anomalous pulmonary artery from the aorta via a patent ductus arteriosus: repair in a premature infant. Ann Thorac Surg 2000;69(4):1259–1261

WuL. Isolated left pulmonary artery in absent pulmonary valve syndrome. Pediatr Cardiol 2008;29(6):1129–113018685800

Case 87 Double aortic arch

Alsenaidi K, Gurofsky R, Karamlou T, Williams WG, McCrindle BW. Management and outcomes of double aortic arch in 81 patients. Pediatrics 2006;118(5):e1336–e1341

Lima JA, Rosenblum BN, Reilly JS, Pennington DG, Nouri-Moghaddam S. Airway obstruction in aortic arch anomalies. Otolaryngol Head Neck Surg 1983;91(6):605–609

Case 88 Double aortic arch

Alsenaidi K, Gurofsky R, Karamlou T, Williams WG, McCrindle BW. Management and outcomes of double aortic arch in 81 patients. Pediatrics 2006;118(5):e1336–e1341

Cerillo AG, Amoretti F, Moschetti R, Murzi B, Chiappino D. Sixteen-row multislice computed tomography in infants with double aortic arch. Int J Cardiol 2005;99(2):191–194

Lowe GM, Donaldson JS, Backer CL. Vascular rings: 10-year review of imaging. Radiographics 1991;11(4):637–646

Pickhardt PJ, Siegel MJ, Gutierrez FR. Vascular rings in symptomatic children: frequency of chest radiographic findings. Radiology 1997;203(2):423–426

Schlesinger AE, Krishnamurthy R, Sena LM, et al. Incomplete double aortic arch with atresia of the distal left arch: distinctive imaging appearance. AJR Am J Roentgenol 2005;184(5):1634–1639

Case 89 Circumflex right aortic arch

Blieden LC, Schneeweiss A, Deutsch V, Neufeld HN. Right aortic arch with left descending aorta (circumflex aorta): roentgenographic diagnosis. Pediatr Radiol 1978;6(4):208–210

McLeary MS, Frye LL, Young LW. Magnetic resonance imaging of a left circumflex aortic arch and aberrant right subclavian artery: the other vascular ring. Pediatr Radiol 1998;28(4):263–265

Case 90 Isolated left subclavian artery

Sun AM, Alhabshan F, Branson H, Freedom RM, Yoo SJ. MRI diagnosis of isolated origin of the left subclavian artery from the left pulmonary artery. Pediatr Radiol 2005;35(12):1259–1262

Victorica BE, Van Mierop LH, Elliot tLP, Elliott LP. Right aortic arch associated with contralateral congenital subclavian steal syndrome. Am J Roentgenol Radium Ther Nucl Med 1970;108(3):582–590

Case 91 Pulmonary artery sling

Berdon WE. Rings, slings, and other things: vascular compression of the infant trachea updated from the midcentury to the millennium—the legacy of Robert E. Gross, MD, and Edward B. D. Neuhauser, MD. Radiology 2000;216(3):624–632

Berdon WE, Baker DH, Wung JT, et al. Complete cartilage-ring tracheal stenosis associated with anomalous left pulmonary artery: the ring-sling complex. Radiology 1984;152(1):57–64

Gikonyo BM, Jue KL, Edwards JE. Pulmonary vascular sling: report of seven cases and review of the literature. Pediatr Cardiol 1989;10(2):81–89

Newman B, Meza MP, Towbin RB, Nido PD. Left pulmonary artery sling: diagnosis and delineation of associated tracheobronchial anomalies with MR. Pediatr Radiol 1996;26(9):661–668

Case 92 Azygos continuation of intrahepatic interruption of the inferior vena cava (IVC)

Applegate KE, Goske MJ, Pierce G, Murphy D. Situs revisited: imaging of the heterotaxy syndrome. Radiographics 1999;19(4):837–852, discussion 853–854

Brueckner M. Heterotaxia, congenital heart disease, and primary ciliary dyskinesia. Circulation 2007;115(22):2793–2795

Kennedy MP, Omran H, Leigh MW, et al. Congenital heart disease and other heterotaxic defects in a large cohort of patients with primary ciliary dyskinesia. Circulation 2007;115(22):2814–2821

Winer-Muram HT, Tonkinl LD. The spectrum of heterotaxic syndromes. Radiol Clin North Am 1989;27(6):1147–1170

Case 93 Ebstein anomaly

Everett AD, Lim DS. Illustrated Field Guide to Congenital Heart Disease and Repair. 2nd ed. Charlottesville, VA: Scientific Software Solutions; 2005:68, 69.

MacLellan-Tobert SG, Feldt RH. In: Moller JH, Hoffman JIE, eds. Pediatric Cardiovascular Medicine. Oxford: Churchill Livingstone; 2000:461–467.

Reemtsen BL, Fagan BT, Wells WJ, Starnes VA. Current surgical therapy for Ebstein anomaly in neonates. J Thorac Cardiovasc Surg 2006;132(6):1285–1290

Case 94 Acute coronary syndrome due to RCA thrombosis, LAD atherosclerosis

Schoepf UJ, Becker CR, Ohnesorge BM, Yucel EK. CT of coronary artery disease. Radiology 2004;232(1):18–37

Case 95 Partial congenital absence of the pericardium (PCAP)

Gassner I, Judmaier W, Fink C, et al. Diagnosis of congenital pericardial defects, including a pathognomic sign for dangerous apical ventricular herniation, on magnetic resonance imaging. Br Heart J 1995;74(1):60–66

Gatzoulis MA, Munk MD, Merchant N, Van Arsdell GS, McCrindle BW, Webb GD. Isolated congenital absence of the pericardium: clinical presentation, diagnosis, and management. Ann Thorac Surg 2000;69(4):1209–1215

Raman SV, Daniels CJ, Katz SE, Ryan JM, King MA. Congenital absence of the pericardium. Circulation 2001;104(12):1447–1448

Scheuermann-Freestone M, Orchard E, Francis J, et al. Images in cardiovascular medicine. Partial congenital absence of the pericardium. Circulation 2007;116(6):e126–e1291

Case 96 Interatrial lipoma or lipomatous hypertrophy of the atrial septum

Heyer CM, Kagel T, Lemburg SP, Bauer TT, NicolasV. Lipomatous hypertrophy of the interatrial septum: a prospective study of incidence, imaging findings, and clinical symptoms. Chest 2003;124(6):2068–2073

Nadra I, Dawson D, Schmitz SA, Punjabi PP, Nihoyannopoulos P. Lipomatous hypertrophy of the interatrial septum: a commonly misdiagnosed mass often leading to unnecessary cardiac surgery. Available at: http://www.heartjnl.com. Accessed July 9, 2008.

O'Connor S, Recavarren R, Nichols LC, ParwaniAV. Lipomatous hypertrophy of the interatrial septum: an overview. Arch Pathol Lab Med 2006;130(3):397–399

Case 97 Lung cancer metastases to the LV apex

Chiles C, Woodard PK, Gutierrez FR, LinkKM. Metastatic involvement of the heart and pericardium: CT and MR imaging. Radiographics 2001;21(2):439–449

Reynen K, Köckeritz U, Strasser RH. Metastases to the heart. Ann Oncol 2004;15(3):375–381

Case 98 Aortic sarcoma

Akiyama K, Nakata K, Negishi N, Henmi A. Intimal sarcoma of the thoracic aorta; clinical-course and autopsy finding. Ann Thorac Cardiovasc Surg 2005;11(2):135–138

Böhner H, Luther B, Braunstein S, Beer S, Sandmann W. Primary malignant tumors of the aorta: clinical presentation, treatment, and course of different entities. J Vasc Surg 2003;38(6):1430–1433

Mohsen NA, Haber M, Urrutia VC, Nunes LW. Intimal sarcoma of the aorta. AJR Am J Roentgenol 2000;175(5):1289–1290

Case 99 Ectopia cordis

Effmann E. Chest wall. In: Kuhn JP, Slovis TL, Haller JO, eds. Caffey's Pediatric Diagnostic Imaging. Philadelphia: Mosby; 2004:822–830

Moore KL. The Developing Human Clinically Oriented Embryology. 4th ed. Philadelphia: WB Saunders; 1988:309

Case 100 Metastatic cardiac calcification secondary to chronic renal failure

Jing J, Kawashima A, Sickler K, Raval BK, Oldham SA. Metastatic cardiac calcification in a patient with chronic renal failure who was undergoing hemodialysis: radiographic and CT findings. AJR Am J Roentgenol 1998;170(4):903–905

Kloeppel R, Luebke P, Mittag M, et al. Acute hypercalcemia of the heart ("bony heart"). J Comput Assist Tomogr 2001;25(3):407–411

Raggi P, Boulay A, Chasan-Taber S, et al. Cardiac calcification in adult hemodialysis patients: a link between end-stage renal disease and cardiovascular disease? J Am Coll Cardiol 2002;39(4):695–701

Rostand SG, Sanders C, Kirk KA, Rutsky EA, Fraser RG. Myocardial calcification and cardiac dysfunction in chronic renal failure. Am J Med 1988;85(5):651–657

Index

Note: Locators refer to case number. Locators in **boldface** indicate primary diagnosis.